Inner Presence

Inner Presence
Consciousness as a Biological Phenomenon

Antti Revonsuo

The MIT Press
Cambridge, Massachusetts
London, England

MIT Press books may be purchased at special quantity discounts for business or sales promotional use. For information, please email special_sales@mitpress.mit.edu or write to Special Sales Department, The MIT Press, 55 Hayward Street, Cambridge, MA 02142.

This book was set in Times Roman by Graphic Composition, Inc.
Printed and bound in the United States of America.

Library of Congress Cataloging-in-Publication Data

Revonsuo, Antti.
Inner presence : consciousness as a biological phenomenon / Antti Revonsuo.
p. cm.
ISBN 0-262-18249-1 (alk. paper)
1. Consciousness 2. Consciousness—Psychological aspects. 3. Sleep—Research. 4. Dreams—Research.
I. Title
BF311.R396 2006 126—dc22 2005050467

10 9 8 7 6 5 4 3 2 1

Contents

Acknowledgments

The roots of this book can be traced back to the early 1990s. In 1992 I delivered a talk entitled "In Search of the Science of Consciousness," published as a book chapter in 1994 (Revensuo 1994b). That paper was perhaps the starting point of my search for a more unified science of consciousness, the line of inquiry that I continue in this book. The first outlines for *Inner Presence* were sketched in 1997, but it has taken rather longer than I expected to bring this project to an end.

Throughout this project I have been privileged to enjoy financial support from the Academy of Finland, in the form of various grants and research fellowships (grants #36160 [1996–1999] and #45704 [1999–2004]). The writing of this book has also been supported by a grant from the Signe och Ane Gyllenbergs Stiftelse in 2004. Furthermore, I have enjoyed the continuous institutional support of the Department of Philosophy and the Center for Cognitive Neuroscience, University of Turku, and toward the end of the project, also from the Department of Psychology, University of Turku. I am extremely grateful for the long-lasting support of these various sources, as it has enabled me to fully concentrate on the problem of consciousness in a friendly and multidisciplinary environment. I also very much appreciate the hospitality that I have enjoyed during my regular visits to the Program for Consciousness Studies, University of Skövde, Sweden, since 1997.

I am deeply indebted to a number of individuals who have helped and supported me in various ways during the project. My PhD students and members of our "Consciousness Research Group" in Turku: Sakari Kallio, Katja Valli, Maria Wilenius-Emet, Sari Laatu, Ville Ojanen, Valtteri Arstila, Mika Koivisto, Mirja Johanson, Levente Moro, Monica Bergman, Jay Fournier, and many others have shared with me the excitement, the fun, as well as the hard work involved. I have also gotten useful comments from them on the manuscript at various stages during the writing process. My special thanks go to Niina Salminen and Valdas Noreika who read through and commented on the penultimate version of the manuscript, leading to considerable improvement thereof. Furthermore, several people outside my group, in particular Lennart Karlsson, Tuula Tanska, Paavo Pylkkänen, Ron Chrisley, and the students attending my seminars at the

University of Skövde, Sweden, were kind enough to read different parts and versions of the manuscript, presenting detailed comments and challenging criticisms. I am especially grateful to the late Dr. Francis Crick, who read through an earlier version of the manuscript and gave me helpful advice, criticism, and inspiration during my visit to the Salk Institute, La Jolla, California, in 2002. Sadly, the news of his death reached me just as I was finishing the manuscript for publication.

I also want to give thanks to my editors at The MIT Press, Barbara Murphy, and Kate Blakinger for valuable advice on how to improve the manuscript, and for the anonymous reviewers who provided me with thoughtful comments and constructive criticism. A number of colleagues that I have had the privilege to get acquainted with through the Association for the Scientific Study of Consciousness, as the European Editor of the journal *Consciousness and Cognition,* at the "Toward a Science of Consciousness" conferences, at the meetings of "Agora for Biosystems," Sigtuna, Sweden, and at the "Nordic Network for Consciousness Studies" have provided me with invaluable discussions, comments, and criticism on the various topics dealt with in *Inner Presence.* My special thanks go to Bernie Baars, Bill Banks, Thomas Metzinger, Yves Rossetti, Max Velmans, Dan Lloyd, Steve Lehar, Talis Bachmann, Oliver Kauffman, Morten Overgaard, Luiz Lopez, and Hans Liljenström.

In my private life I am most indebted to my wife Satu, without whose love, patience and caring both I myself, as well as this book project, would have collapsed long ago. I also want to thank my mother, Eira Revonsuo, who continues to help me to express myself more clearly and correctly in the English language. She read through many parts and versions of the manuscript; however, I am of course fully responsible for any errors that remain. Finally, I am deeply indebted to my late father Teuvo Revonsuo, who passed away in 1996. It was he who originally led me to see the importance of a biological approach to science, and this book is therefore dedicated to his memory.

For a long time my aspiration was to write a book on consciousness that would combine philosophy and empirical inquiry into one fairly coherent "big picture." Now that this project is nearing its end, consciousness still strikes me as the most wonderful invention that nature ever came up with. Yet, the philosophical problem of consciousness no longer looks quite as intractable as it did when I began the project, and it seems as if the science to solve the problem is gradually emerging.

Whether or not the problem of consciousness will eventually be solved, I hope that the readers of this book will be able to share with me the excitement of exploration and the sense of wonder that I have experienced while exploring the largely uncharted realms of subjective phenomenal consciousness.

Antti Revonsuo
Turku, September 2004

Prologue: The Most Fundamental Question

Why is there something rather than nothing? I expect that many share my bafflement, a true sense of wonder, in the face of this ultimate question. But what, precisely, is it about? The conventional interpretation is that it is about the origin of the physical universe. Everyone acknowledges that had the big bang been called off, there would have been nothing rather than something.

There seems to be, though, an alternative way in which there would have been nothing rather than something. Consider the question, Why is there something rather than nothing, *for me*?

That seems to be a mystery at least equally fundamental. It is, at bottom, the problem of consciousness. When your consciousness first emerged from subjective nothingness, what happened was a kind of psychological big bang. Your consciousness had been absent from the physical universe for a respectable while—about 14 billion years or so—but then suddenly there was light *for you.* As a matter of fact, until recently we all had been dead since the dawn of the physical world. Our subjective existence is a kind of life after death; indeed, life after billions of years of being entirely devoid of subjective consciousness. Sadly, it looks like each and every one of us will once again return to that state of impenetrable darkness, probably far sooner than any of us would care to.

Without your consciousness ever coming into being, there would have been nothing rather than something (*for you*). Without the phenomenon of consciousness emerging in some place at some point in the history of the physical universe, there would have been nothing rather than something *for everyone,* and consequently, nothing rather than something, across the board. The physical universe, if deprived of us conscious subjects, has absolutely no way of sensing or knowing its own existence; it simply couldn't care less. The physical universe in itself, then, leads a pretty boring life, at least compared to us sentient creatures. If you don't even know whether or not you exist, and you cannot care, is there any way in which things could get more indifferent for you?

So maybe the importance of the most fundamental question, if taken as the mystery of the physical universe, has been somewhat overestimated. *Why is there something rather than nothing?* A few bits of dead physical matter and energy hovering about in an otherwise empty space-time would be enough to bring up the mystery of the physical universe in its entirety, but even if that mystery could be solved somehow, would the solution make much difference anyway?

The mystery of consciousness is a horse of another color. Consciousness *matters.* It makes a difference whose significance it is difficult to overstate. Just think about it: What if you, that is, your *consciousness,* had never existed? What if there had never been anything *for you*? Surely that is not a minor difference. For whom? Well, the universe doesn't care anyway, so it is pointless to envisage things from its point of view. Of course it would not have noticed if you had not existed, but, then, it would not have noticed even if half of itself were missing. So why ask the universe in the first place? Let's ask you instead. Had you not existed, the *world-for-you* would not have existed either. Your subjective psychological reality, the world-*for-you,* would never have been. It is not a world of space-time, force fields, or subatomic particles we are talking about now, but a world of joys and sorrows, colors and sounds, thoughts and memories, embodiment and movement: a reality of lived experience and sensation. It is a world that, at the very least, *senses its own existence,* though it may not understand it or have the ability to conceptualize it *as* sensed existence. Nevertheless, existence it is, a subjective existence that matters in a way that the objective existence of an entire universe of physical substance, if devoid of consciousness, could never matter.

In the light of the above considerations, it is no wonder that the problem of consciousness has been regarded as perhaps the most significant question that still remains unsolved by science. Consciousness is literally a matter of life and death: you exist only insofar as your subjective psychological reality exists. When it is wiped out for good, the world-for-you will be gone, and so will you.

Thus, it would be really nice, wouldn't it, to have a clear scientific theory about consciousness that explains, once and for all, what these subjective worlds-*for-someone* are really all about; what the place of the subjective psychological reality is in the physical universe? Although the final answers will be certainly hard to come by anytime soon, it seems to me quite clear what the fruitful scientific approach to this problem should consist in. It should take very seriously both the subjective psychological reality of consciousness and the objective neurobiological reality, found in specific regions, called "brains," of the physical universe. Somehow, these two realities, although seemingly worlds apart, must be intimately connected.

If we can make any sense of that connection at all, it would seem that, one way or another, those two realities simply *must* lie along a single integrated continuum in the seamless order of nature. Perhaps such a continuum could be discovered by following—at least for the time being—the working hypothesis that consciousness is just another biological phenomenon in the brain. Not, I gather, an entirely ordinary biological phenomenon; instead, a very special one with several puzzling and amazing features, but a natural biological phenomenon all the same. Therefore, treating consciousness as a real biological phenomenon in the brain seems to me a reasonable approach to the scientific study of consciousness.

I call this approach *biological realism* about consciousness. Biological realism treats subjective consciousness as a *real* phenomenon instead of denying or eliminating it as some sort of grand illusion or intellectual error. Biological realism regards consciousness as a *natural* phenomenon, one that requires a fully naturalistic explanation, instead of treating it as some sort of supernatural or mystical phenomenon entirely beyond the reach of human science. It takes consciousness as a *biological* phenomenon, which means that consciousness is realized at spatial and temporal scales, and levels of complexity in nature, similar to other biological phenomena. That is to deny that consciousness is basically a phenomenon found at the microscopic level of subatomic particles or quantum effects, for example.

Biological realism assumes that the biological phenomenon of consciousness is tightly anchored to, indeed literally located within, the confines of the biological reality found in the brain. Therefore, it denies the philosophical idea according to which consciousness, in some form at least, is present all over the physical universe, even in such unlikely places as electrons, stones, or thermostats (panpsychism). Biological realism also denies the position that consciousness has *no* definable spatial location or spatial properties whatsoever. It further denies the currently fashionable view of "embodied cognition" according to which consciousness is not confined to the brain, but in some unfathomable manner pervades the whole human body (or even extends beyond the body to the surrounding environment).

Biological realism treats the empirical biological sciences and the explanatory strategies applied to them as the best tools we have when trying to understand the place of consciousness in nature. Consciousness should be seen as a biological phenomenon in the brain, located at a particular level of organization in the overall hierarchical structure of nature. A biological research program on consciousness should build its philosophy, methodology and empirical approaches on these kinds of basic assumptions.

Cognitive neuroscientists may have taken for granted that something like biological realism must be the mainstream philosophical approach to the study of consciousness. After all, there is nothing terribly radical or inherently implausible about it—as a matter of fact, it is just our conventional scientific worldview extended to the problem of consciousness. Perhaps something like biological realism is tacitly assumed by most of the neuroscientists who try to uncover the neural basis of consciousness in the brain. But, strangely enough, most of the current philosophical approaches to consciousness seem to be in serious conflict with biological realism. The reason for the dominance of antibiological approaches in philosophy would be somewhat less of a mystery if the biological approach to consciousness had been already thoroughly examined by philosophers and found to be wanting. But, unfortunately, that does not seem to be the case.

Apart from the philosophical contributions of John Searle (1992, 2000), the theoretical and empirical implications of biological realism remain largely unexplored.

Therefore, my main task in this book is the following: To depict a *biological research program on consciousness* that accepts biological realism as its basic principle. A research program should incorporate a coherent global view of its subject domain. In the following chapters, I attempt to bring the study of consciousness under the unifying theoretical framework of biological realism.

This undertaking involves the following tasks. First, to get an idea of what the explanation of consciousness requires, consciousness must be placed in the same boat with other complex biological phenomena: the framework of multilevel explanation. Second, the currently available theories and empirical methods must be evaluated by asking what they can reveal about the levels of biological organization in the brain, where consciousness resides. Third, the wealth of results from different experimental approaches to consciousness should be placed in the context of the biological research program. Only in such a way will it be possible to understand how the different types of experiments and findings contribute to the overall understanding of consciousness.

The explanation of consciousness, in this view, is a slowly progressing scientific effort, an empirical and theoretical puzzle to be solved piece by piece; a biological mechanism to be elucidated gradually and piecemeal by empirical science. I fear that the problem of consciousness will never be resolved all of a sudden by constructing a single philosophical argument, no matter how witty, nor by running a single brain-imaging experiment, no matter how ingenious. Instead of such isolated attempts, an overall scientific research program is needed that provides a general philosophical and empirical framework, the big picture, to which the problem of consciousness can be firmly anchored, and, consequently, taken apart bit by bit and thereby solved, step by step. After all, that is how biological science has succeeded in solving other great mysteries of nature which once seemed eternal and irreconcilable.

So far the field of consciousness research has been quite a mess just because it lacks the big picture or an overall unifying theoretical framework. In the course of this book, I explore the major theoretical and empirical issues in consciousness research and relate them to each other under the framework of biological realism. I shall proceed in this task as follows.

The first, introductory part of the book opens with the observation that, despite frequent references to a "science" of consciousness, the field of consciousness research is still a long way from constituting a true science in the sense of a unified research program. In chapter 1 I delineate what would be required of a unified scientific research program on consciousness. I argue that any such research program must be committed to some shared fundamental assumptions concerning the nature of the *explanandum,* and I propose that biological realism provides us with a theoretical starting point from which to launch the hard core of a promising research program. Other types of fundamental assumptions (e.g., panpsychism, functionalism, and representationalism) lead to research programs dissimilar from biological realism in important respects. Many find the alternative approaches more plausible or acceptable than biological realism. In the course of this book I explain why I do not find the alternatives all that inviting.

Biological realism necessarily anchors the explanation of consciousness in the context of other biological sciences, especially cognitive neuroscience. Recent work in the philosophy of science has shown that the proper explanatory strategy in the context of the biological sciences is not the traditional idea of "theory reduction" or "deductive-nomological explanation" but rather an approach that may be called "multilevel explanation." I will demonstrate how consciousness as a biological phenomenon can be fruitfully placed in the framework of multilevel explanation.

This explanatory framework of the biological sciences greatly clarifies what it means to "explain" consciousness. Consciousness can be placed in the multilevel framework if it is treated simply as one particular level of biological organization: the *phenomenal* level in the brain. In the multilevel framework the overall explanation of consciousness then breaks down into several smaller tasks: the downward-looking, backward-looking, and upward-looking explanations. Different sorts of questions and evidence are relevant for illuminating each of these explanatory dimensions. The downward-looking explanation should answer the question, What are the neural microlevel mechanisms of consciousness? The backward-looking explanation illuminates the causal history of consciousness, How are the contents of consciousness modulated by external stimuli?, When does consciousness emerge and how does it develop in the brain of a newborn baby?, and Why was consciousness selected for during evolutionary history? The upward-looking explanation tells us what the functional role of consciousness is in the brain and in guiding external behavior: How does consciousness contribute to adaptive behavior? In the rest of the book these different explanatory dimensions are systematically charted.

Chapter 2 begins with the observation that before an *explanation* of any biological phenomenon is feasible, the explanandum must be clearly and unambiguously *identified.* This requires a systematic description of the phenomenon. One way to this end is to clarify the conceptual mess surrounding consciousness. The biological research program needs a detailed *conceptual map* of the territory. Only then is there a real possibility for conceptual integration so that most people would use the fundamental concepts of the field in the same way. I present an initial map of the conceptual territory by introducing the most central concepts and conceptual distinctions that I believe a research program on consciousness should include.

Part II of the book describes the theoretical and philosophical foundations of the research program. As evidenced by the history of biology, a useful strategy to make initial theoretical progress in a relatively new area of empirical research is to utilize *metaphors* and *model systems.* In chapters 3, 4, and 5 I explore the model systems and metaphors of consciousness. Visual awareness has been proposed by many to be the most promising model system for consciousness research. I suggest that in addition to visual awareness, *the dreaming brain* also constitutes an excellent model system for the study of consciousness. During dreaming, the full range of subjective experiences is brought about by a brain that is effectively isolated from stimulus input and motor output. The dreaming brain thus creates a kind of "pure" consciousness, which has wide-ranging theoretical and philosophical implications. By exploring the phenomenology of dreaming we end up with a particular metaphor of consciousness that captures the phenomenon — the explanandum—purely from the first-person point of view: *the world-simulation metaphor* of consciousness.

In chapter 6 the theoretical foundations of the world-simulation metaphor are explored. The basic feature of phenomenal reality is *the sense of presence:* The contents of consciousness form *the world now present for me,* a kind of virtual reality in the brain. Thus, the theoretical explanation of consciousness requires a philosophical account of *inner presence* and *presentation* (rather than *re*presentation).

The epistemological and metaphysical implications of the world-simulation metaphor are analyzed in chapter 7. I argue that the biological research program requires a philosophical account of "presence." This concept has a respectable philosophical background in old discussions of "acquaintance." A few current philosophers have reintroduced the concept of "presence" in some form into modern discussions on consciousness, but these writings seem to have appeared in isolation from each other, not accumulating as a serious alternative in the philosophy of consciousness. One reason for this may be that many philosophers still seem to think that this type of view will necessarily lead to a hopeless metaphysical and epistemological cul-de-sac where an internal homunculus must be postulated who infallibly perceives private mental objects or sense-data. I will show that it is not all that difficult to avoid those outdated philosophical traps and to construct a coherent and plausible way of thinking about consciousness as inner presence.

There are several lines of philosophical thought that resist biological realism or the internalism inherent in the world-simulation metaphor. In chapter 8 I try to expose the reasons why many reject the view that consciousness is a biological phenomenon residing within the confines of the brain, or the view that inner phenomenal presence is the most fundamental aspect of consciousness. I suggest that alternative ways of characterizing and localizing consciousness, advocated by such approaches as direct realism, representationalism and content externalism, embodied cognition, neurophenomenology, projectivism, and panpsychism, are not entirely convincing as the philosophical basis of a progressive scientific research program on consciousness.

Part III concentrates on the task of "empirical phenomenology": the description of consciousness on its own terms. In chapter 9 I describe the basic principles of such phenomenology. I end up arguing for the view that the most fundamental ingredient of the phenomenal level is some sort of a unifying spatial coordinate system—which I call "virtual space"— in which the rest of the phenomenal contents must be embedded to be directly present in subjective experience. Virtual space is the invisible but unifying framework that underlies the global unity of consciousness. It explains why there is at any one time exactly *one* world-*for-me* in which all my phenomenal experiences occur in a fundamentally interrelated fashion. In chapter 10 I apply empirical phenomenology to illustrate how the multifarious contents of consciousness are constructed out of dissociable phenomenal parts and features. This exploration leads to insights about the nature of "virtual objects" and the "virtual self," fundamental components of phenomenal consciousness during both dreaming and wakefulness.

The phenomenological observations thus suggest that, on the one hand, consciousness is fundamentally unified—it forms a single phenomenal *world-for-me*—but on the other hand, the diverse phenomenal features and contents of consciousness must be based on a number of different underlying mechanisms. In part IV I concentrate on the *unity of consciousness* and on the problem of its mechanisms: *the binding problem.* In chapter 11 I show that the binding problem is not a single problem, but a set of related problems that need to be disentangled from each other. "Binding" refers to three distinct problems in three different disciplines: neuroscience, cognitive science, and consciousness research. Once these distinctions are made clear, we can see how the binding of phenomenal consciousness, or the unity of consciousness, relates to research at the cognitive and neural levels of description. Chapters 12 and 13 then apply this analysis to several neuropsychological disorders and other related phenomena in which the normal phenomenal unity of consciousness breaks up. The complexity and independency of several different binding mechanisms that must be at work when our normal unified phenomenal consciousness is constructed in the brain is thus dramatically exposed. Chapter 14 describes how the mechanisms of binding fail in the dreaming brain, producing bizarre combinations of phenomenal content in dream images. However, the failures to bind the dream world together coherently seem to follow interesting regularities which will be revealed with the help of a systematic exploration of dream phenomenology.

Chapter 15 explores the binding problem as it appears in cognitive science and cognitive psychology. Although the discussions in those fields hardly ever mention consciousness, it is possible to find interesting theoretical relations between phenomenal unity and cognitive unity. In fact, I argue that some of the data structures or representations identified in cognitive theories are none other than the subjective phenomenal contents of consciousness in disguise. In cognitive theories, selective attention and binding are closely coupled. Therefore, in cognitive science consciousness is often confused with (or even equated with) attention. I believe this is a mistake. Therefore, I try to clarify how exactly visual consciousness is related to the cognitive concept of visual attention.

Chapter 16 explores the neural mechanisms of binding. A large body of empirical evidence from neuroscience shows that the unity of phenomenal consciousness is closely related to neural synchronicity and coherence. These results have important implications also for the search of the neural correlates of consciousness (NCC), a topic to be discussed in greater detail later in the book.

Part V moves downward from the phenomenal level to explore the microlevel mechanisms of consciousness. To define those mechanisms is to give a *downward-looking* or *constitutive explanation* for consciousness. The fundamental problem related to this project is known as the *explanatory gap.* I suggest that the biological research program will be able to build bridges that cross the gap from neuroscience to phenomenal consciousness. In chapter 17 I first point out that the explanatory gap and the possibilities for a reduction between the neural and the phenomenal realities have been discussed traditionally in the context of the deductive-nomological framework of explanation. I argue that it is an inappropriate explanatory framework for the biological sciences and therefore the explanatory gap should be placed in the context of multilevel explanation. The history of science shows that the existence of an explanatory gap in some domain most likely is a sign not of an irremovable mystery nor of the sudden, inexplicable emergence of nonphysical entities, but that there are levels of natural organization involved that have not yet been discovered by empirical science.

The task of the biological research program is to uncover all the levels of organization in the brain that will be crucial for the explanation of consciousness. This task is primarily a challenge for cognitive neuroscience and functional brain imaging. Chapters 18, 19, and 20 deal with the NCC or the experimental search for consciousness in the brain by using the methods and theories of neuroscience. The core question here is, If we find the neural correlates of consciousness in the brain, will we then be able to explain consciousness in neural terms? The view recently defended by several philosophers is that even perfect empirical neuroscience will never be able to explain consciousness, while the view among many cognitive neuroscientists appears to be that the currently available brain-imaging methods are already revealing the neural mechanisms of consciousness in colorful images produced by positron emission tomography (PET) and functional magnetic resonance imaging (fMRI), and that those methods will eventually provide us with theoretical explanations of consciousness. In contrast to these views I argue that, if biological realism is taken seriously, it follows that the currently available methods of functional brain imaging, though useful up to a point, are not adequate to truly discover the phenomenal level of organization in the brain. However, more sophisticated methods might take us to the point where empirical neuroscience is capable of putting forward genuine explanations of consciousness. Since we do not yet have such methods available, we need to stretch our imagination a little to catch a glimpse of the possible future of cognitive neuroscience.

In chapter 21 I speculate how the phenomenal level and its constitutive mechanisms might eventually be discovered in the brain, thereby transforming the cognitive neuroscience of consciousness into "phenomenal" neuroscience. Such a development is not going to be a simple matter because of severe methodological limitations in the measurement, observation, and modeling of higher levels of neural organization in the brain. Although the speculative scenario I delineate may sound like a science-fiction story, we should remember that for the neuroscientists of past generations, our current neuroimaging technology (such as PET, fMRI, magnetoencephalography [MEG], and transcranial magnetic stimulation [TMS]) would have been nothing but far-fetched science fiction.

In the final part VI, (chapters 22, 23, and 24) I explore the *causal powers* of consciousness and the threat from *epiphenomenalism.* The causal role of consciousness is defined at a higher level, where consciousness is itself a part or subsystem of the whole organism behaving in its environment. Thus, in the multilevel framework, defining the causal powers and higher-level roles of consciousness constitutes the *upward-looking* or *contextual explanation* of consciousness.

The *dissociation between explicit and implicit*—or *conscious and nonconscious*—information in the brain is considered first (chapter 22): What exactly do we learn about the causal powers of the phenomenal level from the studies on blindsight, implicit perception, nonconscious visually guided actions, and similar phenomena? The data on implicit processing reveal what the brain can do with purely nonconscious stimulus representations when phenomenal content—the subjective experience—normally elicited by the stimulus is selectively carved off, leaving the brain with only nonconscious information to live on. The evidence suggests that these nonconscious input-output transformations of sensory information in one way or another bypass the sphere of consciousness entirely, thereby revealing complex information-processing mechanisms in the brain that in themselves realize no phenomenal level of organization. These nonconscious zombie systems seem to have only limited causal powers in guiding organism-environment interaction, whereas the contribution of the phenomenal level seems to be decisive for meaningful interactions with our environment.

In chapter 23 I explore a variety of fascinating disorders, such as epileptic automatisms and sleepwalking, which temporarily seem to carve off the entire state of being conscious. Thus, these disorders turn the whole person into a nonconscious zombie that continues to roam about in the world, totally oblivious of the fact that within, there is nobody home. A careful examination of such zombies, however, reveals the crucial role of the internal world simulation in guiding external behavior. If the causal contribution of consciousness is wiped out, the remaining nonconscious organism-environment interaction, even if sometimes remarkably complex, is rather pointless all the same. Conversely, other types of disorders show that the simulated phenomenal world in the brain has unique causal powers in determining the behavioral trajectories of our physical bodies. In the light of evidence from these disorders, consciousness surfaces as a causally potent biological system with unique causal powers. Therefore, we need not worry about epiphenomenalism any longer.

In chapter 24 I explore *the biological function of dreaming:* Why does the brain bother to construct a subjective world-*for-me* during sleep, when the internal world simulation can in no way influence behavior? I propose that the dream reality in the brain was originally a nocturnal simulation of adaptively important events that our ancestors repeatedly were exposed to during the course of evolutionary history. This theory explains most of the conspicuous statistical properties of phenomenal dream content; among other things, why nightmares, bad dreams, and other unpleasant recurring dream themes exist and why they are a universal feature of human dream life; why we all easily fall prey to posttraumatic nightmares after going through life-threatening events in the real world; and why we all frequently dream about being late, failing in studies or work, or about our other everyday worries. The threat-simulation theory postulates that our dream-production system is originally an *evolved biological defense mechanism.* Once we know what to look for in the content of dreams, we find that the dreaming brain still shows clear and abundant traces of its evolutionary function.

All in all, the biological research program on consciousness, based on the core assumptions of biological realism and the world-simulation metaphor, integrates the philosophy, methodology, and empirical study of consciousness into one unified big picture which guides empirical research in new and fruitful directions. I have tried to present the big picture in this book as clearly and in as much detail as possible. The treatment covers philosophy, psychology, and cognitive neuroscience in an attempt to integrate their independent contributions to the study of consciousness and to incorporate the emerging overall view of consciousness into the biological research program.

Still, I am afraid that in many places the treatment remains rather sketchy or superficial, at least for specialists working within the particular disciplines involved. I have had to trespass into the territories of at least the following disciplines: philosophy of mind, philosophy of science, biology, neuroscience, dream research, evolutionary psychology, neuropsychology, and cognitive science. The issues I have included in the book I have judged as being absolutely crucial for understanding consciousness, no matter which disciplines they fall into. Undoubtedly, most of the issues deserve a book of their own for a more detailed treatment. My goal, however, was not to write another purely philosophical book about consciousness for professional philosophers (and most likely almost incomprehensible to empirical scientists), or another purely scientific review of the neural basis of consciousness for neuropsychologists and cognitive neuroscientists (without any discussion of the philosophical issues involved). By contrast, my goal is to cross the traditional disciplinary borderlines to paint with broad strokes a general multidisciplinary picture of consciousness. I hope that the broadness of the overall treatment is sufficient compensation for the unavoidable lack of detail and depth at some points.

The problem of consciousness, the most fundamental question, if ever solved, will be solved in the context of some sort of systematic empirical research program that takes phenomenal subjectivity very seriously. Biological realism looks to me like a respectable candidate for establishing exactly such a research program. The big picture that I present in this book is my idea as to how we might reach a more unified science of consciousness. I hope that some of my readers will be able to share this idea with me or, if not, at least point out where I have gone wrong.

I Theoretical Foundations of the Research Program

The central question in this book is: "Can science explain consciousness?" But before it is possible to give any meaningful answer to this question, we need a better understanding of what the question is really all about. What is "science"? What is an "explanation"? And what exactly is the phenomenon called "consciousness" that we are trying to explain? These fundamental theoretical issues are clarified in the first part of the book. The research program that will be developed throughout the book is based on the view that consciousness is a biological phenomenon to be explained in the overall context of the biological sciences, using the strategies of biological explanation. In chapter 1 the fundamental background assumptions of a science that takes consciousness as a biological phenomenon are defined and explored, and in chapter 2 a coherent conceptual basis for such science is outlined.

1 Consciousness as a Biological Phenomenon

The study of consciousness is at a stage where it is finally separating itself from pure philosophy, and rapidly becoming a new branch of empirical science. The motto in this emerging new field seems to be: "Toward a Science of Consciousness." Yet the field is still not sufficiently coherent to count as a genuine science. Therefore, greater unity is essential for the future of the field. In science, the theoretical and empirical coherence of a field is based on a well-established research program. A unified research program delivers the big picture of the order of nature in the respective domain. In this opening chapter of the book, the proposal is put forward that the unified science of consciousness should be anchored to the biological sciences. The big picture of the place of consciousness in nature would best be built on the (philosophically controversial) view that consciousness is a biological phenomenon within the brain. This view leads to a new and much clearer picture of the scientific explanation of consciousness.

The Study of Consciousness: Pretending to Be a Science, but Is It Really?

The official news from the frontline of the study of consciousness has been more or less the same for a number of years: We are steadily progressing *toward* "the science of consciousness." But what exactly is the nature of the progress made? The search for the science of consciousness was launched way back at the beginning of the 1990s, when it became increasingly clear that mainstream psychology and cognitive science had not been able (or even willing) to face the problem of consciousness. How long will it still take before we finally reach the goal, a genuine science of consciousness? A cynical observer, one who is getting impatient with the situation, might go so far as to suggest that no actual progress is being made: the whole field of consciousness studies seems to be nothing but a big philosophical and theoretical mess which is not moving in any particular direction.

I am certainly more optimistic than that about the prospects for a science of consciousness. But even so, much progress is still to be made before it will be possible to go to a bookstore and purchase something like a standard textbook of consciousness science. That would be a clear sign that the science of consciousness is a fact, not a fiction. The transmission of scientific knowledge in established fields of science relies heavily on the advanced textbook (Giere, 1988) which as clearly as possible explains the theoretical and methodological basis of the branch of science in question and presents the central empirical approaches and core findings within one coherent framework, accepted by most of those working in the field. Conversely, the absence of a basic coherent story about the science of consciousness may be interpreted as a sign that a coherent body of scientific knowledge about the subject matter of consciousness is still hard to come by.

Why, precisely, are we still so far away from the science of consciousness? The scientific explanation of consciousness is not an entirely straightforward undertaking. It is difficult to say exactly what the task consists in, and which branches of science are supposed to take the responsibility for solving it. Resolution of the problem of consciousness has been sought in such fields as philosophy of mind, cognitive science, psychology, neuroscience, and even quantum physics. The really hard problem of consciousness—or explaining how *any* physical system could have *any* subjective, qualitative states in the first place—is still mostly thought to fall in the philosopher's domain rather than belong to empirical science. The general agreement appears to be that empirical science and experimentation can at best scratch the surface of the *easy* issues about consciousness (such as the cognitive or neural correlates of subjective experience), but the *really hard* issues (such as why anything in the physical world should have any subjective experiences at all) are best left for the philosopher to ponder. Yet, nobody expects that philosophers would actually *solve* them. The gap between the "hard" philosophical and the "easy" empirical problems of consciousness still remains wide-open (Chalmers, 1996).

Discussions in consciousness studies cover an incredibly large range of topics which leave almost no branch of science or the humanities untouched. Underlying this wide scope appear to be a multitude of dissimilar views about the basic nature of consciousness and about the empirical evidence and methodology most relevant to the theoretical explanation of consciousness.

There are some who think that one of the central issues in consciousness studies is whether consciousness is algorithmic or nonalgorithmic (e.g. Penrose, 1989), which is essentially a topic for mathematics and computational science. Some have suggested that consciousness is fundamentally related to the notion of information, which, if true, would make consciousness ubiquitous in the universe: consciousness should be present in all kinds of physical systems carrying information, even extremely simple ones (Chalmers, 1996). Some believe that the problem of consciousness is intimately tied to physical phenomena at the quantum level (e.g. Squires, 1998; Hameroff & Scott, 1998): wave-particle duality, nonlocal effects, the collapse of quantum fields, and other elusive microphysical phenomena residing at incomprehensibly small spatiotemporal scales, way below the scales where brains, neurons, or even whole organic molecules reside. Others have argued that the key to consciousness lies at the level of specific receptors at certain types of synapses (e.g., the NMDA receptors at glutamatergic synapses [Flohr, 2000]). Moving towards still higher levels, still others have argued that there are specific "consciousness neurons" whose biophysical and neurophysiological properties differ from other neurons (Crick & Koch, 1998). Contrary to this view, some believe that consciousness cannot be defined as a property of specific single neurons but depends on the synchronized, coherent activity of large neural populations (Singer, 1994). Others have presented evidence that consciousness is associated with specific neural pathways in the brain, whereas the rest function in the absence of consciousness (Milner & Goodale, 1995). Then there are those who are reluctant to attribute consciousness to any part of the brain, but would say that consciousness is a property of the whole brain or the whole person rather than any of its parts. Consciousness is not viewed as based on particular biological phenomena in the brain, but instead on organism-environment interaction or even language and social communication (Dennett, 1991; O'Regan & Noë, 2001). The doctrines of "embodied cognition" and "enactive cognitive science" go so far as to say that mind and consciousness are not in the head but embodied in the whole organism embedded in its environment (Thompson, 2001; Thompson & Varela, 2001).

This wild variety of views, theories, and evidence argued to be relevant to the explanation of consciousness gives the impression that there are few, if any, fundamental theories or empirical findings that would form a *shared* core of the study of consciousness. If a novice enters the field and would become a consciousness researcher—a true professional in this fascinating new field—he might wonder what exactly it is supposed to include. What is the *philosophical* view of the nature of consciousness that the empirical *science* of consciousness is based on? What are the basic theories to be learned and mastered? What are the empirical results that every consciousness researcher is expected to know about? In any other field of established science, say biology, it is perfectly clear what the shared philosophical view is (and is not, say, vitalism or creationism). It is also rather obvious what a newcomer is expected to learn to become a professional in the field (simply observe which topics the standard advanced textbooks in the field cover), and what is only peripheral or totally irrelevant. One can furthermore be sure that any professional in the field will know about certain basic theories and phenomena (say, evolutionary theory, protein synthesis, or the structure of DNA), no matter what the exact specialization of that person is. But not so in the field of consciousness science. After taking a look at the massive literature published on consciousness since the early 1990s, the novice would have to wonder whether she should study quantum theory and learn about double-slit experiments, Schrödinger's cat, and the like? Or would she be better off studying the neurochemistry and neurotransmitter systems of the brain? What about single-cell response properties in the visual system of the monkey? Or the synchronization patterns of human scalp electroencephalography (EEG) during visual perception or rapid eye movement (REM) sleep? Then there is a huge amount of data on neuropsychological patients: how important is that? What about the phenomenology of altered states of consciousness: hypnosis, dreaming, meditation, religious or aesthetic experience? Or the experimental psychology of change blindness or implicit learning? And then there are all the ancient and mysterious religious and contemplative practices of the East: perhaps they hold the key to the secrets of consciousness?

The difficulties of the would-be consciousness researcher are a reflection of the heterogeneity and incoherence that currently dominate the field of consciousness studies: there are neither any universally accepted basic theoretical principles nor any well-defined empirical core or database of consciousness science that most people working in the field would agree about and everybody would be required to master in order to be taken seriously as a professional in the field. Different people emphasize entirely different, often idiosyncratic theoretical principles and selected empirical findings; therefore, the field seems to have failed so far in establishing a shared "big picture" of consciousness. The big picture about the scientific study and explanation of consciousness would put the various theories and empirical findings into context and thereby indicate what the relative importance of different sorts of evidence is for the overall explanation of consciousness. Since such a big picture seems to be missing, consciousness studies do not (yet) have enough coherence to be called a "science" (in the sense that, say, biology or neuroscience deserves the label).

However, at the same time it appears that the study of consciousness would very much *want* to become a true, respectable science. There are large conferences being arranged that strive toward a *science* of consciousness; there is a professional organization for the *scientific* study of consciousness; there is an academic journal, *Consciousness and Cognition,* promoting a *natural-science* approach to consciousness; there have been several books published recently about the *science* of consciousness.

The Explanation of Consciousness Requires a Unified Research Program

To be worthy of the label "science" unfortunately requires more than just the frequent use of the words "science" and "scientific." It requires a *unified research program* that establishes the theoretical, philosophical, and methodological foundations of the particular science in question. Phenomena that are scientifically explained (or explainable) are explained within the context of some specific research program. Thus, to truly strive toward a science of consciousness is to seek the appropriate foundations for a coherent scientific research program on consciousness. Conversely, as long as no genuine research program on consciousness exists, no amount of throwing around the word "science" will help (in fact, too much talk might only raise the suspicion that the scientific status of the field must be somehow questionable). Instead, it might be wise to figure out what sort of thing a research program is and what would transform the mere study of consciousness into a genuine research program.

What does a coherent, systematic research program typically consist in? Philosophers of science have attempted to explicate what sort of an entity a scientific research program is supposed to be. While there have been considerable disagreements among them about this, there is also substantial agreement on the general characteristics of research programs (I will here mainly follow the ideas of Larry Laudan and Imre Lakatos).

A research program is a set of background assumptions shared by the community of researchers within that program. The background assumptions involve significant ontological and methodological commitments. These commitments can be thought of as general assumptions concerning the substantive entities and processes in the domain of study, and the appropriate methods to be used for investigating the phenomena and constructing the theories in that domain. The research program outlines the domain of application of the theories belonging to it, indicating which empirical questions are regarded as central to it and which belong to foreign domains or are only pseudoproblems. There are often several competing specific theories within a research program which present more detailed hypotheses of the ontology of the basic entities and their interaction. However, despite the variety of competing theories within a program, there is also significant integrity. The basic assumptions of the research program prevent any scientist working within the program from adopting theories that are incompatible with the metaphysics or methodology of the program. To adopt a view or to advocate a theory that is inconsistent with the core assumptions of the research program is to put oneself outside that program and to reject it.

A research program in many ways guides the research around the phenomena that fall into its domain. It constrains the interpretations that can be given to empirical findings, suggests promising lines of research, and points out suspicious lines of explanation. It allows the empirical results from a wide variety of empirical subdomains to be integrated into a coherent big picture of the subject matter.

A unified research program on consciousness would thus tell us what the relevance of the different philosophical approaches, theories, and empirical findings is to the scientific explanation of consciousness. Most importantly, it would provide us with a coherent, integrated big picture of the place of consciousness in the order of nature.

A Research Program Must Be Committed to Some Fundamental Assumptions: Not Anything Goes

Any research program needs to make *some* assumptions concerning the basic metaphysical and ontological status of the phenomena that are the objects of study. If we want to move toward a science of consciousness by aiming to establish a unified research program on consciousness, then some criteria have to be set for what sort of claims about consciousness can be made within the program, and what cannot be accepted because they are inconsistent with the core assumptions of the program.

The sad truth about the current state of consciousness studies appears to be that there is nothing even remotely resembling a unified scientific research program on consciousness. The field of consciousness studies includes a colorful variety of rival philosophical theories as well as a heterogeneous assortment of empirical studies of consciousness. While this may be a prosperous starting point on the way toward the science of consciousness, it cannot be the ultimate destination. A coherent science cannot be built on an incoherent and messy theoretical basis.

To establish a science of consciousness in the form of one widely shared and internally unified research program, at first several competing empirical research programs should emerge in the field. They will embrace dissimilar background assumptions, but each will try to develop a plausible overall account of consciousness that guides further research into, and theory about, the topic. Each program should be internally coherent and explicitly committed to some specific first principles that are both philosophically plausible and empirically fruitful. While empirical fruitfulness may be a feature that can be assessed in some objective manner in the long run, the plausibility of particular metaphysical commitments often comes down to subjective intuitions and tastes rather than objective facts, once internal conceptual coherence is established. Thus, what is plausible to one may be outrageous to another. In any case, coherent and plausible fundamental commitments—whatever their precise content may be—will pave the way for a true science of consciousness. The research program that in the long run shows the greatest overall explanatory power should be the most inviting candidate to develop into a unified science of consciousness.

Hence, if we want the diverse studies of consciousness to become a unified science in the long run, some degree of philosophical and theoretical freedom must be given up, at least by those who practice empirical research and commit themselves to a particular research program. Furthermore, any research program is associated with a specific empirical context. The phenomena under study must lie on some specific spatiotemporal scale and at some particular level of complexity in the world. The sciences that study phenomena at those scales and levels, or close to them, must be the ones most relevant to the study of consciousness. I am inclined to believe that if there is any proper place for a scientific research program on consciousness, it will be found in the empirical sciences that directly study the interface between neural and mental phenomena. Any viable research program on consciousness should build primarily on the phenomena, vocabulary, and methodology relevant and acceptable to those sciences, and try to connect the empirical study of consciousness with them.

This cognitive neuroscience approach to consciousness seems to me almost self-evident, but many others seem to have taken a different course. There have been serious attempts to show that the brain and neuroscience are irrelevant for explaining mind and consciousness (argued by classical cognitive science, and more recently by some forms of philosophical representationalism) or that quantum physics is highly relevant (argued by several researchers recently in consciousness studies).

The point here is not that we could somehow know in advance that, say, quantum mechanics, shamanism, or robotics is not going to be relevant for the explanation of consciousness. They could well be, but so could a myriad of other somewhat far-fetched fields of human knowledge. The point is, rather, that we do not know in advance that they *would* be highly relevant or, indeed, relevant at all. Any claim for their relevance must be empirically anchored to actual phenomena of consciousness and to actual data, experiments, testable hypotheses, and predictions.

Consciousness: A Theoretical Problem for the Biology of the Mind

Until recently, the neural-mental interface was relatively untouched by the psychological and biological sciences, save for the isolated attempts in neuropsychology and physiological psychology to cross the borderline. During the 1990s, a new overall approach changed it all. Cognitive neuroscience is the branch of science that explicitly operates at the interface between the biological and the mental realms, and seeks global theoretical integration between these domains. Cognitive neuroscience has been characterized as the empirical science invented to close the explanatory gap and to solve the most fundamental problem of modern science: the gap between biological processes and the processes of mind (Gazzaniga, 1995a). Remarkably, in this spirit cognitive neuroscience has been boldly declared to be "the biology of the mind" (Gazzaniga, Ivry, & Mangun, 2002).

If there already exists an empirical field of inquiry devoted to the biology of the mind, then the mind-body problem (or the brain-consciousness problem) can no longer be the sole property of an empirically isolated philosophy of mind. I suggest that consciousness should primarily be regarded as a theoretical problem of those special sciences where it *must* figure in, where it simply cannot be avoided or ignored. Therefore, the problem of consciousness is now becoming a central problem in the *philosophy of cognitive neuroscience.* Consequently, questions about whether or not science can explain consciousness should be understood as fundamental questions about the scope and limits of cognitive neuroscience.

The Hard Core of the Biological Research Program

If the philosophical mind-body problem is built into the very foundation of cognitive neuroscience, then the scientific research program on consciousness should have its roots in the same terrain. It should be a *biological* research program above all.

A research program is a metatheoretical entity that includes a set of paradigmatic assumptions, sometimes called the "hard core" of the program. What might be an appropriate pretheoretical assumption for a biological research program on consciousness? What kind of ideas should constitute the hard core of the program? I propose that the biological research program on consciousness should start with a few very simple, crystal clear, empirically plausible basic assumptions that are consistent with the overall approach in cognitive neuroscience as a branch of the biological sciences. Those assumptions should include some general metaphysical commitments as to the nature of the phenomenon, and a clear idea of where in the physical world the phenomenon can be found. My suggestion is the following:

Subjective phenomenal consciousness is a real, natural biological phenomenon that literally resides within the confines of the brain.

Let me explain briefly what these assumptions imply. To say that consciousness is a *real* phenomenon is, first, to deny that consciousness is a mere illusion (i.e., to deny that we are zombies or that there is no important difference between us and nonconscious zombies—the notorious Dennettian view), and second, to deny that consciousness is merely some sort of causally impotent epiphenomenon. To say that consciousness is *real* implies the following claims: (1) consciousness exists, (2) it exists in time and space (i.e., conscious phenomena have temporal duration and spatial location), (3) it has some causal powers. I adopt the philosophical view that *to be real is to have causal powers* (Kim, 1992; a defense of this definition of "real" is, however, outside the scope of this book). The fundamental assumption that consciousness is a real phenomenon thus entails the claim that the phenomenal realm is causally potent, and that it has causal powers distinct from the nonphenomenal (e.g., purely neurophysiological) realm.

To say that consciousness is a *natural* phenomenon is to deny that consciousness is a supernatural or mystical phenomenon, in principle beyond a natural-science approach. It is also to deny that consciousness is only an observer-relative interpretation or social construction whose existence is dependent on conditions external to the biological organism to which the phenomenon is attributed. Consciousness exists in its own right, and the fact that there are conscious phenomena in the world is not ontologically dependent on any other facts apart from ones concerning the biological systems—brains—in which consciousness is realized. To have a fully functional human brain is a sufficient condition for having consciousness, regardless of what else there is in the world or what the causal history or surrounding context of the fully functional brain happens to be.

To say that consciousness *literally resides within the confines of the brain* is to characterize the spatial location of the phenomenon in the natural world; to determine unambiguously where we should look for the principal explanandum in the science of consciousness. Note that this statement by no means implies that consciousness is localized in a *single* area or point inside the brain (which is very unlikely); it only postulates that consciousness is somewhere within the confines of the biological reality of the brain rather than anywhere outside that reality. There are many who reject this view because their fundamental background assumptions are different from mine. To accept this internalist view is to deny that consciousness resides in, or is necessarily dependent on, any physical or logical relations between the brain and its surroundings (a claim defended by externalists, e.g., Dretske, 1995; Tye, 1995), and it is to deny that consciousness resides only at the "personal" level of organism-environment interaction (a position defended by Dennett [1991] and O'Regan & Noë [2001]); it is to deny that consciousness is somehow "projected" or "reflected" by the brain into the ordinary physical or some ill-defined nonphysical space (cf. Velmans, 1996, 2000; McGinn, 1999; J. Smythies, 1994b, 2003) and to deny that consciousness somehow pervades the whole body or is literally embodied in the physical body outside the brain (Thompson, 2001). Like other biological phenomena, say protein synthesis or postsynaptic potentials, consciousness is, according to biological realism, located within the confines of the very biological system in which it is realized; it has no supernatural powers to escape from within the depths of the brain.

I suggest that these fundamental assumptions could establish the core of a unified biological research program on consciousness. This research program is consistent with the biology of the mind, but may have implications concerning the general metaphysical commitments of future cognitive neuroscience. Whatever the commitments might turn out to be, they should be worked out in such a manner as to be consistent with the core assumptions of the biological research program on consciousness. Cognitive neuroscience cannot turn its back on consciousness anymore; therefore, the theoretical and philosophical commitments of cognitive neuroscience have to accommodate the reality of consciousness.

The task for us now is to follow the implications of the proposed fundamental assumptions and thereby work out the theoretical foundations of the science of consciousness.

Explanation in the Biological Sciences Is Different from Explanation in Physics

If consciousness is a theoretical problem in the biology of the mind, and the proper research program is a biological one, then the question about explaining consciousness should be placed in that particular context. Thus, to understand what it takes to explain consciousness, we should find out what scientific explanation in biology requires. How are complex biological phenomena in general explained in the biological sciences? In other words, what constitutes an "explanation" in these branches of science? If that can be figured out, then it is possible to place the problem of consciousness in the proper explanatory context and ask, Could consciousness be explained by using a similar explanatory strategy? That is the appropriate question to be asked as far as the explanation of consciousness is concerned. Only by incorporating the problem of consciousness into the biology of mind will it be possible to evaluate whether consciousness constitutes some sort of inexplicable anomaly for science. Only by seeing consciousness in the proper explanatory context can we begin to understand whether consciousness is explicable, to what extent it is explicable, and, if some of its aspects must remain mysterious, why exactly that might be the case.

In current philosophy of science there are two somewhat opposing views of scientific explanation (Salmon, 1989): the *unification approach,* which is mostly based on how explanation works in physics; and the *mechanistic approach,* which applies especially to the biological sciences. The unification approach is a descendant of the classical deductive-nomological (or D-N) view in the philosophy of science. It seeks laws of nature that are as universal as possible. Universal physical laws would provide the basis of a systematized, coherent overall picture of how the world works. According to this framework of explanation, scientific knowledge consists of language-like representations in theories and laws (such as equations, mathematical formulas, or expressions and propositions in some other types of exact formal languages). Consequently, the reductive explanation of a phenomenon consists of a deduction of the phenomenon from a lower-level explanatory theory or general law, with the help of "bridge principles." These bridge principles connect the vocabulary of two theories by identifying a term in an old theory (say, "water") with a term in the new, lower-level explanatory theory ("H_2O").

The D-N view of explanation is closely related to the standard model of theory reduction which has not only been popular in the philosophy of science but has also dominated the philosophical discussions of mind-body reduction (Kim, 1998). The bold idea behind the reductive explanation of mental phenomena is that every term describing psychological phenomena could be identified with a term in (future) neuroscience, and thus psychology would reduce to neuroscience. Hence, in modern philosophy of mind it has been deemed as of utmost importance to establish whether there are "laws" or "bridge principles" that connect the mental and physical domains in a reductive manner, as required in classical D-N explanation. If reductive psychophysical laws cannot be found, then perhaps there are "fundamental" psychophysical laws that link psychological terms with biological terms without reducing the former to the latter. Or perhaps no laws between the physical and the psychological are to be found—perhaps the psychological domain is "anomalous," that is, not to be connected to the biological domain by any "lawlike statements."

This traditional view of scientific explanation and theory reduction seems to have little to do with actual scientific practice in the biological sciences, including the neurosciences. When neurobiologists explain complex biological phenomena found in the nervous system (which they are perfectly capable of doing, at least once in a while), they do not construct deductions or logico-mathematical derivations of laws, or connect predicates of two theories with bridge principles. Explanation in neurobiology is not a logical proof procedure; nor is explanatory knowledge represented in a purely propositional or linguistic form. Furthermore, universal laws of nature comparable to those found in physics are virtually unheard of in the biological sciences.

Still, philosophers of mind almost invariably accept the D-N approach and apply it to the explanation of consciousness. But if consciousness belongs in the scope of the biology of the mind, then there is every reason to believe that the appropriate explanatory strategy for consciousness is going to resemble the successful explanations in the biological sciences rather than the physical sciences. Unless we have a deep understanding of the nature of explanation in the biological sciences, we are in no position to evaluate whether science could or could not explain consciousness. A more naturalistic conception of explanation in biology is urgently needed. Such a conception is provided by the framework of the so-called mechanistic approach. The term "mechanistic" is slightly misleading, though; thus, I shall call this explanatory framework by the more proper term, *multilevel explanation.*

Multilevel Explanation: The Proper Explanatory Strategy for the Biology of the Mind

Multilevel explanation sees explanatory knowledge not clothed in language-like representations, laws, or logical deductions, but as an understanding of the *hidden mechanisms* by which nature works. Proponents of this view (e.g., Bechtel, 1994; Machamer, Darden, & Craver, 2000) have pointed out that the traditional notion of a universal law of nature has few, if any, applications in neurobiology and molecular biology. Biological knowledge is not primarily represented in universal laws, or other propositional expressions in formal languages and mathematical symbols. Biologists typically first *identify* and *describe* an interesting system or phenomenon at one *level of organization* in nature and then try to figure out what the *components* of this system are, how they interact, and how they produce the effects that can be observed at the level of the whole system. When they go about doing this task, they try to take the system apart, or visualize it better with the help of various research instruments, in order to figure out what the components and microstructures of the system are. From these data biologists attempt to build *an idealized multilevel model* of the system, the purpose of which is to show the general structure and function of the system across several levels of organization. The model may be only partially if at all clothed in linguistic representations. Instead, all kinds of visualizable diagrams and figures, scale models, and graphical representations such as charts, maps, and computer simulations can often best depict the component structures of, and their mutual interactions within, the biological system in question (Bechtel, 1994; Bechtel & Richardson, 1992).

The biological research program on consciousness should utilize the same explanatory scheme that applies to the multilevel explanation of other complex biological phenomena. Placing consciousness, the most fascinating of all biological phenomena, into the multilevel framework would then reveal what kinds of questions must be resolved in order to explain consciousness. One big—and seemingly unanalyzable—problem would be thus decomposed to a set of smaller explanatory subproblems, each of which could then be attacked separately. Furthermore, the framework might help the researchers to see which subproblems can be studied by a particular method or experimental approach, and how the different subproblems connect to the big picture of the subject domain. It would also help the researchers to evaluate which phenomena are central and which peripheral, and what the role of a particular empirical phenomenon is in contributing to the big picture. A general explanatory scheme on consciousness would thus serve the function of integrating the various empirical approaches and relating them to each other in a meaningful way.

The Hierarchical Structure of the World: Levels

The mechanistic view in biology depicts natural phenomena as parts of complex hierarchical causal networks. A central notion in this framework is the notion of "levels." Biological phenomena are realized at different levels of complexity in nature. The notions I will use to capture this structure, inherent in nature, are *levels of organization* and *levels of description.*

Hierarchical structure is evident in the case of biological systems. Thus, before we try to fit consciousness into this scheme, let us take a brief look at some of the levels of complexity elsewhere in biology.

We may start at the level of biochemistry which is concerned with the compounds, their chemical properties, and the multitude of chemical reactions involved in the building of living organisms. Small organic molecules are first built by autotrophs, using simple natural oxides. The molecules are then further assembled into macromolecules: amino acids into proteins, monosaccharides into polysaccharides, and so on. At the level of molecular biology, there are macromolecules and the complexes they form inside living cells. Macromolecules are capable of combining into multimacromolecular complexes, out of which the structural components found inside cells (e.g., filaments, tubules, and membranes) are built. Macromolecules, by way of their complex three-dimensional (3D) structure, are capable of causally contributing to the correct performance of otherwise highly unlikely chemical reactions within the cell. Enzyme molecules, almost all of which are proteins, catalyze thousands of chemical reactions by binding only the molecules that are the natural substrates of a specific reaction. Despite all this complexity already found at the level of the building blocks of life, we have to move to a higher level of organization in order to find an actual living system. That is the level of the complete cell, the basic unit of life. A single cell has all that is needed for life (DeDuve, 1991). At this level, we find a complex system that is separated from its environment by a boundary, the cytomemb[illegible]ains a multitude of subsystems such as the nucleus, the cytoskeleton, [illegible] various organelles and so on. These subsystems carry out the various fu[illegible]nstitute life: biosynthetic manufacturing of the constituents of the cell, extracting energy from the environment and converting it to work; multiplying, and so on. Pluricellular living systems such as trees, moths, and humans are composed of huge numbers of specialized cells joined together and organized into systems at levels higher than the individual cell (e.g., tissues and organs).

A Hierarchy of Levels of Organization

Thus, biological organisms can be seen as consisting of a multitude of distinct but interconnected levels. Phenomena at different levels in the hierarchy reside at different spatiotemporal scales or grains. I call the different levels of complexity in nature the *levels of organization.* These levels are taken as *ontological,* that is, as real, causally potent natural phenomena that exist out there, independent of our scientific practices or conceptual systems. A level of organization has a specific orderly structure of entities and it realizes specific activities or functions. The structure appearing at one level can be understood as composed of parts that reside at a lower level of organization. However, the interrelationships between parts and wholes are not always simple or straightforward, for a process or function thought to take place entirely at one level (e.g., a specific chemical reaction chain) may in fact be possible only in the context of structures that reside at higher levels of organization (macromolecular enzymes, membrane properties) (Bechtel & Richardson, 1992). For the sake of simplicity, we may think of the levels of organization in biological systems (such as ourselves) as composing a *hierarchical* system, with basic physical phenomena residing at the bottom levels, chemical and biochemical phenomena at the intermediate levels, and biological and physiological phenomena at the higher levels (Bechtel & Abrahamsen, 1991).

The entities and properties in this multilayered model of the world can be thought of as forming a micro-macro hierarchy (figures 1.1 and 1.2). Entities and properties reside at specific levels of organization. The same properties and entities cannot be realized at levels lower or higher than where they actually reside. Cells reside at one particular level of organization. Parts of cells are not themselves cells (but organelles, macromolecules, etc.); wholes formed by a multitude of cells are not cells themselves (but tissues, organs, and multicellular organisms).

Higher-level properties and entities can be called *macro*properties and *macro*entities, emphasizing that they reside at a higher level of organization than their *micro*constituents. But because they are in such a way constituted by lower-level phenomena, we may also say that they are *micro-based* properties and entities. An important point about *micro*-based *macro*phenomena at higher levels of organization is that *they have their own causal powers that go beyond the causal powers of their microconstituents;* they have novel causal powers not had by any of the lower-level phenomena that constitute them (Kim, 1998).

The idea of the world as a hierarchy of levels of organization is a fundamental assumption in the multilevel explanatory framework. Therefore, if this is the framework that applies to the explanation of biological phenomena in general, then also consciousness as a biological phenomenon should be seen as residing at a specific level of organization in nature. And if consciousness is a biological phenomenon within the confines of the brain (another fundamental assumption of the research program), then there must be some specific level of organization and some specific spatiotemporal grain in the brain where consciousness resides. Furthermore, if consciousness is a micro-based

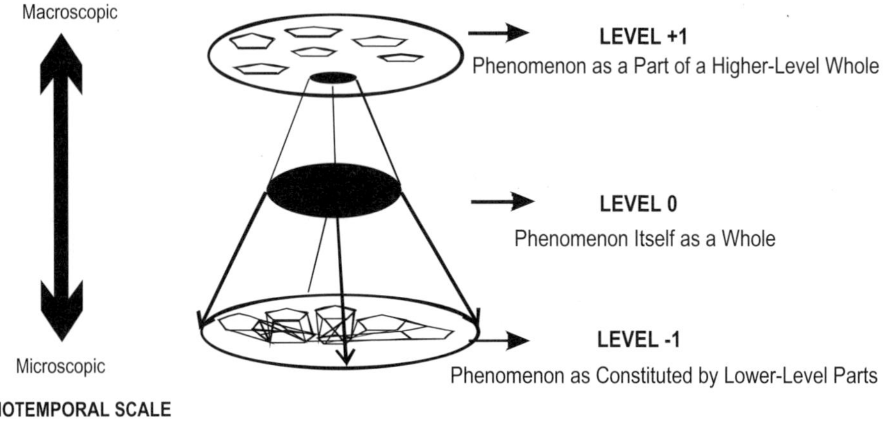

Figure 1.1
The hierarchy of levels of organization. The framework of multilevel explanation depicts biological phenomena as residing at different spatiotemporal scales in the overall micro-macro hierarchy of nature. Entities at contiguous levels bear part-whole relations to each other.

macrophenomenon along with other biological phenomena, it is bound to have unique causal powers not had by other phenomena in the brain, not even by those neural systems that are the microconstituents of consciousness itself.

A key idea that runs through this book is the following: We should adopt the working hypothesis that consciousness is a part of the hierarchical structure of the biological world. More precisely, consciousness constitutes one particular level of organization among all the other levels in nature. Thus, we may *reconceptualize* consciousness as *the phenomenal level of organization* in the brain. The characterization of consciousness as one particular biological level of organization is in harmony with the core assumptions of biological realism. Furthermore, it would clarify several problems that have surrounded consciousness. Most of them can now be reconceptualized in terms of "levels": How does the phenomenal level of organization relate to other levels of organization in the brain? How could the phenomenal level be measured or observed empirically? How could it be conceptualized or modeled theoretically? What are the causal powers of entities and properties residing at the phenomenal level of organization? I explore possible answers to these questions in the course of this book.

Note that the reconceptualization I propose above is not a *reduction* of consciousness to something else. I am not proposing that consciousness, this subjective world-*for-me,* would be anything other than what it is: a world of subjective experience. My proposal simply tries to find the proper place for the subjective world-for-me in the wider context of the physical world, by placing it among other biological levels of organization. This working hypothesis guides our further research efforts when we try to figure out how it is possible that a biological level of organization in the brain manifests itself as a sub-

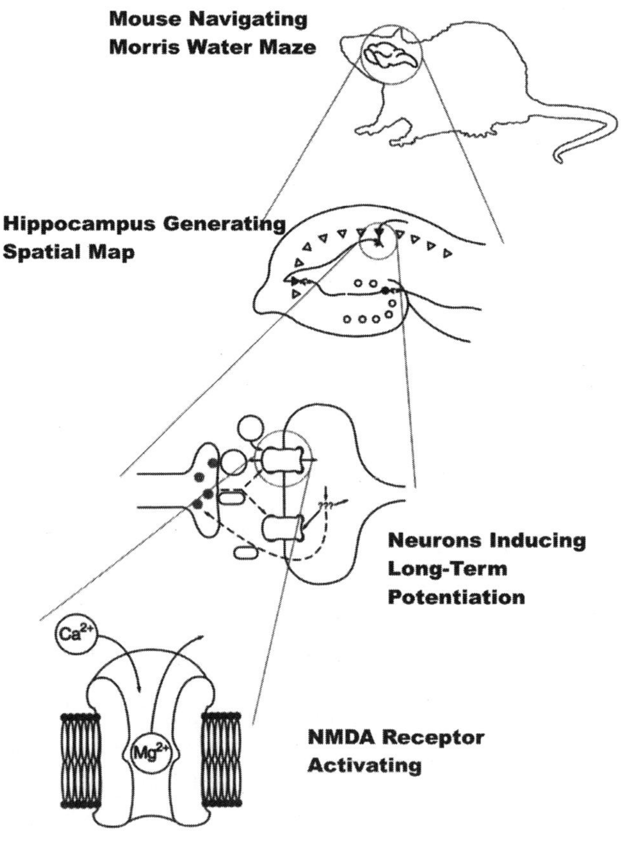

Figure 1.2
A hierarchy of levels in neuroscience. This concrete example from neuroscience shows the levels of hierarchical organization involved in the mechanism of spatial memory. (From "Discovering Mechanisms in Neurobiology: The Case of Spatial Memory" by Carl F. Craver and Lindley Darden from *Theory and Method in the Neurosciences*, Peter K. Machamer, Rick Grush, and Peter McLaughlin, Eds., © 2001 by University of Pittsburgh Press. Reprinted by permission of the University of Pittsburgh Press.)

jective world-for-me. By applying the multilevel framework I am not trying to get rid of consciousness; on the contrary, I am trying to preserve it in all its glory, only exposing its proper place in nature.

The Structure of Biological Science: Levels of Description

We should now define another notion of "levels" that is central to multilevel explanation, but that should not be confused with the levels of organization in nature. Multilevel explanatory models of natural phenomena are human constructions believed to *reflect* the hierarchical structure of the levels of organization in nature. There are different scientific disciplines and subdisciplines specialized in describing the phenomena that reside at distinct levels of organization in nature: for example, quantum physics, particle physics, inorganic chemistry, organic chemistry, biochemistry, molecular biology, cell biology, histology, and so on. Let us call the conceptual and theoretical systems, produced by humans to describe nature, the *levels of description.* These levels, unlike the levels of organization, are dependent on and constructed by human activity and mostly clothed in linguistic representations (as in mathematical equations or laws or as verbal descriptions in textbooks) or graphical representations (as in models or visualizations or computer simulations of complex systems).

If biological realism is on the right track in assuming that consciousness is a biological level of organization in the brain, then the science of consciousness should deliver the corresponding *phenomenal level of description.* This description should first systematically capture the central features of the phenomenal domain. Next, the entire phenomenal level should be placed in the context of a multilevel explanatory model. The multilevel model should show how the phenomenal level is related to biological phenomena at other levels in the causal-mechanical networks of the brain.

The Network of Biological Explanation

To explain a biological phenomenon is to make its existence and behavior intelligible within the framework of biological levels of description. A full multilevel explanation of a biological phenomenon requires that the explanandum be located within the overall causal network that (metaphorically speaking) "surrounds" it. The network has several dimensions or pathways, involving different spatial and temporal directions in the causal network (Craver & Darden, 2001). The different dimensions of a full multilevel explanation include at least the following (figure 1.3): a downward-looking explanation, describing what constitutes the phenomenon; an upward-looking explanation, describing how the phenomenon acts as an element of higher-level mechanisms; a backward-looking explanation, specifying the causal pathway that brought about or modulated the phenomenon; and a black-box description, specifying at an abstract level the input-output functions that take place at the interface between the phenomenon and its surroundings.

Constitutive Explanation

Constitutive explanation involves moving downward in the hierarchy and looking at a smaller-scale spatiotemporal grain or a lower level of organization. It is accomplished by showing that the phenomenon appearing as an integrated whole at one level can be decomposed to its constituent parts and their causal interactions at the immediately underlying, lower levels of description. Constitutive explanations describe the lower-level mechanisms that the entity is composed of, or whose activity, when taken as a whole, simply *is* the phenomenon to be explained by the description of the mechanism.

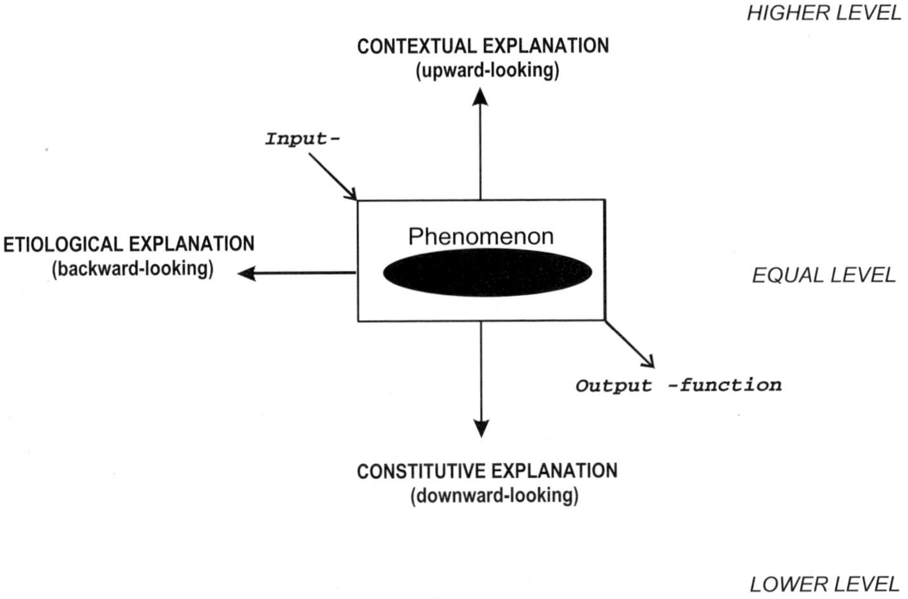

Figure 1.3
The dimensions of the causal-mechanical network. The full mechanistic explanation of a biological phenomenon involves different subtypes of explanation. The *downward-looking* and *upward-looking* explanations move across different spatiotemporal scales to lower and higher levels of organization, and the *backward-looking* explanation moves backward in time, tracing the causal chain of events that modulated or causally interacted with the phenomenon to be explained. These different, partial explanations correspond to different spatiotemporal directions in the causal-mechanical network that surround the phenomenon. The explanandum becomes intelligible when the phenomenon itself and its connections to the causal network surrounding it can be described in detail, without gaps.

An illuminating example from biology is the cell. A single cell, taken as a whole, is an independent living unit. The constitutive explanation revealing what makes the cell tick descends to the immediately lower levels of organization where the different parts of the cell and their causal interactions are to be found.

When the same strategy is applied to the explanation of consciousness there is, first of all, the phenomenon to be explained (the explanandum): consciousness. It resides at some specific level of organization in the brain (the *phenomenal* level). The lower-level, nonconscious neurophysiological mechanisms, whose activity as a whole constitutes consciousness, reside at a lower level of organization in the brain (figure 1.4).

The current search for the direct NCC appears to be the empirical approach to the constitutive explanation of consciousness. However, the notion "neural correlates of consciousness" requires considerable clarification. The relationship between an explanandum and its lower-level constituents must be stronger than mere correlation, for correlation is not an explanatory relationship. The cell membrane, the nucleus, chromosomes, cell

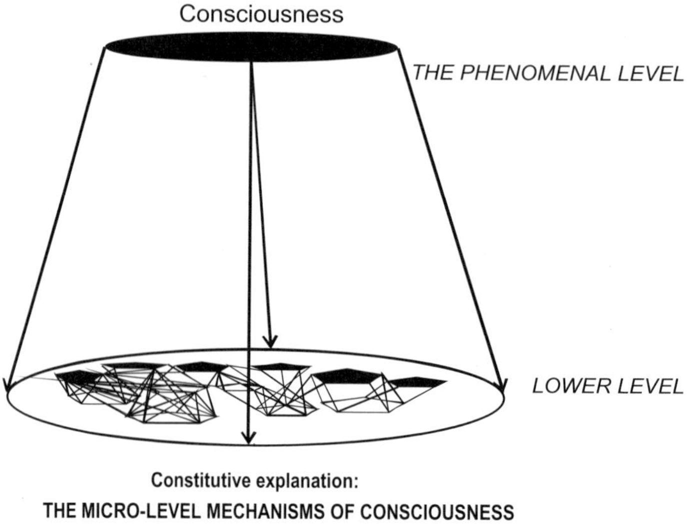

Figure 1.4
Constitutive explanation. This direction of explanation moves *downward,* to a smaller spatiotemporal scale than the scale where the explanandum lies as a whole. Constitutive explanation describes the immediately lower levels of organization (the microlevel constitutive mechanisms). Those mechanisms themselves lack the holistic features of the explanandum (in this case, consciousness). Nonetheless, when the constitutive explanation is completed, then the lower-level mechanisms can be seen to nonmagically form the higher level of organization where the explanandum itself resides.

organelles, and other microscopic parts of the cell are not merely the biological *correlates* of life, but crucial *microlevel constituents* that explain *why* the whole system is alive. In the same vein, the constitutive explanation of consciousness should describe such part-whole or mereological relationships between the lower- and higher-level phenomena that make their hierarchical connection truly explanatory.

Etiological Explanation

An *etiological explanation* is an account of the causal history of the explanandum (figure 1.5). It starts with the phenomenon to be explained, then looks backward in the temporal dimension along the causal chain to figure out what the preceding causes are that brought the phenomenon about. A distinction should be made, however, between the etiological explanation of the immediate (or proximate) causes of the phenomenon, the ontogenetic (or developmental) causes, and the evolutionary (or ultimate) ones.

In the case of visual consciousness, for example, the etiological story about the immediate causes of visual experiences—say, my perception of Orion's Belt in the night sky—would have to describe how the light (after traveling through space for years) entered my eyes, striking at the retina, causing a sequence of electrophysiological changes

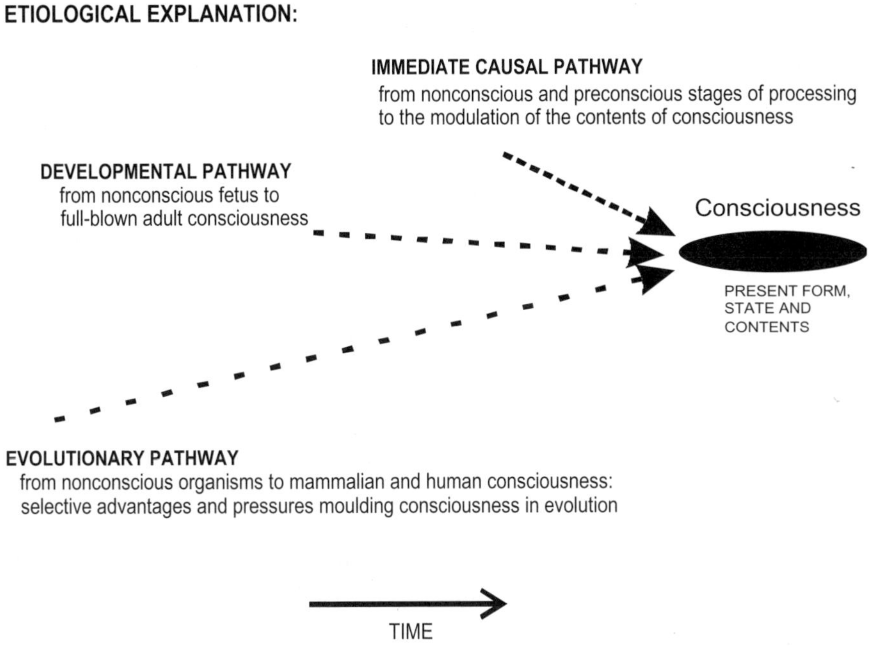

Figure 1.5
Etiological explanation. In this type of explanation, the causal chains that led to the occurrence of the explanandum are traced back. Etiological explanation looks *backward* in the temporal dimension to describe the causal pathways that *preceded* the current state of the explanandum and *causally modulated* it. Three different etiological explanations can be demarcated on the basis of how far backward in time these explanations look: (1) The short or immediate causal pathway describes how phenomenal content in consciousness was brought about by the immediately preceding external stimuli that brought about changes in sensory organs and sensory input pathways, eventually leading to changes at the phenomenal level in the brain. (2) The developmental (ontogenetic) pathway describes how the nervous system is being wired during ontogeny, at some point giving rise to the phenomenal level in the infant brain, and then developing toward full-blown adult consciousness. This story will be enormously complex, involving accounts of genetic expression in the fetal brain and of the modulatory influences of internal and external stimulation to the developing brain. (3) The evolutionary (phylogenetic) pathway looks even further backward in time and describes how, at some point during evolutionary history, the emergence of nervous systems that included the phenomenal level solved a greater number of adaptive problems than nonconscious neural systems were able to solve. Furthermore, the etiological story also describes how the organization of the phenomenal level gradually became a finely tuned species-specific adaptation (at least in mammals). The phenomenal level promoted the reproductive success of different species by constructing exactly the kind of subjective world that was useful for guiding behavior in the particular type of behavioral environment and ecological niche where each species evolved.

in the pathway from retina to V1 and from there to other parts of the visual cortex and into complex feedforward-feedback loops of neural activity, eventually causing the emergence of a well-organized visual percept in my visual consciousness.

The field known as *psychophysics* provides sorts of etiological explanations for subjective sensations by describing the lawlike relationships that obtain between physical stimulus characteristics and subjective experience: say the principles or "laws" involved when a proximate stimulus at the retina is transformed into (or rather how it causally modulates) visual phenomenology. The full story about the immediate etiological pathway should explain how the regularities and laws of stimulus-sensation relationships are physiologically implemented within the sensory input channel.

It should be made clear that the entities and activities themselves that participate in the chain of the immediately preceding causes are *not* conscious or even parts of consciousness. They are nonconscious entities and activities either entirely outside the organism, or nonconscious (preconscious) biological events inside the organism but entirely outside consciousness. *Consciousness does not and could not leak backward to its own immediate etiological pathway;* if it did, that pathway itself would be a part of consciousness rather than a chain of preceding causes leading to changes in consciousness.

The confusion between what constitutes consciousness itself and what constitutes its (nonconscious or preconscious) etiological pathway is one of the most frequent sources of error in the explanation of consciousness. Here is one way to define their difference accurately: The *constitutive* basis of consciousness includes those lower-level entities on which consciousness is *ontologically dependent;* consciousness could not exist without them existing.[1] By contrast, the *etiological* pathway includes entities on which consciousness is *causally dependent:* entities which can causally modulate, influence, and interact with consciousness. Causal dependence does not entail ontological dependence, however: I can causally interact with a stone without being ontologically dependent on it. Thus, consciousness can in principle exist even in the absence of the entities and activities that make up its etiological pathway, while it cannot, even in principle, exist without the entities and activities that make up its constitutive basis.

Again, let us consider an illuminating example from biology. First, the double helix DNA molecule could not exist without the nucleotides and the base pairs (A-T) (G-C) existing: they are microlevel constituents of the DNA double helix. Thus, DNA is *ontologically dependent* on them: it is impossible to find or synthesize (or even imagine) a DNA molecule without nucleotides and base pairs. Second, all the DNA in my cells and yours is *causally dependent* on mitosis (or meiosis): every single DNA molecule in our cells was originally constructed in one of those processes. Yet, DNA in general is not ontologically dependent on mitosis or meiosis. We can imagine that a thread of DNA could be synthesized in the laboratory through some entirely different method. There could in principle be DNA molecules without mitosis or meiosis being involved in their causal history. Therefore, DNA is not ontologically dependent on mitosis or meiosis. Just like the DNA molecule, consciousness also depends ontologically only on its constitutive mechanisms, not on the preceding etiological pathways where the mechanisms happened to have come about or by which consciousness happened to have been causally modulated.

The etiological story that tells how the constitutive mechanisms of consciousness came about during individual development, or *ontogeny* describes (in the case of visual consciousness) how the basic neuroanatomical structure of the visual pathways and cortical areas was constructed in the fetus by an immensely complex sequence of gene expression and how the system then matured in interaction with the actual visual environment after birth. Consciousness is causally but not ontologically dependent on this etiological pathway. A brain equipped with consciousness could conceivably result from some other type of process than normal development (I will have more to say about such philosophical thought experiments later, especially in chapter 8).

The etiological account of the *ultimate evolutionary causes* of visual consciousness would have to describe the adaptational, evolutionary story that describes how sensitivity to light increased the fitness of distant ancestral species millions of years ago, leading among other things to the emergence of the primate visual system. It answers the question, Why does visual consciousness exist in the first place; why was it selected for? In biology these evolutionary explanations are sometimes called "accounts of the ultimate causation of the phenomenon."

I shall call the first type of etiological explanation *the immediate causal pathway* to consciousness; the second type, the *ontogenetic etiological pathway* to consciousness; and the third type, the *evolutionary pathway to consciousness.* A full explanation of consciousness should make it possible for us to trace backward on each of these types of etiological pathways that lead to the phenomenon to be explained.

Contextual Explanation

Contextual explanation describes the role of the entity at a higher level of description (figure 1.6). It answers such questions as: How is the phenomenon related to other ones at higher levels of organization where the phenomenon is just one element or subsystem in a complex mechanism? What role does it fulfill in the overall functional economy of the higher-level system?

DNA molecules in the chromosomes of the cell are not themselves "alive" in any manner whatsoever. "Life" does not exist at the level of single molecules. Still, the DNA plays a crucial role at the higher level of organization, in interaction with RNA and amino acids, thus contributing to the higher-level processes that render the cell as a whole a living system. The contextual explanation of DNA literally puts the molecule in the context of the causal networks in which the molecule is involved. In a similar vein, a DNA sequence becomes the gene for some phenotypic feature only in the context of the whole organism.

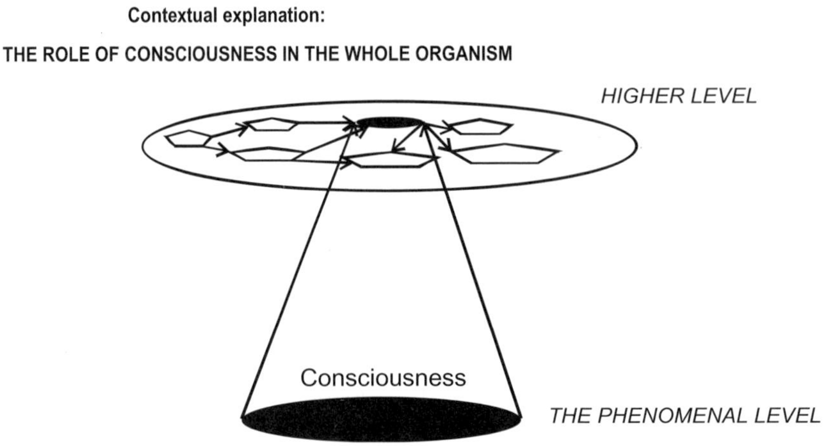

Figure 1.6
Contextual explanation. This dimension of explanation zooms *upward,* away from the level of organization where the explanandum itself lies, to higher levels of organization at coarser spatial and temporal scales. Thus it describes how the explanandum relates to and interacts with other phenomena at the higher levels. In the case of consciousness, the contextual explanation describes the special role that the phenomenal level plays at the behavioral level of organism-environment interaction, in interaction with several nonconscious sensory, cognitive, and motor systems. Although the phenomenal level alone cannot realize sensory perception or externally observable behavior but needs to interact with many nonconscious mechanisms, the contribution of the phenomenal level to the higher level of organism-environment interaction appears to be absolutely crucial.

The contextual explanation of consciousness should place the phenomenal level in the context of the causal networks in the brain. How does the phenomenal level causally interact with various nonconscious phenomena "surrounding" it in the network? Say, preconscious sensory processing that modulates the phenomenal level by providing input to that level, or "postconscious" motor programming that is influenced by conscious intentions to initiate actions. In a multilevel explanation, consciousness should be connected to various nonconscious biological systems in the brain and in the whole physical body of the biological organism, which, together with consciousness, enables coherent sequences of adaptive behavior and successful organism-environment interaction.

Input-Output Description

Sometimes it is useful just to describe the operation of the phenomenon from start conditions to finish conditions without yet specifying the micro-level mechanisms. Such descriptions are called *input-output functions* (figure 1.7). They focus on some specific activities that take place at the boundary between the phenomenon and its environment. Such activities may be represented at an abstract level, mathematically for example, and at that level the input-output function can be described explicitly and computationally.

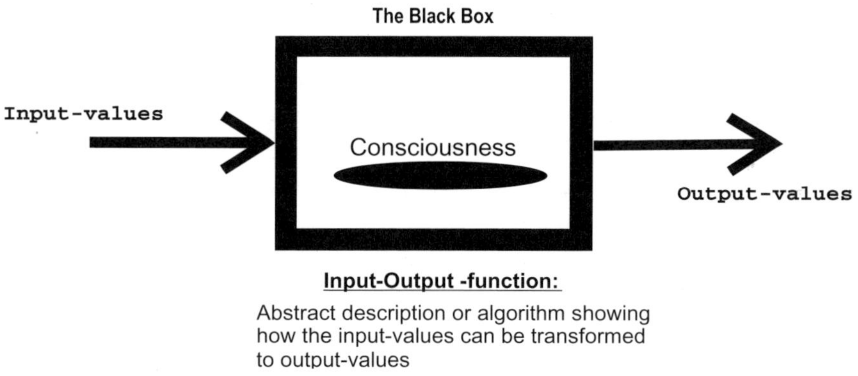

Figure 1.7
Input-output function. This description captures, at an abstract level, the formal features of the input-output transformations performed by the explanandum. These transformations may be described computationally, in an explicit computational model, by determining the algorithms that carry out the transformations.

An algorithm describing a particular input-output function may be realized in a computer program as a *simulation* of the function. It should be noted, however, that the algorithm itself is an abstract entity, not identical to the phenomenon, and in fact, the algorithm becomes a very different kind of mechanism when it is written in a programming language and instantiated in computer hardware (Machamer et al., 2000). Computational modeling and simulation in biology, neuroscience, and cognitive science depend on our ability to provide explicit input-output descriptions of biological and psychological phenomena.

The input-output function of (some aspect) of consciousness describes, at an abstract level, the activities that take place at the conscious-nonconscious interface. It specifies the algorithm or function which transforms the input values (describing sensory stimulation) to the output values (standing for some features of the conscious sensation or perception). An example that perhaps comes rather close to something like this concerns the relationship between stimulus luminance (the physical intensity of visible light striking the retina) and perceptual brightness (a feature of subjective visual experience). The input values of the function represent physical luminance, the output values represent perceived brightness, and the task is to describe an algorithm that transforms the input values to the output values in a manner closely matching empirical data from psychophysical experiments. When an accurate simulation of the brightness-from-luminance transformation is developed, some might go so far as to say that now the algorithms "used" by the brain to solve this problem have been found.

Even if we had an accurate input-output function available for some aspects of consciousness, it would be unwise to treat it as *the explanation* of the phenomenon. An input-output function treats the phenomenon as a mere black box and reveals nothing about its internal constitution or microlevel mechanism. An algorithm that simulates the transformation from luminance to brightness does not tell us what the conscious visual experience of brightness is, or what its underlying biological mechanisms are. Certainly, an explicit function or algorithm will constrain the set of mechanisms that would be regarded as acceptable constitutive explanations for the phenomenon, but it cannot replace the microlevel explanations, or supersede the full multilayered model of the phenomenon. [2]

Multilevel Models and Consciousness

The explanation of a phenomenon is completed with the construction of a multilevel mechanistic model of the phenomenon. Such a model describes the explanandum across several different levels. The conceptual structures (theories and models) in neurobiology are really descriptions of such multilevel causal networks forming complex hierarchies of mechanisms (figure 1.8).

In a multilevel mechanistic model the phenomenon is situated at some specific level of description within the multidimensional causal network. An important part of the task is the *identification of the correct level of organization* at which to understand par-

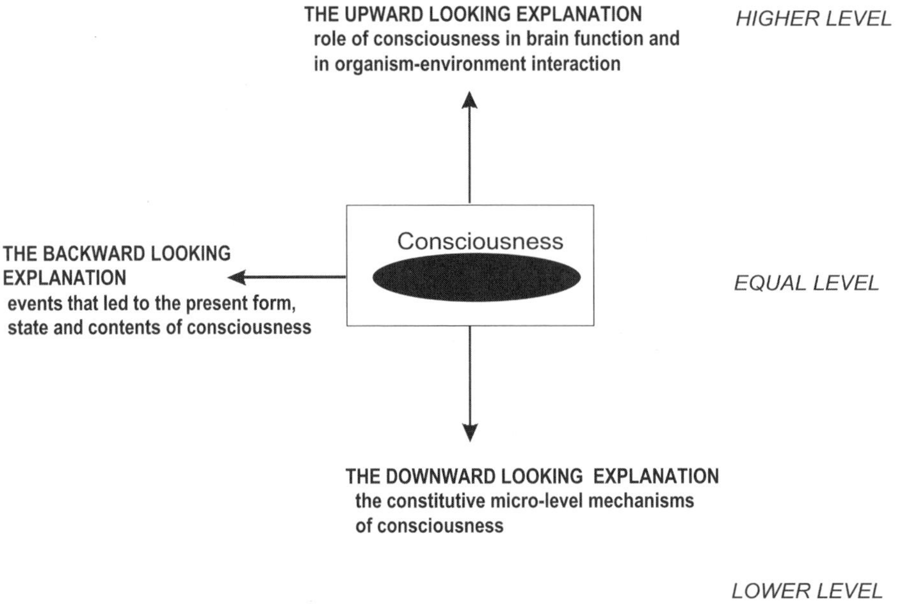

Figure 1.8
The multilevel model of consciousness. The complete explanatory model should include a description of consciousness itself (the explanandum) and then link it to the causal networks surrounding the explanandum.

ticular causal interactions: how the explanandum interacts with other phenomena, what the lower-level components of the explanandum are and how they interact at the microlevel (Bechtel, 1994). To achieve this goal, the multilevel model should include three types of explanation. These different types of explanation correspond to three different directions with respect to which the phenomenon can be situated in the mechanical reticulum: (1) The *downward-looking explanation* specifies the *constitutive mechanisms* of the phenomenon at the lower levels of description; (2) the *upward-looking explanation* specifies *the role function of the phenomenon at the higher levels of organization;* (3) the *backward-looking explanation* (the immediate or proximal causes, the ontogenetic or developmental causes, and the ultimate or evolutionary causes) specifies the etiological causal pathways or the temporally preceding events that led to or causally modulated the phenomenon.

The point of the above discussion is this: the explanation of consciousness should be seen in the context of multilevel explanation. As far as cognitive neuroscience is concerned the problem of consciousness boils down to the questions: Is it possible to locate consciousness within the multilayered causal-mechanical networks that reside in the brain? Can we find a level of organization in the brain to which consciousness naturally corresponds? Can we discover and fully describe the constitutive mechanisms, the etiological pathways, and the contextual role functions of consciousness?

If there is a place to be found for consciousness within the multilevel framework of biological phenomena, and if the causal network surrounding consciousness can be reconstructed, then consciousness can be scientifically explained by the biological sciences. If not, then we must either give up the basic assumption that consciousness is a real, natural biological phenomenon belonging within the scope of biological science, or at least the view that it can be explained by such science. The aim of this book is to find out whether this sort of multilevel explanation of consciousness is philosophically and empirically feasible.

Summary

The current state of confusion in the study of consciousness can be overcome only if theoretically and empirically unified research programs emerge in the field. One potential candidate for a unified research program, based on the philosophy called "biological realism," has been outlined in this chapter. It treats consciousness as a biological phenomenon: a particular level of organization in the brain. It ties the study of consciousness to the context of the biological sciences, especially cognitive neuroscience. Thus, consciousness should be explained in the same manner as other complex biological phenomena are explained. The explanatory framework that applies to the biological sciences appears to be significantly different from the traditional concepts of "explanation" in the philosophy of science. In the biological context, the overall explanation of consciousness consists of several smaller subtasks that all contribute to building a multilevel model of the explanandum. This picture of the explanation of consciousness confers new unity to the field, as it sorts out and defines the different questions that we should try to answer when seeking an explanation of consciousness. Thus, the biological approach might be able to establish a unified research program in the study of consciousness.

2 A Conceptual Map of the Territory

Science in general provides us with more or less accurate maps of the world. The subjective realm of consciousness is one of the last wholly uncharted areas on the scientific map. Consciousness research constitutes an exploration of that scientifically exotic territory. At the start of the exploration some sort of rough map of conscious phenomena must be outlined so that we get an initial idea of the scope of the domain. The purpose of this chapter is to offer just that: a rough conceptual map of the subjective world of consciousness. The most basic concepts that are needed to describe that world will be defined as clearly as possible. Their interrelations will also be pointed out, so that gradually an entire interconnected vocabulary will develop with which it will be possible to navigate in the realm of consciousness without getting immediately lost in a conceptual jungle.

The First Stage of Explanation: Systematic Description

An empirically based scientific discipline must start with a systematic description. That is the indispensable foundation of all explanatory research in biology too (Mayr, 1996). In the framework of multilevel explanation the descriptive stage is called the *identification* of the *explanandum.* It makes sense to invoke the lower levels of explanatory *mechanisms* only after there is a clear conception of the phenomenon that the mechanisms are supposed to explain. In science, phenomena come first, mechanisms and explanations later.

It is not difficult to see why consciousness research still largely lacks the level of systematic description: there is no well-established empirically based conceptual framework to turn to. In the history of experimental psychology, introspectionists tried to discover the basic elements of consciousness and describe them systematically, but their project eventually failed. Consequently, an empirically based, scientific phenomenology is still regarded by many as an outright impossibility. The purely philosophical variety of phenomenology, as practiced in the continental tradition initiated by Franz Brentano and Edmund Husserl, seems to be too obscure and conceptually isolated from current cognitive neuroscience to tempt the empirically minded scientist all that much.[1] Furthermore, many philosophers are not optimistic about the prospects for an "objective phenomenology" (Nagel, 1974).

Thus, it is no wonder that in consciousness research conceptual frameworks are primarily borrowed from the empirically respectable and well-established branches of cognitive science and neuroscience. The problem, however, is that the science of consciousness is not just another trivial outgrowth of those fields. Mainstream cognitive science and neuroscience have largely ignored consciousness. They will not automatically provide us with adequate levels of description for handling phenomenal experience. Therefore, the phenomenal level of description cannot be imported from any already existing branch of science—it must be contributed by the science of consciousness itself.

The Diversity of Consciousness

The first serious challenge to developing a systematic description of consciousness is this: We do not seem to have any clear idea, any widely shared understanding, as to what the concept "consciousness" even refers to. What is the phenomenon in the real world that this concept picks out? *Is* there any coherent phenomenon there that deserves the label "consciousness"?

Consciousness was not originally a scientific concept—it was not introduced in the context of experimental psychology to name some novel mental process discovered in the laboratory. By contrast, its origin is in everyday language and folk psychology. Hence, it is no wonder that "consciousness" involves multifarious forms and meanings. It means different things to different speakers, yet none of those meanings seem to be clearly defined anywhere, or universally shared. The concept of consciousness undoubtedly is a heterogeneous concept, which suggests that there is no single, unified real-world phenomenon to be found behind the concept. Does this imply that there can be no unified science of consciousness either?

That line of argument is taken by *eliminative materialism.* Its supporters suggest that the diversity and obscurity of the concept of consciousness is a sign that there is no real phenomenon there that science could or should take seriously, even if it wanted to. Similar eliminations have taken place in the history of science. Scientists (and laypersons) have believed in a number of things that were later found to be nonexistent. Detailed theories and concepts have been put forth to describe phenomena that turned out not to be there; therefore the concepts did not pick out anything in the real world after all.

In the nineteenth century it was believed by astronomers that irregularities in the movements of the planet Mercury were caused by another, unknown planet hidden from our view—the planet Vulcan. The main advocate of this idea was the French astronomer Leverrier. But later on this concept had to be eliminated; no such celestial body was found to exist, and the observations supposedly revealing Vulcan had to be explained in a different manner. The detailed descriptions and careful calculations characterizing this planet were thoroughly mistaken and did not refer to *any* heavenly body at all. Around the same time another concept mesmerized both astronomers and the general public: the canals of Mars. Intricate maps were published of a system of canals on the surface of Mars. The origin of the canals was believed to be intelligent design: an intelligent Martian form of life, an alien culture, that had built an advanced system to manage the scarce water resources of the barren planet. Keen observers of the planet, first and foremost Percival Lowell, believed they could actually *see* through their telescopes the canals crisscrossing the planet's surface. But that was just an illusion. Now we know that the concept "the canals of Mars" refers to nothing at all: there are no canals there, there is nothing that even remotely resembles canals, and there never was anything like that. Around the same time, it was believed that there is an invisible stuff filling every last corner of empty space. This stuff was called "ether" and it was believed to be the medium that carries waves of light or radio waves through empty space. Now we know that no such mysterious physical substance exists—the concept of ether has been eliminated from science.

The above is just a small sample of things that do not really exist, but in whose existence a number of intelligent people used to believe. In the history of science such things are not uncommon: animal spirits, élan vital, phlogiston, animal magnetism. . . . Is the concept of consciousness going to be next in line?

The current state of confusion in the study of consciousness is all grist to the mill of the eliminativist, who argues that the conceptual and descriptive obscurity is a sign of the fact that there is no coherent phenomenon there, underlying all the confusion. Perhaps consciousness does not exist. Perhaps it also is just a grand illusion; therefore there can be no valid description or explanation of it. Eliminative materialism is, however, a rather unreasonable solution to the problem of consciousness (Revonsuo, 1993, 1994b). It advises us to give up the science of consciousness, as any such project is necessarily doomed to failure. Giving up would hardly make the problematic data and the mysterious phenomena disappear, however. Eliminative materialists have no alternative explanation to offer for the phenomena discussed in consciousness studies. Just saying that they are "illusions" or that we are "mistaken" when using the concept of consciousness is hardly sufficient. If indeed we are deeply mistaken and consciousness is but a grand illusion, then the eliminativist's burden is to show us how the illusion is generated so that the trick is plain for anyone to see, just like it is now plain for anyone to see that the canals of Mars were an illusion.

So far no eliminativist has been able to explain how the illusion of consciousness, the illusion of there being a *world-for-me*—if indeed it is an illusion—is brought about.

Therefore, instead of just giving up the science of consciousness at this rather early point, we should start to systematically develop a clearer idea of the concept of consciousness and find out how much progress can be made.

I believe that the diversity of the concepts of consciousness is a sign that we are dealing with several different but closely interrelated phenomena, rather than a sign that nothing deserving the label "consciousness" exists. Thus, in consciousness science a conceptual map is needed that names the basic phenomena and makes the distinctions between them crystal clear. In the following, I present the first sketch for a conceptual map that aims at clarifying the conceptual basis of empirical consciousness science.

I shall try to accomplish the clarification without venturing too deeply into the endless philosophical controversies surrounding many of these topics. The reader should be aware, however, that *any* definitions and distinctions concerning the concept of consciousness are bound to be deeply controversial (particularly among philosophers), and so are the ones I am putting forward. I am not implying that the conceptual map I offer is the only way, or the correct way, of defining consciousness and related phenomena. My definitions certainly are not free of philosophical presuppositions (but neither are anyone else's). My interest is to delineate concepts that respect the phenomena as we know and experience them, that can be clearly distinguished from each other, and that I have personally found helpful in the empirical study of consciousness. These are the most important principles, then: respect of the first-person perspective, maximal clarity, and usefulness for empirical science.

Basic Concepts of Consciousness

In this section I define the most fundamental concepts of the science of consciousness. They name the basic phenomena, hopefully clearly enough to allow empirical research to build more detailed theories and experiments on them.

Phenomenal Consciousness

The study of consciousness is, first and foremost, the study of the world-for-me, or, more generally, *worlds-for-someone:* the subjective psychological realities within which all of us live our lives. That is the principal explanandum for the science of consciousness. Accordingly, the most fundamental concept in the study of consciousness should capture the essence of the world-for-me. What kinds of facts are the basic facts describing the world-for-me?

The facts of the world-for-me are the immediate and undeniable facts of experience. In psychology, such facts have been called simply *phenomena.* Phenomena are all the indisputable facts concerning seeing, hearing, touching, feeling, embodiment, moving, and thinking *as subjective experiences that happen to you right now.* The *world-for-you* is

constituted by such subjective experiences, and a description of the world-for-you should capture the undeniable facts of your experience.

The concept of consciousness that refers to the world-for-you as the seat of subjective experiences is called *phenomenal consciousness.* The adjective "phenomenal" here is of course derived from the above-mentioned psychological conception of "phenomena," and thus refers to something concerned with phenomena, the immediate, undeniable facts of experience. In the same vein, "phenomenology" refers to the study of the facts of experience; the "phenomenal level" refers to the level of organization in nature and the level of description in science which deal with the undeniable facts of immediate experience.

Thomas Nagel's (1974) famous formulation of the essence of consciousness obviously refers to phenomenal consciousness, too: "An organism has conscious mental states if and only if there is something that it is like to *be* that organism—something it is like *for* the organism" (p. 436).

The facts concerning subjective experience, the phenomenal facts, define *what it is like to be* the biological entity, here and now. The phenomenal facts define what it is like *for* it. That is, it defines the *world-for-it.* An organism's *entire momentary sphere of subjective experiences* is the world-for-it.

Now that we have defined a concept of consciousness that incorporates the world-for-me, we should say something more precise about the inhabitants of this world. What *are* the undeniable facts of experience? At the beginning of our mission it would be most useful if we could find some *universal characteristics of experience,* some facts that hold for any experience, no matter what type of experience or who or what entity the experiencing subject is.

To simplify matters a little, let us treat sensory-perceptual experiences as the paradigm cases of experience. These include, but are not limited to, visual experiences such as colored shapes or objects in the subjective field of view; auditory experiences such as musical tones or sounds of nature, bodily experiences such as pain, touch, or itch; and olfactory and gustatory experiences such as smells and tastes. Although these experiences in some ways differ from each other as night differs from day, yet in other ways they share some characteristics that seem to be universally shared by all kinds of experiences.

Presence Perhaps the most fundamental feature of all the elements in phenomenal consciousness is their direct *presence.* Anything that counts as an experience at all, anything that enters the world-for-me, must possess the feature of presence. To be a part of the world-for-me is to be something that is directly *present-for-me.* Presence-for-me is both *spatial* and *temporal.* For a sensation to be present-*for-me* it must manifest itself directly before my mind, somewhere within my perceptual space. The visual experience of seeing a color or the auditory experience of hearing a melody, take place somewhere

within my perceptual space. With regard to presence, there is no difference between experiences caused externally (perception) and internally (hallucination, dreaming): the experiences themselves are present in my subjective perceptual space, no matter how they were produced or what caused them. Presence is also temporal: to be present for me, an experience must happen right *now.* Only for a passing moment does an experience remain in the momentary window of presence. The stream of consciousness flows ever on, never ceasing to change. When a momentary window of presence is gone, the experiences it contained are gone forever.

All in all, for a sensation to be a part of the world-for-me is for the sensation to be present-for-me in some part of my subjective field of perception *right now.*

Location If presence-for-me implies spatial presence, spatial presence in turn implies location. Thus, all experiences have a spatial location somewhere within the sphere of my subjective experiences, within the world-for-me. A point of brightness, an expanse of blueness, the sound of ticktock, the sharp pain, the soft touch—all of them have *some* more or less definable location within the overall context of the world-for-me; they occupy some places rather than others within the sphere of subjective experience. Although the location may not be exactly definable in all cases, there is always something to be said about the spatial features of an experience. Furthermore, some experiences, say visual experiences of colors, also have spatial *extension* within the sphere of subjective experience. Colors occupy not just a general direction or a single point within the sphere of experiences, they may fill in entire spatially extended regions within the sphere. In some circumstances the blueness of the sky fills the visual space in its entirety, for example.

Duration If presence-for-me implies temporal presence, temporal presence in turn implies duration. An experience comes into existence at some point in time (which may not be sharply definable on a millisecond scale) by manifesting itself within the current window of presence; it ceases to exist at some later point when it disappears from the then current window of presence (which may be the same or a different time window from the one where it appeared). Note that we are now talking about experiences, not external physical stimuli. It may well be that the stimulus has a different duration than the experience it causes. A rapid sequence of several discrete stimuli may be experienced as one temporally extended phenomenal entity, for example.

Intensity Experiences vary along a dimension of strength. Two sounds or two lights may appear in the same spatial position in the sphere of experiences and have the same temporal duration, and yet vary radically in intensity. The sound or light may be barely distinguishable (and in that case barely present-for-me at all) or it may be extremely loud or blindlingly bright.

Quality Experiences not only exhibit intensity, spatial position, and temporal duration in the subjective psychological reality, they also have *identity:* a qualitative feature that makes them the *kinds* of experiences they are, and that tells them apart from other kinds of experiences. All the other features of two different experiences might be identical, yet the experiences could differ radically in their qualitative features, say one being red and the other being green; or one taste being salty and the other sweet; or one sensation being itchy and the other painful. The quality of experience is perhaps its most fundamental feature, for we can construe the other features as characterizing the occurrence of qualities. Whenever a quality occurs in the sphere of subjective experience, it has position (and perhaps spatial extent), duration, and intensity. Qualities are thus the "stuff" that experiences per se are made of. They come into existence within the sphere of subjective experience in some particular spatiotemporal coordinates and they display some particular level of strength.

Although qualities are usually discussed by taking their simplest forms as examples, such as single patches of color, points of lightness, simple tones, pains and itches, yet the sphere of subjective experiences as a whole amounts to much more than simple, isolated qualities. The sensory-perceptual world we normally enjoy involves immensely complex, ever-changing dynamic combinations of qualities. The qualities are carefully organized to make up shapes and forms, surfaces and objects, melodies and words, aromas and caresses: the entire world-for-me.

Qualia

Philosophers use the term *qualia* (singula "quale") to describe approximately the same thing that I call the quality of experience above. This philosophical concept was first defined by C. I. Lewis ([1929] 1956) as the qualitative characters of "the given." The given he understood as a presentation of something, and the quale as a qualitative character of this presentation. Any presentation was either a specific, pure quale or could be analyzed into a complex combination of different qualia. Qualia he took to lie at the elementary level of experience, so they could not be analyzed any further.[2]

The philosophical literature includes a number of terms that have been used to refer to qualia or to phenomenal consciousness: the subjective or qualitative character of experience, raw feels, what-it-is-like, qualitative consciousness, the internal illumination, and so on. In this book I will stick to the terms *phenomenal consciousness* and *primary consciousness* when I talk about the subjective sphere of experience as such. The name in itself is not important, however; much more important is to grasp what it is that we are talking about. Stubenberg (1998) characterizes the fundamental facts of phenomenal consciousness in the following way:

> At every moment of our waking and dreaming lives we are immersed in a sea of colors, sounds, smells, tastes, tickles, pains, and the like. Throughout our lives we are subject to a ceaseless barrage of such qualities. At every moment an abundance of such qualities confronts us. Nothing

seems more obvious to me. . . . [p.18] It is in virtue of this fact that it is like something to be me. . . . Without my qualia I am, as far as *I* am concerned, dead [p. 24].

I can only agree with this characterization. Still, I should point out that the sea of qualia in which we are immersed is far from a mere kaleidoscope of qualities hurrying about chaotically. The qualities we confront in our waking and dreaming lives are for the most part organized into coherent perceptual wholes in the context of the entire sphere of experiences. We rarely (if ever) experience just a pure and simple quale, out of all context. By contrast, our consciousness usually includes extremely complex patterns of subjective experience that are well organized as a sensory-perceptual world.

The relation between primary, phenomenal consciousness and qualia is that the notion of "primary (or phenomenal) consciousness" refers to the entire *sphere* or *field* of subjective experience; the totality of experiences that are currently present; the totality of "what it is like" for the subject at this very moment. The notion of "qualia," by contrast, refers to the elementary phenomenal features. A quale characterizes a restricted part or region of the sphere of subjective experience. Combinations of various qualia form the more complex patterns of subjective experience and ultimately fill in the entire sphere of subjective experience.

Let me illustrate this difference with the following example (Revonsuo,1994a). Imagine that you are admiring a sunset from the top of a hill. Your conscious experience involves a variety of relatively simple qualia, yet they are organized as a global sphere of subjective experience. Your color vision allows you to enjoy a pallet of different tints and shades: the sky and the clouds near the western horizon burn in purple as the red-orange sun slowly sinks behind the skyline. If you look further up, you can see how the shades of the sky at dusk change from purple to violet, to light blue, and eventually to very dark, velvet blue, revealing the first diamond-like stars against the dim background. Maybe you can hear the sound of the waves and the screech of seagulls from the distance, and smell the salt air rising from the ocean. The rock on which you are sitting feels hard and still slightly warm, but the chilling wind sends cold shivers down your spine and, eventually, you feel how you are getting goose pimples all over your skin. It is exactly these kinds of basic sensory components of subjective experience—defining what it is like to have those experiences—that philosophers call qualia.

Of course, your experience of the night falling and the stars coming out is much more than a kaleidoscope of chaotic patterns of phenomenal features. Most of your perceptions are carefully organized, thus forming meaningful wholes. Some patterns of qualia form a carefully organized body image and the various bodily sensations located within it or at the surface of the body image. Other patterns of qualia form the visual and auditory space surrounding your body image. These organized patterns of qualia are of course not thought of as "patterns of qualia" in our everyday thinking. On the contrary, they are instinctively taken as meaningful, familiar objects. It is almost impossible for you to see the red-orange circle in your visual field as an uninterpreted or meaningless patch of color or as just a pattern of qualia—instead, you instantaneously categorize it as "the sun."

Definition of Phenomenal Consciousness

Now we may formulate a simple definition of our explanandum. Phenomenal consciousness is the current *presence* of subjective experiences, or the *having* of subjective experiences. An organism possesses phenomenal consciousness if there is any type of subjective experience currently present for it. The mere occurrence or presence of any experience is the necessary and minimally sufficient condition for phenomenal consciousness. For any entity to possess primary phenomenal consciousness only requires that there are at least *some* patterns—any patterns at all—of subjective experience *present-for-it.* It is purely about the *having* of *any* sorts of patterns of subjective experience, whether simple or complex, faint or vivid, meaningful or meaningless, fleeting or lingering.[3]

In the current literature other terms have also been used to refer to the most fundamental aspect of consciousness, the presence of subjective experience. "Phenomenal" and "qualitative" consciousness are often contrasted with the *functional* aspects and causal roles of consciousness, also called "access" consciousness (Block, 1995; see discussion later in this chapter). The term "core consciousness" (Damasio, 1999) emphasizes the here-and-now nature of experience, its immediate, direct presence (as opposed to "extended consciousness," which includes awareness of the temporal continuum of a self and its past and future experiences). The notion of "primary consciousness" (Farthing, 1992; G. M. Edelman, 1989) emphasizes the primacy of subjective experience—experience comes first, thought and other higher cognitive operations later. The pure having or presence of patterns of experience (primary consciousness) thus must be sharply distinguished from higher-order forms of consciousness (e.g., reflective consciousness, introspection, self-awareness) which involve further processing of selected features or contents of primary consciousness (say thoughts about them). Higher-order forms of consciousness are discussed in more detail later in this chapter. Philosophical views that totally deny or eliminate phenomenal consciousness are discussed in chapter 8.

The Phenomenal Contents of Consciousness

Any pattern of phenomenal experience that is included in the phenomenal level—whether a pattern of sensations, perceptions, mental images, emotions, inner phonological images, or some combination of the these—is a content of consciousness. I use the word "content" here in its literal meaning: it refers to something that is literally contained within another, larger entity (a container). In the case of consciousness, the "container" is the phenomenal level of organization in the brain, and the contents are the patterns of subjective experience that occur at that level. When I talk about the contents of consciousness, I mean the variety of experiences that are now literally contained within the phenomenal level of organization, within the sphere of subjective experience. The total contents of consciousness constitute the phenomenal level as a whole, and a single specified content of consciousness is a proper part of what is contained within the phenomenal level as a whole.

A word of caution is in place here. In philosophy of mind the term *content* is not understood in this concrete sense, but in quite another sense in which symbol systems, signs, and representations have content. For example, the content of a printed word or picture is not the patterns of ink literally contained within it, but here "content," paradoxically, means something *external* to the thing that has or carries the content (it could mean such things as "reference," "reliable indication of," or "causal covariation with"). Thus, the "content of consciousness," as standardly used in the philosophy of mind, refers to the "intentional content," "semantic content," or "representational content" of consciousness.

Hence, there are two almost directly opposite notions of "content": the first, intuitive notion where, if Y is a content of X, then Y is located *inside* the confines of X. "Content of X" refers to something internal to X. According to the second (the philosophical) notion, the "content of X" refers to something *outside* of X itself, something *external.*

Philosophically, much depends on whether one understands "the content of consciousness" in the first or the second way. Most theories in current philosophy of mind embrace the second reading and thus externalize the contents of consciousness from the mind and the brain to the external world. These approaches are discussed in more detail in chapter 8. In biological realism, however, the "contents of consciousness" primarily refers to something *inside* the mind and the brain rather than outside of it.

To keep these two opposite notions of "content(s)" strictly apart, I will use *phenomenal* content(s) of consciousness as referring to that which is literally contained within the phenomenal level of organization, and *representational* content(s) of consciousness as referring to that with which the phenomenal content of consciousness reliably covaries, or what it indicates, or refers to, in the world external to the mind-brain. When no specification is made, I mean by the content of consciousness the phenomenal content of consciousness.

Focal and Peripheral Consciousness

If primary consciousness is metaphorically depicted as a sort of "sphere" or "bubble" that includes the "here-and-now" of momentary subjective experience at the phenomenal level of organization, then the borders of this bubble should be depicted as relatively fuzzy, in both the temporal and the spatial dimension. The fuzzy areas contain what can be called *peripheral consciousness* (Farthing, 1992) or *fringe consciousness* (James, [1890] 1950; Mangan, 1993) or the *phenomenal background* (Dainton, 2000). The clearly articulated center of phenomenal experience can be called *focal consciousness* or *focal awareness,* or *the center of consciousness* (figure 2.1).

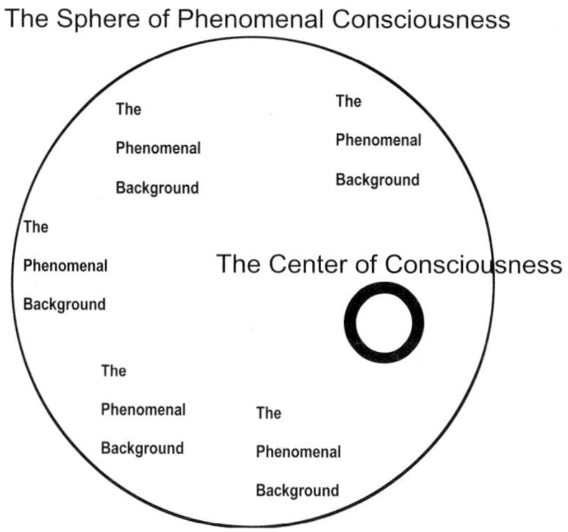

Figure 2.1
The internal structure of phenomenal consciousness. Phenomenal consciousness involves a "center" of clearly defined experiences, surrounded by a wide phenomenal background that contains a rich variety of more vaguely defined experiences.

Every definite image in the mind is steeped and dyed in the free water that flows around it. With it goes the sense of its relations, near and remote, the dying echo of whence it came to us, the dawning sense of whither it is to lead. (James, [1890] 1950, p. 78)

The patterns of phenomenal experience gradually fade away from the vivid experience of the here-and-now when they become spatially or temporally more distant from the focus. Thus, the total content of primary consciousness does not consist of a multitude of perceptual objects that can be clearly and distinctly experienced all at once. The phenomenal world is clear and distinct only where the focus of attention is; the rest is more or less vague. I can never catch the vagueness itself by focusing my attention on it. Focusing on a vague experience on the phenomenal background will bring the experience to focal consciousness and render the experience clearer, but then the experience is no longer part of the phenomenal background. Wherever I turn the focus of attention there the mists of phenomenal background immediately dissolve and the phenomenal contents become clear and distinct. The vagueness necessarily remains in the background. But the immediacy with which the contents of the unclear background clear up when attention is turned to them creates a powerful illusion that the perceptual world is clear and distinct all the time everywhere around me, even when or where I am not currently focusing.

The global sphere of subjective experience thus has an internal structure and organization in terms of a clear, vivid center and a vague background. The mechanisms that underlie this structure are closely related to selective attention. William James ([1890]

1950) described selective attention as the taking possession of the mind, in clear and vivid form, of one out of what seem several simultaneously possible objects; out of all the sensations yielded, attention picks out certain ones as worthy of its notice and suppresses all the rest. Thus, what appears in focal consciousness and what remains in the phenomenal background is the result of selection.

The center-surround structure of primary consciousness and the ability to select among a multitude of patterns of subjective experience are involved in the construction of higher-order forms of consciousness, such as reflective consciousness and introspection. The patterns of subjective experience to be reflected upon have first to be demarcated from other experiences. Without the ability to selectively attend to some experiences to the exclusion of others, reflection upon any particular experience would be impossible.

Reflective Consciousness

Reflective consciousness is a higher-order form of consciousness. It cannot exist without primary consciousness: one must first have some phenomenal experiences in order to reflect upon them. Primary consciousness thus is a necessary condition of reflective consciousness.

How should we understand the term *reflective*? What kind of activity is that supposed to involve? Here is one way to define reflective consciousness: When we have reflective consciousness, we deliberately focus on some feature or element of our experience in primary consciousness: some content in primary consciousness becomes the *object* of our attention in an act of reflection. The act of reflection may include, say, the questioning, evaluation, comparison, or description of the elements found in primary consciousness. We may wonder why we have a certain emotion, whether our perception is veridical or illusory, whether our toothache is getting better or worse, or we may produce a verbal description of the contents of primary consciousness.

A cognitive model could explicate the difference between primary and reflective consciousness in the following way: Some contents of primary consciousness become selected by attentional mechanisms and thereby they *serve as input for further conscious cognitive processing* in working memory.[4] That is, some further cognitive operations can be carried out where the selected phenomenal content is involved: a judgment or evaluation of some sort may be passed, or the percept may be categorized or named, for example. What philosophers vaguely call "reflective thought that takes the mental content as an object," the cognitive psychologist can analyze into conscious cognitive processes of various sorts, which take phenomenal experience as their input (figure 2.2).

The cognitivist way to define reflective consciousness is to say that it is any voluntary cognitive operation that takes the contents of phenomenal consciousness as its *input*, and as an *output* produces an analysis of the experience in terms of such things as category, name, course of action, verbal description, preference, similarity, and so on.

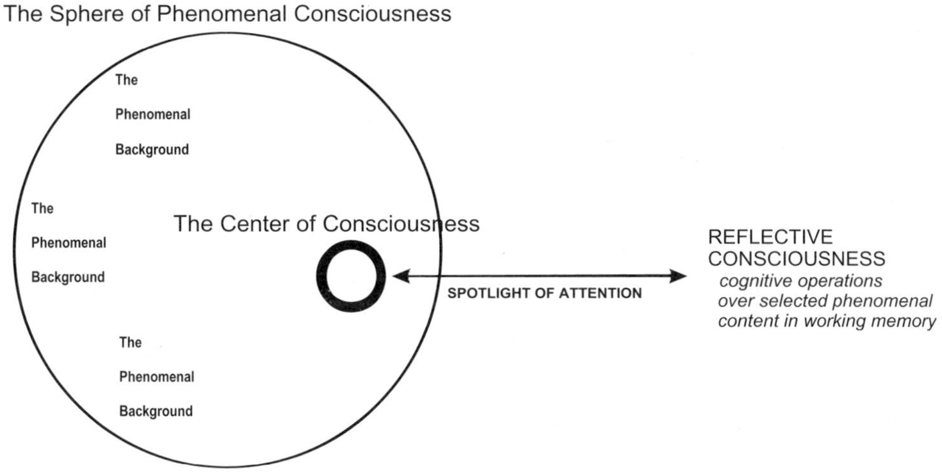

Figure 2.2
Phenomenal and reflective consciousness. Phenomenal contents in the clearly defined center are channeled to reflective consciousness by the narrow gateway of selective attention.

Reflective consciousness involves a cognitive operation that *adds something to* and is *separable from* the phenomenal content itself. The phenomenal content of consciousness per se may be subjectively experienced at the phenomenal level without the (reflective) cognitive operation being involved at all. The contents of phenomenal consciousness are thus not dependent on reflective consciousness. Reflective cognitive operations are not necessary for phenomenal contents, whereas phenomenal contents are necessary for reflective consciousness. Furthermore, since reflective consciousness involves an operation that takes phenomenal content as its input, the phenomenal consciousness involving a particular content must temporally precede the reflective consciousness involving the same content. Phenomenal content must itself first come into existence before it can be reflected upon. Let us look at some concrete examples of the interplay between phenomenal and reflective consciousness:

Imagine that you are presented with two highly similar-looking patches of color and your task is to tell if they are the same color or if there is some discriminable difference. To accomplish this, you will have to reflect upon your color experiences. You are actually trying to figure out whether the quality of your visual experience when you focus on *this* patch is exactly the same as when you focus on *that* patch (or if they are side by side, whether there is a borderline of qualitative difference). The phenomenal color experience in primary consciousness is taken as input to cognitive operations of similarity judgment. In psychophysics, the minimal differences between sensory stimuli that can be detected are called "just-noticeable-differences" or JNDs. Noticing a difference between two stimuli is an act of reflective consciousness.

Imagine that you are presented with a display of twenty letters (five letters in four rows) for a very short time, say 100 milliseconds. Your visual experience is of seeing all the letters for a fleeting moment. The phenomenal trace of the display may remain visible for 1 or 2 seconds at most. In cognitive psychology, such persistence of visibility is called *iconic memory*. It can hold virtually complete visual information for a very short time (Palmer, 1999). The content of iconic memory holds information about the location, color, size, and shape of items in the phenomenal visual field. Thus, we may say that the complete visual information is for a fleeting moment in primary phenomenal consciousness. Imagine further that immediately after the display is gone an arrow appears, pointing at one of the rows that just disappeared. Your task is to report the letters that were in that row. Now you focus attention quickly on that row and select the items there for reflective consciousness and formulate an introspective verbal report about the content of visual consciousness. In such a task, you will be able to report the five letters in any single row although the stimulus is already gone, but you will not be able to report all the letters in all the rows during any one trial. After you have reported one row, all the rest have decayed from iconic memory and thereby also from phenomenal consciousness. Thus, your selective attention cannot focus on them anymore or transport them into working memory for reporting; the objects of reflection in phenomenal consciousness or the phenomenal input to higher-order consciousness is already gone.

In such iconic memory tasks it is easy to differentiate the total contents of phenomenal consciousness (the entire visual display with a multitude of distinct visual objects) from the more restricted contents of reflective consciousness (the four or five letters that can be reported). Iconic memory experiments show that the momentary contents of phenomenal consciousness are immensely richer and wider than the contents of focal attention, reflective consciousness, or our verbal introspective reports.

The concept of *pseudohallucination* refers to hallucinations that the subject recognizes as hallucinations and treats as such. The phenomenal content of the hallucination, say an elephant in your backyard, is taken as input to reflective processes that judge, with the help of your semantic and episodic knowledge about elephants and about your own mental condition, whether the vision is real or likely to be a hallucination.The recognition of the percept as a hallucination thus takes place through reflective consciousness. In fact, people diagnosed with a neurological disorder called Charles Bonnet syndrome suffer from various types of recurring visual hallucinations (faces, objects, textures, or colors may appear in their field of vision) due to neurological damage to the visual system and an overactivation of the visual brain areas. Typically they are well aware that the things they see are not real. Hence, whenever they experience a hallucination, they can reflect upon their experience and judge it as unreal and nothing to worry about.

A dramatic example of reflective consciousness is the prelucid stage in lucid dreaming, when the veridicality of the whole perceptual content of primary consciousness is questioned in reflective consciousness by asking, "Is this a dream?" "Am I dreaming?" In the face of such a question, one attempts to pass a reflective judgment concerning the entire sphere of subjective experience, as well as one's own current mental (and physiological) condition. I once had a dream in which something quite peculiar happened and, consequently, I started to wonder whether I was dreaming or was perhaps awake but had gone mad. I tried to find some definite empirical proof of the unreality of the dream world by touching and feeling its objects and by visually observing them very carefully. Unfortunately it all seemed much too real, and I ended up with the conclusion that I was awake but had gone mad!

My definition of reflective consciousness is quite broad; hence, reflective consciousness is a ubiquitous feature of subjective mental life in humans. Our conscious mental life is all the time seamlessly fluctuating between the mere having of experiences (phenomenal consciousness) and the further cognitive elaboration of those experiences (reflective consciousness). In my definition of reflective consciousness, no special status is given to the reflection of the inner, subjective aspects or qualities of the experience. But some would be inclined to define reflective consciousness in a more restricted way.

According to a more narrow definition of reflective consciousness, the subject turns his attention to the experience *as an inner experience* and reflects upon such questions as "What is it like for me to have this experience?" "What was the inner quality of the experience?" "How did the experience come about in my mind and how did it evolve through time?" I call this narrower sense of the term *self-reflective consciousness* because there phenomenal experience is reflected specifically *as* phenomenal experience. Normally we do not think about the contents of perceptual consciousness *as* experiences, but as objects and events in the surrounding world. When we see a flying object flashing by (phenomenal consciousness) and think "that was a bird" (reflective consciousness), we engage phenomenal and reflective consciousness without thinking about them specifically in terms of subjective experience. Self-reflective consciousness goes beyond this natural attitude and asks such things as "What was the visual quality of the flash in my subjective visual field?" "How exactly did I become conscious of the rapidly moving object?" "How exactly did I attach the interpretation that it is a bird to the experience?" And so on. This is consciousness specifically reflecting upon itself. This type of reflection rarely happens in everyday life. It comes close to certain forms of introspection, to be discussed next.

Introspection

Reflective consciousness is closely related to the concept of *introspection.* When we introspect, we use reflective consciousness with the intention to deliberately observe and report or communicate the contents of primary consciousness—at least to ourselves for the record, if not to outsiders. The dividing lines between the mere presence of contents of primary consciousness, the reflection on those contents, and the introspection of the contents could be illuminated with the following story. Imagine that you are in the middle of something when a loud, irritating noise suddenly sounds close by. Your automatic orienting reaction immediately selects the noise and its perceived source and communicates them to focal consciousness. Almost simultaneously you start to wonder about and reflect upon the noise, trying to find an explanation for it, trying to find a category in which the source of the noise could be fitted (alarm clock, fire alarm, cellular phone, gunshot, explosion, etc.). Let us suppose that then you wake up and notice that it was just your alarm clock intruding into your dream. You start to deliberately recall the dream events; you revive the vivid dream images of what happened just before the noise intruded into your dream. You translate the sequence of complex, multimodal dream images into a propositional form and then write them down or tape the whole story. While you go about doing all of this, you *introspect* and as a result produce an *introspective verbal report.*

As the above examples show, primary consciousness includes the mere presence of phenomenal experience; reflection on this experience involves focused attention and an attempt to categorize, conceptualize, evaluate, or think about the experience. Introspection on this experience furthermore involves the deliberate attempt to translate some aspects of the experience into a reportable form. The form may be propositional or linguistic if a verbal report is needed, pictorial if a graphical representation is required, or just a keypress if an explicit categorization of the experience is to be reported in a laboratory experiment.

Introspection was once considered the special method typical of psychological science. Here is how Titchener described the method of introspection in a textbook in 1896:

> The special method employed by psychology is that of introspection or self-observation. We "look into" the mind, each for himself. . . . This "looking into" one's mind or observation of one's own mental processes must not be understood literally, however, as if consciousness were one thing, existing of itself, and the "I," the observer, could stand apart and watch it from the outside. (p. 32)

As the observing "I" cannot be separate from the conscious phenomena observed, the process of observation necessarily changes the original experience. This methodological problem was recognized by Titchener:

> [A] method of observation which involved an alteration of the facts to be observed would not be worth much. Direct introspection—observation of a process which is still running its course—is, as a matter of fact, entirely worthless; it defeats its own object. (p. 33)

Therefore, introspection should not be direct, but always rely on memory:

> Psychological introspection, however, does not consist in the effort to follow up a process during its course. The rule for introspection, in the sphere of sensation, is as follows: *Be as attentive as*

> *possible to the object or process which gives rise to the sensation, and, when the object is removed or the process completed, recall the sensation by an act of memory as vividly and completely as you can.* . . . We avoid any interference with the workings of consciousness by postponing our observation of the process which we wish to examine until after it has run its full course . . .We then call it back, look at it from all points of view, and dissect it. Introspective examination must be a *post mortem* examination. (p. 33–34)

It is worth noting that introspection as a method in experimental psychology is not just a historical curiosity. Most current psychological experiments on, say, visual perception not only involve primary consciousness but also reflective consciousness and introspection, for they typically require some judgment to be passed and communicated about the experience caused by the stimulus. Experimental psychology has gotten rid of the *concept* of introspection, but it seems impossible to get rid of the phenomena of reflective consciousness and introspection as parts of the methodology, even if they are not called by those names.

There are different varieties of introspection. *Descriptive introspection* is used when a report of subjective experiences *exactly as they were experienced* is required. The report is usually verbal and propositional, but it could be partly or even wholly graphical, or a categorical keypress that means "I saw X" (as opposed to seeing Y, for example). In dream research, researchers collect dream reports from subjects who are instructed to practice careful descriptive introspection in order to obtain detailed accounts of experiences during sleep. The immediately past contents of consciousness as remembered are reported (it could thus be called *retrospection* rather than introspection).

Interpretive introspection refers to an attempt to discover the preceding causes of our own behavior by looking for the possible motivations for it within our own experiences and thoughts. The central question in interpretive introspection is *Why?:* "Why did I choose this course of action rather than that?" or "Why do I feel nervous today?" However, empirical research has shown that the accounts we come up with are surprisingly often ad hoc confabulations that merely rationalize our actions for ourselves after the fact. We are extremely good at constructing plausible stories that we ourselves believe, but such stories do not necessarily reveal the real causes of our behavior.

Analytic introspection refers to a method used by structuralism in the history of experimental psychology (around 1880–1920). Structuralists believed that some sort of atoms of experience exist, and that the complex experiential world is really built out of a limited number of these elementary atoms. They tried to uncover the elements or atoms of perceptual experience by analyzing experiences into simple features that make up the complex wholes we are directly aware of. Unfortunately the method did not produce converging results from different laboratories and therefore it has not been used since the days of introspectionism. Furthermore, Gestalt psychologists criticized the approach for its unnaturality: conscious experiences are integrated wholes, not decomposable aggregations of simple elements.

Reflective consciousness and introspection are also closely connected to the concept of *metacognition:* awareness or knowledge of our own mental capacities. We gain metacognition by selectively focusing our attention on our mental capacities and forming judgments about them. "I have a poor memory" or "I am quick at learning new skills" are metacognitive judgments concerning one's own cognitive capacities, in this case memory and learning.

Can Introspection Be Trusted?

In psychology, introspection as a method for collecting scientific data has a bad reputation. Does this mean that the science of consciousness would commit a serious mistake if it were to take introspection seriously as a method? I do not think so. The bad reputation of introspection has several roots. First, *analytic* introspection as practiced by structuralists does not produce reliable results, and it includes a questionable atomistic theory about the structure of consciousness. Second, *interpretive* introspection is also quite suspect as a method for collecting data about the actual causes of behavior. Third, much of the bad reputation of all forms of introspection was due to the behaviorist propaganda whose purpose was to wipe out all subjective phenomena from the domain of psychology (Baars, 2003). Consequently, consciousness and introspection constituted a taboo in experimental psychology until the late 1990s.

But psychology never got rid of subjective experiences or reports of them. Even in a laboratory setting, the subject is usually instructed to select a response and press a key based on what he sees or hears or perceives, that is, based on his subjective phenomenal experience caused by the stimuli. The keypress is thus an introspective report, a message that communicates to the researchers what the experience of the subject was like. These facts are obscured by the technical terms in experiments, often only mentioning stimuli and responses, hits and misses, detection and discrimination performace, but never consciousness or introspection. Other areas of psychology, such as dream research, are of course totally dependent on introspective verbal reports: that is the only way (at least for now) to find out about the phenomenal content of dreams.

Even though (descriptive) introspection does not quite deserve the bad reputation the legacy of behaviorism has left it with, surely caution is needed when introspective data are collected. The introspective method, although not as hopeless as behaviorists made it look like, certainly is not without its pitfalls. When reliable descriptive reports are sought for, factors that may interfere with their reliability should be carefully taken into account. The most important intervening factors are forgetfulness, censorship, the demand characteristics of the task (telling the researcher what you think she wants to hear), difficulties in the verbal description of ineffable experiences, filling in the gaps by inferences to the best explanation, and changes in the experience due to observation of the experience (Farthing, 1992). All of these factors are possible sources of error in any research where subjective reports are collected, but with appropriate precautions their influence on the results can be minimized or controlled. In the following I describe how these problems emerge in the context of dream research.

Forgetfulness is a serious problem in dream research. Our memory for dreams is particularly fragile, and unless dream experiences are recorded immediately after awakening, they will be lost or at least seriously impoverished. Immediate recollection and recording of dream experiences is thus necessary to obtain reliable data in dream research. Subjects are also instructed to rehearse their memory for dreams by reminding themselves of the task just before going to sleep.

Another related problem is the *selectivity of memory:* we tend to remember unusual, bizarre, and highly emotional experiences much better than dull, mundane, or emotionally neutral experiences. This restriction applies not only to dream reports but to all episodic and autobiographical memory of our real-life experiences. The longer the delay between the original experience and the reporting of it, the more likely it is that only the emotionally charged contents will be remembered and most of the mundane features forgotten.

Censorship may also distort the data in dream research. When people have highly personal or aggressive or sexual or bizarre dream experiences, they may be reluctant to share them with anyone, especially if they cannot deliver their reports anonymously to the researchers.

The *demand characteristics of the task* may influence the results, especially if the participants in the research know what the researchers would like to find in the reports. Most people would like to be "good subjects" and therefore knowledge of the researchers' expectations and hopes will function as an indirect suggestion to have particular types of dreams, and to pay more attention to particular types of dreams and dream elements when reporting dreams. Thus, the data and the results may be biased toward fulfilling the researchers' expectations, compared to a situation where the subjects have no idea what the researchers expect or would like to find.

Difficulties in the verbal description of ineffable experiences sometimes occur in dream research: a subject may see or hear or feel something so unusual or bizarre in the dream that no words can accurately describe her experiences. There may be no adequate concepts available to transform the complex qualitative experience to a string of linguistic symbols. Even quite ordinary dream experiences are difficult to describe in words in a way that would preserve the richness of the original experience. The dream is a complex sensory-perceptual world. How could the richness of the events in this world—all the colors, shapes, movements, emotions, objects, places—be translated into plain words so that the verbal report would preserve all the experiential richness?

Filling in the gaps by inferences to the best explanation may take place when a dream suddenly jumps from place to place, and it remains unclear what happened in between (if anything). We have a natural tendency to invent a plausible story describing how the earlier events led to the later events, and how we proceeded from one place to another.

But while in real life, time and space always are continuous and something always must have happened in between two events, in dreams the time and space experienced may be discontinuous, and there may have been nothing in between two successive scenes. Then we easily resort to inventing a story of what probably happened in between, although we may not have any actual recollection of the events. In such cases we infer something that was not part of the original experience at all, and the dream report becomes more logical and continuous than the original experience ever was.

Changes in the experience due to observation of the experience do not occur very often in dream research, for the simple reason that we are normally unable to reflectively observe the dream while it unfolds. But sometimes subjects who are overly motivated to recall their dreams (or perhaps trying to induce lucid dreams) feel they must resign from the research because they are unable to sleep normally. They say that they are so eager to remember their dreams that whenever they start to dream they remember that *now* they should be especially attentive (or if trying to induce lucidity, that *now* they should try to become aware that it is just a dream). This causes them to immediately wake up due to excitement. In these cases the attempt to observe and recall one's dreams interferes with normal sleep patterns and actually causes loss of sleep and dreaming.

During the era of classical introspectionism the researchers were well aware of the shortcomings of the introspective method. Titchener wrote in 1896:

> But this introspection, it may well be said, cannot furnish very reliable results. The individual can apply the method to one consciousness only—his own; and we all know how easy it is for a single observer to make mistakes, and how necessary to have more witnesses than one, if a fact is to be securely established. There is no guarantee that other individuals would come to the same conclusion, from an examination of their consciousness; and no means of comparing the conclusions reached by different individuals under similar circumstances. (p. 34)

Nevertheless, the shortcomings of introspection may be overcome if exactly the same experimental conditions are applied to large numbers of individuals who are careful and skilled in their use of attention, memory, and language when they report their experiences.

> The "facts" of the psychology of sensation are, then, average results obtained from observers trained in introspection under experimental conditions of both a general and a special character. (pp. 41–42).

In this way it has been possible to learn facts about the typical content of dreams (e.g., see Domhoff, 1996). Such facts can only be obtained through the systematic use of the method of descriptive introspection.

Self-Awareness

An important type of higher-order form of consciousness is self-awareness.[5] It is in fact a special form of reflective consciousness. The necessary conditions for self-awareness are the following:

1. The system must have a conception or an internal representation of itself.
2. The system must have the capability for reflective consciousness.
3. Current self-related experiences (e.g., one's reflection in a mirror) must be connected with the more permanent internal representation of the self.

Self-awareness is manifested when the internal representation of the self (say one's own body image as perceived in a mirror) is consciously updated, evaluated, or described. In this process some self-related experiences (say perceptions or memory images of one's self) first enter primary consciousness and are then taken as an object by reflective consciousness. In reflective consciousness they are connected to the permanent internal self-representation, with the understanding that both the current experience and the permanent representation refer to the same entity, oneself. Thus the creature becomes self-aware. In a nutshell, self-awareness is the ability to become aware of one's own phenomenal experiences (bodily experiences, thoughts, memories) as *one's own* phenomenal experiences.

There are several different types of self-representation. The most elemental may be the representation of one's own body or physical configuration as the center of the egocentric space in consciousness ("first-person perspective"; see below). There is no doubt that many animals have this kind of self-representation; what most animals seem to lack is the ability to become aware of it as their *own* body. They cannot reflectively realize that the body representation is a representation of the animal itself. They cannot make the crucial connection between the current experience and a permanent self-representation. A much more sophisticated self-representation is the *autobiographical self* that we humans build in our long-term memory. It contains the entire history of the self (as remembered). Human self-awareness connects particular contents of phenomenal consciousness (say the image seen in the mirror) with the enduring self-representation in autobiographical memory. To be aware of seeing myself in the mirror is to realize that *that* person seen *out there* in the mirror is basically the *same* person who I call "me" *in here,* in whose shoes I am right now, and about whom I have a detailed life history recorded in my autobiographical memory in the first-person perspective.

Primary consciousness without self-awareness is devoid of the identity and continuity of the self. Sometimes in dream experiences we may not be aware of our identity and continuity at all because we are fully engaged in the dream events. Sometimes in intensive mental or physical activity (e.g., sports) a similar (temporary) loss of self-awareness may take place. These moments of total absorption are sometimes described as "flow" or "peak" experiences.

People who suffer from devastating global amnesia are trapped inside a discontinuous moment of here-and-now primary consciousness, and they often feel as if they had only just regained consciousness anew, because they have to constantly reorient themselves to the place and time where they are. Their sense of self may be seriously limited or regressed to a point in the past after which all autobiographical memories have been destroyed. Oliver Sacks (1985) describes one such patient, a gray-haired man in his fifties, who believed that he was 19 years of age, because that's where his autobiographical memory stopped. When Sacks told the man to look into a mirror and tell what he sees, the poor patient could not believe his eyes, but thought it was a joke or a nightmare (fortunately, he forgot the incident in a minute).

The variety of consciousness related to knowledge about our own personal history (autobiographical memory) has been described as involving "mental time travel." In autobiographical memories we literally see ourselves as subjects in another spatiotemporal context and we understand that the subject of that past experience is continuous with the subject of our present experience: it is the same subject or the same "me" who then was there and now is here. Thus, mental time travel necessarily involves a conception of the self as an entity that endures and extends through time, from personal past to personal future. It requires a complex form of self-awareness. The memory researcher Endel Tulving (1985) calls this form of consciousness *autonoetic* consciousness and suggests that only humans have it. Damasio (1999) introduces the concept *extended* consciousness to refer to the type of consciousness that escapes the immediate moment of primary consciousness. Extended consciousness is consciousness colored by the sense of self, the sense of temporal continuity of the self from the past to the future; it is primary consciousness colored with long-term episodic memory and the capability of full self-awareness.

Perhaps the most dramatic demonstration of a loss of extended consciousness was recorded by a 51-year-old professional musician who became very severely amnesic. He was encouraged to write a diary in order to gain a sense of continuity through time, but to no avail. His diary read line after line like this (Kapur, 1997):

7.50 a.m.	I wake up for the very first time
8.20 a.m.	I am totally awake for the very first time
8.52 a.m.	I am really awake for the very first time
10.03 a.m.	I am completely awake for the very first time
10.36 a.m.	NOW I am perfectly awake (very 1st time)
4.49 p.m.	All other claims to be awake are rubbish
4.54 p.m.	Time for my first conscious walk + TV, all systems work, I AM alive
6.15 p.m.	I return after dinner, now I am totally alive (1st time)
7.08 p.m.	I am really perfectly awake (1st time). First conscious walk.
7.19 p.m.	I return and now my senses work (1st time). First conscious walk.
7.30 p.m.	First conscious walk: all my senses do work (1st time)
7.54 p.m.	I return completely awake. I've suffered from amnesia.

Most of the lines were crossed out because every time he read the previous lines he had no sense of ever having written them and therefore felt that the claims to have been conscious before now must be incorrect and therefore should be crossed out. For every momentary self, the previous lines in the diary were totally alien, as if written by some-one else. The diary did not help him to gain a sense of continuity. In the same vein, when requested to think about yesterday or tomorrow, the amnesic patient reported by Tulving (1985) experienced a total blank: there was nothing there.

First-Person Perspective and Third-Person Perspective

First-person perspective (1PP) refers to a structural feature of the sphere of conscious experience: the centeredness of experiential space upon one's own body image. 1PP involves a special egocentric reference frame, in which the locations and distances between perceptual entities in space are represented in relation to a personal agent and his physical configuration (body image). This egocentric structure involves the entire sphere of primary consciousness, whereas self-awareness is intimately connected to the body image in the center of this coordinate system. In our everyday thinking, we locate our "self" within the boundaries of the body image, or simply identify the two.

By contrast, the third-person perspective (3PP) describes objects or persons in space as they are related to each other (this is called an allocentric reference frame). In such a description there is no observer or subject to whom the location of objects would be related.

We can illustrate the difference in the following way: If you are playing football or ice hockey, you see the field (or rink) and the other players from 1PP and you act accordingly. There is a subject or a self whose spatial relation to the other players and to the ball (or puck) is immediately clear. By contrast, a camera placed right above the field or the rink captures an image where all the players are seen in relation to each other, but no single player's viewpoint of the situation can be seen. If you are shown a videotape of the game, you might not even recognize which one of the players is you. Your body is just one more moving object among others in the field. In some rare occasions (out-of-body experiences, autoscopy) consciousness may temporarily lose its egocentric frame of reference. In such altered states of consciousness the self (the body image identified as "me") is seen as from an external point of view.

3PP is the external or "objective" viewpoint that is regarded as typical of scientific descriptions of phenomena. They may even assume a viewpoint that would not be physically possible for any human subject, say, describing the Milky Way galaxy as it would be seen from a point located somewhere in intergalactic space. Sometimes the maximally objective 3PP is described as the "God's-eye view," a perspective from which the entire universe, its history and future, can be seen all at once. The critical question is whether science can describe and explain the existence of 1PP if the standard scientific description of all phenomena is from 3PP (Nagel, 1974).

Confusing Conceptions of Consciousness

The concepts of consciousness discussed above form the theoretical cornerstones of the science of consciousness. However, they are not the only ways to understand the concept.

In this section, a few alternative concepts that might be extremely confusing are outlined. While there are contexts in which these concepts might also be useful, in the present context they create confusion as they are directly in conflict with some of the definitions given above. To avoid the confusion, it is useful to understand how these concepts define consciousness and why they are at odds with the concepts chosen as fundamental in this book.

Consciousness as Responsiveness to Stimuli

There are fields of clinical medicine where, for practical purposes, the concept of consciousness has been defined operationally as behavioral responsiveness to external stimuli. This is because it is clinically important to estimate the so-called level of consciousness (or the "depth" of unconsciousness) of a brain-injured or otherwise unconscious patient. The "depth" of unconsciousness is taken to be a function of the strength and amount of stimulation that is needed to make the patient respond to the external world. It is estimated by formally checking the tendency of the patient to respond to different types of external stimulation or the possibility of waking him up. If the patient responds to verbal questions or calls, his level of consciousness is not very low, but if he does not respond to even very painful stimuli in any way, he is in a deep coma.

The assessment of the level of consciousness has been standardized by using formal coma scales. The most widely used of these is the Glasgow Coma Scale. Three different types of responses are evaluated: eye opening, best verbal response, and best motor response. In the deepest forms of unconsciousness, none of these responses are elicited, even by painful stimuli. This scale allows the clinician to compute a score that reflects the "level" of consciousness and helps in the follow-up of the development of the patient's condition.

It should be noted, though, that a definition of the level of consciousness in terms of responsiveness has its difficulties, because responsiveness and primary phenomenal consciousness may be (and in some cases in fact are) dissociated from each other. For example, a nonresponsive patient may have subjective conscious experiences, while a responsive patient may be only undergoing complex but nonconscious behavioral automatisms. Hence, it should be remembered that the clinically useful concepts of consciousness are not necessarily adequate for the theoretical and philosophical explanation of consciousness.

Wakefulness and "Awareness of" the Surrounding World

Another conceptual confusion occurs easily if "consciousness" is taken to mean the same as "wakefulness." This usage must be clearly differentiated from the use of consciousness as phenomenal experience. Wakefulness may be dissociated from subjective experience in epileptic absence seizures: the patient is awake, but apparently is not having any subjective experiences for a few seconds at a time (Damasio, 1999). Furthermore, while it is true that when we are in the state of wakefulness we normally have subjective phenomenal experience, it is not true that when we are asleep we do not have any experiences. Our experiences during sleep typically do not inform us about external events—we are not *aware of* the external world that surrounds our biological body—but that does not mean that the experiences do not exist. On the contrary, the phenomenal level of organization tends to be fully realized during rapid eye movement (REM) sleep and it often exists in some form also during sleep onset and nonrapid eye movement (NREM) sleep. There is an abundance of subjective experience during sleep, in the absence of wakefulness, although we usually cannot remember most of it when we wake up.

Consciousness thus need not be an *awareness of* something real or external. If consciousness were defined in that way, it would exclude all types of hallucinations from the domain of consciousness. *Awareness of* is closely related to *representation of* the external world and the representational contents of consciousness. But we should note that representation and phenomenal consciousness have no necessary relationship. There are lots of accurate representations (or cortical sensory "maps") of the external world in the brain, some accessible to consciousness, many completely nonconscious. Conversely, although much of our waking consciousness may accurately represent something external, our phenomenal consciousness during dream sleep does not represent the place we are sleeping in. "Representation" and "awareness of" are matters concerning the *relationship* between a mental phenomenon and something *else;* thus phenomenal consciousness per se is not dependent on them and should not be confused with them.

Access Consciousness

The concept of access consciousness was recently introduced by the philosopher Ned Block. He argues that there is an important distinction between two concepts of consciousness: "phenomenal consciousness" and "access consciousness" (Block, 1995; see also Block, 2001). However, as I see it, "access consciousness" is again a concept of consciousness that involves no necessary connection to subjective experience. Block's definition of access consciousness allows that even a total nonconscious zombie could possess access consciousness (Revonsuo, 1995a).

Access consciousness refers to information in the system that can be used to guide rational behavior in ways that conscious information typically does, but in spite of that the concept of access consciousness has no *necessary* connection to subjective experience. It abstracts the causal role (or the input-output function) that conscious information normally has in the human brain (global accessibility to other cognitive systems, or global broadcasting, for example). Anything that plays exactly *this* causal role in *any* system constitutes access consciousness, regardless of whether or not the system has any subjective experiences, any phenomenal level of organization. Access consciousness is the concept of consciousness one ends up with if one's philosophical theory of mind is metaphysical functionalism (Block, 2001). Biological realism rejects metaphysical functionalism.

In the framework of multilevel explanation the concept of access consciousness could be delineated as the input-output description of the function that consciousness normally plays in the human brain. The question that has interested philosophers is whether this function could be carried out also by some system devoid of the phenomenal level. This issue seems to boil down to the possibility of zombies and the plausibility of the doctrine of philosophical functionalism: Could there be systems functionally indistinguishable from a conscious human being, yet without a trace of subjective phenomenal experience? A zombie fulfilling the function of consciousness in the absence of the phenomenal level of organization does not look like an empirical possibility. Yet, contrary to functionalist theories of consciousness, it remains a *logical* possibility. The fact that a system fulfils the input-output function of consciousness does not logically entail that the system should enjoy any subjective experiences.

Conscious Creatures, Conscious States, and Altered States of Consciousness

In this section we sort out some basic ideas describing the realization of the phenomenal level in the world. Some systems have it, others do not. Even in those systems that have it, it may be realized only intermittently. Furthermore, it may be sometimes realized in an altered form.

Conscious Creature and Conscious State

The concept of primary consciousness can be used to define the concepts of a conscious creature (or system) and a conscious state. Conscious creatures or systems include all those creatures in which primary, phenomenal consciousness is (at least sometimes) realized, or in other words, whose constitution is capable of generating and supporting the phenomenal level of organization.

A conscious creature may, however, be momentarily in a nonconscious state (e.g., deep sleep, anesthesia) during which consciousness is not realized and the phenomenal level is temporarily absent. But as long as this state is reversible and a conscious state can be brought about later, it can still be said that we are dealing with a conscious creature—a genuine subject—as opposed to a mere object that will never have any states of primary consciousness.

Different species of biological organisms can be divided into two categories with respect to their capability for realizing the phenomenal level of organization. Viruses, bacteria, single-cell organisms, and plants are relatively uncontroversial examples of nonconscious creatures, whereas all mammals and birds almost certainly fall into the category of conscious creatures. There is variation across species as to whether the phenomenal level is a level of biological organization in members of the species. There is

also variation across the life span of an individual conscious creature as to whether the creature is in a conscious as opposed to a nonconscious state, or as to whether or not the phenomenal level is at some particular moment realized in the organism.

There are ethical implications about how genuine subjects (i.e., conscious creatures) should be treated as compared to mere nonconscious objects. If a conscious creature is in a conscious state, we can deliberately treat it in ways that may make an enormous difference as to what it is like to be the conscious creature in question. We may cause terrible pain and suffering to it, or intense pleasure, or not interfere in its life at all. If a conscious creature is in a nonconscious state we cannot have an influence on what it feels like to be that creature in the here and now; by definition, it feels like nothing at all. We can, however, through our action (or inaction), deliberately destroy the capability of the system to regain its conscious state ever again. We could transform a conscious creature into a nonconscious system and thereby deprive the conscious creature that once existed of enjoying any further conscious states ever again.

An important practical matter related to the conscious state is to establish some objective marker which would tell us when exactly the phenomenal level is realized in the brain and patterns of phenomenal experience therefore can occur, and when the phenomenal level is absent and no patterns of phenomenal experience therefore can occur. This is a significant practical question for the anesthesiologist who tries to control the presence and absence of the phenomenal level in patients during surgery. He should know exactly when the patient loses consciousness and prevent him from coming back to his senses during anesthesia. Being subjectively aware during anesthesia is regarded as a serious complication in anesthesiology. The ideal anesthetic depth monitor would discriminate in real time between the conscious state (i.e., the realization or presence of the phenomenal level in the brain) and the nonconscious state (i.e., the total absence of the phenomenal level in the brain).

A popular solution to this problem in anesthesiology is to measure the brain's electrical activity and calculate from it the bispectral index (BIS) online. BIS is computed from the relationships between the power at different EEG frequency bands and it is expressed as a numerical value between 0 and 100. BIS is well, though not perfectly, correlated with the presence of the conscious state. Values of BIS below 60 are very rarely accompanied by any subjective experience whatsoever. BIS is, however, merely a predictive empirical tool; it does not provide us with a theoretical explanation or a multilevel model of the conscious state in the brain. No theory is provided to explain *why* BIS correlates with the presence and absence of the phenomenal level.

Animal Consciousness and Machine Consciousness

When we ask the question, Do creatures of type X have consciousness? we must first clarify what we mean by consciousness: primary (phenomenal) consciousness, reflective consciousness, self-awareness, or perhaps something else that none of these concepts

covers. I will first consider the question whether animals and artificial man-made systems have primary phenomenal consciousness, whether animals or machines can at least in some sense subjectively feel that they exist.

As long as we do not have any objective means to verify the presence or absence of subjective experience in any physical system, this question is impossible to answer. We cannot confirm with any absolute certainty that a dog really has conscious experiences or that a thermostat or a virus does not. But if we accept the working hypothesis that consciousness in humans is a biological level of organization in the brain, then perhaps some educated speculation can be based on that foundation. In the context of biological realism the question can be reformulated: Do (other) animals have the phenomenal level of organization as a part of their biological machinery? Could we build a machine that would include the phenomenal level of organization?

For all we know, at least mammals and birds have a central nervous system not very unlike our own. They also manifest roughly similar sleep-wake patterns and have REM sleep (and perhaps also dream), unlike fish and reptiles. Thus, there is no reason why birds and mammals at the very least should not have a phenomenal level of organization in their brain, whereas it looks unlikely that insects and other invertebrates could incorporate any such level of organization. Fish and reptiles land in the twilight zone—perhaps they turn out to be nothing but nonconscious biological zombies, or perhaps they have some kind of rudimentary alien phenomenology. It is too early to tell. (For a discussion, see Seth, Baars, & Edelman [2005], D. B. Edelman, Baars, & Seth [2005]).

The question, Do animals have self-awareness? can be answered through empirical investigations much more easily than the question about phenomenal consciousness. When it comes to self-awareness, experiments such as the mirror self-recognition test can be applied. At least chimpanzees and orangutans have the capability of recognizing themselves in the mirror—evidence of a basic form of self-awareness. Human children acquire this capacity at about the age of 18 months (Parker, Mitchell, & Boccia, 1994). Gorillas and dolphins also show some evidence of being aware of themselves. But the rest of the animal kingdom seem to be restricted to primary phenomenal consciousness and perhaps some simple forms of reflective consciousness.

The concepts "machine consciousness" and "artificial consciousness" have been used in many ways, and it seems that "consciousness" in these contexts is often understood not as phenomenal experience but instead as "awareness of" the surroundings and flexible behavior guided by the information representing the system's surroundings. Sometimes it seems as if "machine consciousness" or "conscious robots" would mean for some people about the same thing that used to be called "artificial intelligence."

But in the context of biological realism, "machine consciousness" should be interpreted as a man-made artificial system (say, a robot) that enjoys subjective phenomenal experiences. If the robot does not enjoy any experiences, then it is just a nonconscious zombie, no matter how accurately it represents its surroundings or how flexibly and

intelligently it guides its behavior. If it does enjoy experiences, then it is a conscious machine, even if it were terribly dumb and clumsy, or even if its experiences were mere hallucinations rather than accurate representations of the environment.

To build a conscious robot requires that the robot's brain is capable of supporting the phenomenal level. If consciousness is a biological phenomenon in the brain and the brain is a biological mechanism, then producing artificial consciousness should be possible to the same extent as producing or synthesizing any other artificial biological phenomenon. Hence biological realism does not deny the possibility of machine consciousness (or "artificial" or "synthetic" consciousness). If consciousness is some sort of electrophysiological or bioelectrical phenomenon in the brain, realized, say, by synchronous activity in large-scale corticocortical and thalamocortical networks, then the question of producing "artificial" consciousness is the question of simulating or duplicating such a phenomenon in a man-made machine.

There is a crucial difference between mere simulation and true duplication, though. Simulation of the input-output functions of consciousness is in principle possible at the purely computational level. A simulation of consciousness could be implemented in a computer without actually producing any phenomenal experiences. A program that simulates consciousness would not necessarily enjoy any phenomenal consciousness, just as a computer-simulated model of a living cell is not alive.

Genuine duplication of the bioelectrical phenomena that constitute the phenomenal level would require a machine implementation that can support large-scale synchronous electrical phenomena resembling those realized in the conscious brain. Thus, the robot that posesses phenomenal consciousness would most likely have to be built from neuron-like elements that have macrolevel electrophysiological properties closely resembling those found at the higher levels of organization in the brain.

Baseline State and Altered States of Consciousness

The paradigmatic baseline state of consciousness is the state where we are awake and perceive the environment and ourselves more or less accurately. In the baseline state the contents of consciousness are modulated by the physical environment and the physical body and therefore consciousness succeeds in accurately representing them. For a state of consciousness to count as an altered state, it must be altered in certain ways in relation to this baseline state (for a comparable view, see Hobson, 2001).

Paradigmatic altered states of consciousness (ASCs) are such that the *background mechanisms* of subjective experience (i.e., the etiological and constitutive mechanisms) are temporarily predisposed to create contents of consciousness that misrepresent or create delusional beliefs about the environment or the self (figures 2.3. and 2.4.).

For example, when we fall asleep, we become functionally blind (even if we could keep our eyes open). Thus, the background mechanisms leading from peripheral sensory organs to subjective experience do not function anymore, as in the baseline condition,

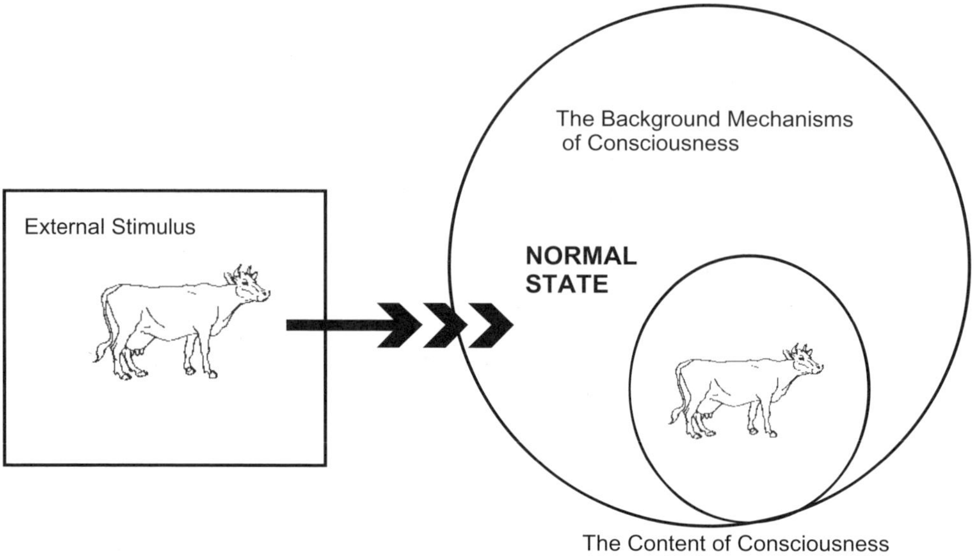

Figure 2.3
A normal state of consciousness. The contents of consciousness represent external stimuli accurately, because the neural background mechanisms mediating between stimuli and phenomenal consciousness operate flawlessly.

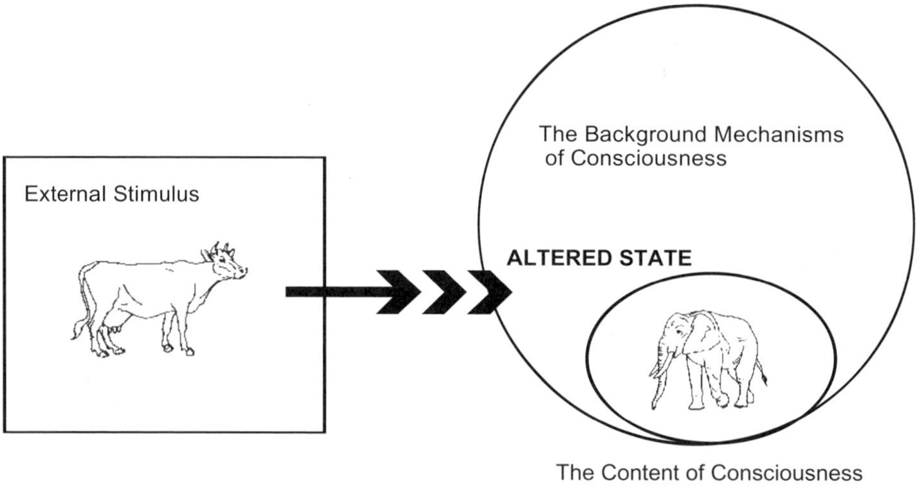

Figure 2.4
An altered state of consciousness. The background mechanisms of consciousness block or distort stimulus information so that phenomenal consciousness is temporarily disposed to carry *misrepresentations* of the external world. In an altered state, at least some aspects of the subject's surroundings or the subject's self tend to be misperceived or hallucinated, or delusional beliefs about them tend to be entertained by the subject.

but now prevent perception of the environment. If we take LSD, there will be micro-level changes in the neurochemistry of the background mechanisms of experience, leading to highly unusual hallucinatory and delusional contents of consciousness. If we reach a deep meditative state where we feel that our self disappears and becomes one with the universe, we have temporarily altered the deep-rooted background mechanisms of phenomenal consciousness and self-representation.

The phenomenal contents of consciousness do not all by themselves directly reveal whether the state of consciousness is an altered state or not. An identical phenomenal content of consciousness (say the experience of seeing an elephant in front of you) may be produced during the baseline state of consciousness (if you are in the zoo) or during an altered state of consciousness (if you are at home and dreaming or under the influence of LSD). The phenomenal content of consciousness (the pattern of subjective experience) does not by itself determine whether the background mechanisms of consciousness function normally or are somehow altered. The relevant alteration in the background mechanisms is a matter of the relation between experiences that are *actually* produced and those that *would have been* produced in the baseline state of normal wakefulness. The alteration in the background mechanisms changes the *relationship* between the phenomenal level and the stimulus environment that causally modulates it.

In brief, an ASC requires that the *representational contents of consciousness are deviated from the baseline.* Accurate representation has become inaccurate, a misrepresentation.

An ASC can be defined as the predisposition of the background mechanisms of subjective experience to process and represent available information inaccurately or delusionally so that the resulting conscious experience will misrepresent reality. When such a predisposition exists, the subject is in an ASC regardless of what the subject's contents of consciousness are and regardless of what circumstances brought about the predisposition in the subject's brain. Dreaming, hallucination induced by drug states, hypnotic suggestions, sensory deprivation, epileptic seizures, all are examples of ASCs where the background mechanisms of experience are temporarily predisposed to produce patterns of experience that misrepresent the world in one respect or another. Although ordinary visual illusions also misrepresent reality, they do not count as evidence for an ASC, because ordinary illusions are not temporary or reversible: certain types of stimuli invariably elicit them. Also, a fleeting misperception that comes about momentarily when the signal contains a lot of noise, is obviously not an ASC.

According to this analysis, the mechanisms that are altered in an ASC themselves reside *outside* the phenomenal level. The important alterations that define a state as an ASC take place in the background mechanisms of consciousness rather than at the phenomenal level itself. The altered phenomenal *contents* of consciousness that the subject experiences are a *consequence* of the altered *state* that prevails in the nonconscious background mechanisms of consciousness.

This conception of ASCs as alterations in the background mechanisms of consciousness clarifies many questions that have remained unclear in the literature on altered states. According to this conception, a subject need not *recognize* that she is in an altered state to be in one; when we dream we usually have no idea that we are not in our normal state of consciousness. Hence, whether or not the subject herself feels or realizes (by using reflective consciousness) that her experiences are different from normal, her own judgment cannot be the criterion of an ASC.

Even an unusual pattern of experience is by itself no guarantee that there is an altered background state of consciousness involved; unusual patterns of experience may be brought about by unusual stimulus environments accurately perceived. In fact, when something very unlikely or bizarre happens during wakefulness in front of our own eyes (like seeing a giant aircraft crashing into a skyscraper), the first reaction for many is to think that this just cannot be real. There is *derealization:* a dreamlike or unreal quality to one's experience, due to the unexpected and incredible nature of the events perceived. Yet, that is not an ASC (although the subject may believe that it must be); it is a perfectly normal emotional reaction to a highly unexpected event.

The proper criterion of an ASC is thus not to be found within phenomenal consciousness as such or even in the reflective consciousness of the subject. Unusual experiences may occur without an ASC, and mundane experiences can occur while in an ASC. ASCs may occur without the subject becoming reflectively conscious that he is in an ASC, and subjects might come to believe that they are in an ASC even if they are not. The proper (and objective) criterion of an ASC is not to be found within the subject's experiences or beliefs, but in the representational relationships between the subject's consciousness and his stimulus environment. If the neurocognitive background mechanisms mediating between consciousness and the world (and consciousness and the body) are disposed to distort the information in some way clearly different from the baseline condition, then the subject is in an ASC.[6]

The ASCs discussed above are temporary and reversible. The paradigm cases of altered states seem to imply *reversibility:* the system will return to the baseline state sooner or later. This raises the question whether the effects of irreversible structural neural pathology should be described as ASCs. Perhaps they would be best described as *permanent* ASCs to discriminate them from the reversible types of ASCs. While reversible alterations in the background mechanisms can take place in the healthy brain, permanent alterations imply pathological damage to those mechanisms. Reversible alterations tell us something about the flexibility of the healthy brain, but permanent alterations tell us about preserved mechanisms in a damaged brain.

Subjective Experiences during Sleep

Sleep is the most commonly occurring ASC. In sleep research, there is a need to describe and classify different types of subjective experiences that occur during sleep. The most important category is "dreaming." There is, however, no agreement on how this category of subjective experience should be defined. There is a theoretical motivation for some dream researchers to define dreaming as "mentation during sleep which has most, if not all, of the following formal features: hallucination, delusion, narrative structure, hyperemotionality, and bizarreness" (Hobson, Pace-Schott, & Stickgold 2000, p. 1019). Although complex, temporally progressing contents of consciousness during sleep often have some of these features, I believe it would be a mistake to regard as dreams only experiences that fulfill these criteria. Dreams that lack some of these features are entirely possible: not all dreams are bizarre, hyperemotional, or have much of a narrative structure. The theoretical motivation behind this definition is that dreams that fulfil these criteria are almost entirely restricted to REM sleep. Hence, if one wants to explain dreaming by referring to REM physiology, one might prefer to define dreaming in a way that excludes NREM dreams.

I suggest that the category of "dreaming" should be defined on the basis of the *complexity* and the *spatiotemporal organization* of subjective experiences during sleep. Experiences reaching a certain degree of complex, dynamical organization should be counted as "dreams" whereas other experiences during sleep should be left out. I suggest the following distinctions:

1. *Dreaming:* Complex, organized, temporally progressing, multimodal contents of consciousness during sleep that amount to a *simulation* of the perceptual world
2. *Sleep mentation:* Other contents of consciousness during sleep that show a lesser degree of complexity and organization (e.g., simple, unimodal, static images or isolated thoughts)
3. *Nonconscious* information processing during sleep

During sleep there is a *continuum* from very simple phenomenal contents to extremely complex ones. The crucial question is: at which point in this continuum should we draw the line between sleep mentation and dreaming? My suggestion is that the concept of "world simulation" defines the theoretically distinctive, special *form* of consciousness that should be used as the criterion. "Dreaming" proper hence requires phenomenal experiences that include many distinct patterns (say sensations, percepts, emotions) that are spatiotemporally well-organized to form an entire dream *world* (i.e., a simulation of the perceptual world). In a world simulation, there is an overall, well-organized spatiotemporal setting where (simulated) objects, persons, animals, and so on interact with each other. By contrast, sleep mentation only includes unimodal simple images, sensations, or thoughts, or repetitive images without dynamics or progression. Sleep mentation never amounts to a simulation of the perceptual world. Both dreaming and sleep mentation are, however, forms of phenomenal consciousness.

Lucid dreaming is sometimes described as "conscious dreaming." Note that according to the concepts used in this book, *all* dreaming involves primary phenomenal consciousness, and is therefore "conscious." Thus, there can be no such thing as "nonconscious dreaming"—that would be a contradiction in terms. Still, lucid dreaming is a special form of conscious dreaming in the sense that it involves *reflective* consciousness. In fact, it involves a special form of reflective consciousness that takes the entire sphere of primary consciousness as its object and, consequently, passes the judgment, *This is a dream!* The reflective consciousness that defines lucid dreaming thus turns the hallucinatory dream world to a pseudohallucination: a hallucination that is recognized as such by the subject experiencing it.

If the definition of dreaming as world simulation is accepted, that might lead to theoretical unification between dream research and consciousness research. As will be argued later in this book, the notion of "world simulation" is fundamental to the theory and philosophy of consciousness more generally. It might also lead to new insights concerning the function of dreaming, because now we may ask, Why should the brain construct an entire simulated world during sleep? What kind of events in particular is the dreaming brain designed to simulate? (For my answer to this question, see chapter 24.)

One widespread misconception about dreaming is that it only happens during REM sleep. A review of a number of studies in which subjective experiences during sleep were correlated with various sleep stages shows that in actual fact, the probability of remembering a dream when waking up from REM sleep is 60 to 90% (Nielsen, 2000). Thus, we may safely say that well over half of the time (yet, not *every* time) when waking up from REM sleep, an average subject will report a dream experience. In NREM sleep, the probability of dream recall is significantly lower, but not nil. Some kind of subjective experiences are reported in 25 to 50% of awakenings from NREM sleep, but the probability of experiences fulfilling the definition of dreaming is lower, perhaps 10 to 25%. Vivid dreaming in NREM sleep is even less likely, with an estimated probability of 7% (for a review, see Nielsen, 2000).

The Absence of Consciousness

We need clear concepts for talking not only about the presence of consciousness but also its absence. The notions "unconscious" and "nonconscious" have been widely used but it is not entirely clear what they refer to and how they can be distinguished from each other. Furthermore, the concept of "zombie" has been used, especially in philosophy, to refer to the absence of consciousness, and the supervenience relation has been applied to explain the possibility of zombies. In this section, we sort out this family of concepts.

The Unconscious and the Nonconscious

On what basis can some phenomenon be counted as an *unconscious* phenomenon? Try to recall, as vividly and in as much detail as possible, the following things: (1) The faces of your closest family members, (2) The place that you visited during your last trip abroad, and (3) your favorite tune. Now, before you followed the instructions, information about all those things existed in your brain as totally unconscious neurally coded patterns of information. They have the capability to modulate the phenomenal content of your primary consciousness in particular ways. The ones in the first example cause specific visual imagery of faces; the second, of places; and the third, auditory imagery of music. Because of this ability, those neurophysiological patterns can be considered as unconscious (rather than nonconscious) phenomena: the information they contain can modulate the patterns of phenomenal experience in highly organized and specific ways. If the unconscious neural patterns are lost, the corresponding patterns of phenomenal experience cannot be reconstructed from memory anymore.

By contrast, patterns of neurophysiological organization in your brain that are incapable of directly transforming the content of your subjective experience can be regarded as entirely nonconscious neurophysiological phenomena. There is biological information coded in the DNA of our brain cells, but that type of information is in a totally nonconscious format and we will never be able to read it out by just reaching into our own minds and trying to retrieve it to consciousness. It is in a format unreadable at the phenomenal level.

Consider an analogy: A music CD not being played right now contains music in the same sense as unconscious memory traces in the brain contain memories even when they are not being retrieved into consciousness at the moment. The CD contains patterns of information that can modulate the stereo system in such a way as to let specific pieces of music flow from the loudspeakers. The music that resides within the CD itself is the analogy of the unconscious phenomena, whereas the music flowing from the loudspeakers is the analogy of conscious phenomena currently experienced. Even if you spill something on the CD that temporarily prevents access to the codes that contain the "unconscious music," the music is still coded there, and after cleaning the surface, it can be reaccessed. Thus, even when we sometimes cannot retrieve a memory because of some psychological or physiological obstacle, the memory trace is still there in the brain as an unconscious mental phenomenon. By contrast, a CD containing no coded information, or only the type of information that cannot be played on a music CD player (e.g. a photo CD), could be called a "nonmusical" phenomenon and is thus analogous to nonconscious phenomena in the brain.

This view of unconscious and nonconscious phenomena derives from those of Searle (1992) and Strawson (1994). I share their view that unconscious mental entities are ontologically dependent on phenomenal consciousness. In a world where phenomenal consciousness does not exist, there can be no unconscious phenomena either. A totally nonconscious creature (such as a behavioral zombie) cannot have any unconscious mental phenomena, whereas a conscious creature has lots of them stored in its brain regardless of whether the creature is currently in a conscious state or not.

The Threshold of Consciousness

The idea of a threshold of consciousness can be interpreted in the following way: There is some minimum duration or intensity of physical stimulation which, when applied to the stimulus field, will trigger a chain of causal events in the immediate etiological pathway that leads to a (minimal) change in the content of primary consciousness. Below that minimum duration or intensity of stimulation, no change in the patterns of phenomenal experience results (but there may be changes at the nonconscious levels of implicit processing).

In experimental research, the subject must additionally give an introspective behavioral report as to whether there was a change in the content of consciousness or not. When such changes are reported, we say that the stimulation has crossed the *subjective threshold* of consciousness. Even when no changes are reported, the stimuli may still modulate some aspects of the subject's behavior. If that is the case, the stimuli are below the subjective but above the objective threshold. When no systematic changes in any aspect of indirect behavior can be measured, the stimulus is below the *objective threshold.* There has been great controversy in experimental psychology over whether subjects are really not conscious of the stimuli that fall between the objective and subjective thresholds (Palmer, 1999). My interpretation is that immediately below the subjective threshold, the stimulus might still cause some extremely feeble changes in the pattern of phenomenal experience, too weak or too fleeting to become the objects of reflective consciousness and introspection. Therefore the subjects do not (or cannot) report such effects as the detection of the stimulus. However, if we want to study the difference between the presence and the absence of consciousness (of some stimuli), then we should only treat stimuli that are clearly above the subjective threshold as indicating the presence of phenomenal consciousness and the rest as indicating the absence of phenomenal consciousness. (In some special circumstances, however, phenomenal and reflective consciousness might be dissociated so that events in phenomenal consciousness escape reflection and reportability; see the discussion on change blindness and inattentional blindness in chapter 15.)

Zombies

In consciousness research, the concept of "zombie" is used to talk about the *opposite* of consciousness: creatures that by definition are totally nonconscious; creatures or systems in which the phenomenal level of organization is permanently absent. It might be useful to present some clarifications about the usage of this concept. The original meaning of "zombie" comes from voodoo culture and was popularized by the horror genre. It refers to a "living dead," a person who has been brought back from the dead by voodoo magic, but who no longer possesses a mind or will of his own. A zombie simply wanders around like a vacant body without a purpose, but it can follow simple orders and be used as a slave. Often zombies turn against their masters or other living humans and take revenge. A typical voodoo zombie is immediately recognizable; it does not look like or behave like a normal human being.

In philosophy, the concept of zombie refers to imaginary creatures that behave like completely normal human beings—zombies are in principle indistinguishable from a normal human being—but nevertheless, mentally, a zombie is a completely nonconscious creature; a mere object that does not have any kind of primary consciousness. By definition, the phenomenal level of organization is not realized in a zombie. In the original thought experiments against behaviorism and functionalism the point was to show that those theories could not distinguish between zombie systems and conscious creatures, which implies that the theories totally ignored phenomenal consciousness.

An imaginary nonconscious creature that interacts with its environment exactly like a normal human being can be called a *behavioral zombie.* It is stipulated to be behaviorally identical with a conscious human being, but its internal constitution need not necessarily resemble human biology (it could be some kind of mechanical robot, for example). For someone who exhaustively identifies psychological reality with externally observable behavior, there is no psychological difference between a behavioral zombie and a normal human being. Thus, behaviorists are forced to say that the postulated difference between the behavioral zombie and us humans is wholly illusory and unimportant—there is no "real" difference. (Just for the record, Daniel Dennett denies that there is any difference between us and behavioral zombies.)

An imaginary nonconscious creature that processes information in the same way as the human brain is a *functional* zombie. It is cognitively and computationally identical to a normal human being, but still just a robot or computer devoid of phenomenal consciousness. Its internal constitution need not resemble human biology; the information processing can be carried out in any other physical implementation just the same. For someone who identifies psychological reality with cognition, computation, and information processing, there is no difference psychologically between this creature and a normal human being. Thus, functionalists are forced to say that the postulated difference between the functional zombie and us is wholly illusory and unimportant; nothing mental can be missing from such a system.

A third type of philosophical zombie is a totally nonconscious creature that is also neurophysiologically indistinguishable from a normal human being (a molecule-for-molecule identical copy; see Chalmers, 1996). It can be called a *neurophysiological zombie.* A dualist would allow even the possibility of neurophysiological zombies, because he supposes that consciousness is something extra that has to be attached to the material brain before the creature can enjoy genuine subjective experiences. (David Chalmers argues that neurophysiological zombies are conceivable.)

For someone who regards psychological reality as a higher level of the biological reality inside the brain, there can be no psychological difference between normal human beings and neurophysiological zombies. Thus, biological realists are forced to deny this kind of zombie, because the microlevel material constitution of a biological system could not be copied without at the same time copying the macrolevels of organization. If consciousness is a macrolevel of brain organization, then neurophysiological zombies are impossible.

The idea of dependence between lower and higher levels is known in philosophy as the *supervenience relation.* Many philosophers accept the claim that consciousness supervenes on the brain (or that patterns of phenomenal experience supervene on patterns of neurophysiological activity). Anyone who accepts that would be inclined to deny the possibility of neurophysiological zombies, although accepting the possibility of behavioral and functional zombies (more on supervenience below).

The concept of zombie has spread from the philosophical community to neuropsychology. Empirical scientists apply the concept to neurocognitive mechanisms that perform complex transformations of sensory input to motor output outside consciousness, nonconsciously or implicitly. For example, Place (2000) proposed that there is a non-conscious automatic pilot system, "the Zombie within," that can respond automatically and appropriately to many stimuli for which there exists a preprogrammed response pattern. The September 1998 *New Scientist* featured research on implicit perception and action with a front cover headline "Zombies: They Are inside You." In that article, the implicit processing systems that can guide actions toward visual stimuli in the absence of consciousness of those stimuli were called "The (visuo-motor) Zombie." Thus, the concept of "zombie" has become the general idiom used to refer to nonconscious systems that handle complex input-output transformations or show complex external behavior.

Supervenience

Supervenience is a useful concept to characterize the relationship between higher- and lower-level features, such as the relationship obtaining between phenomenal consciousness and neurophysiological activities. Anyone who accepts, along with biological realism, that consciousness supervenes on the brain alone is bound to accept the possibility of behavioral and functional zombies, but to deny the possibility of neurophysiological zombies.

The central ideas of the supervenience relationship are *covariance* between higher- and lower-level features, and *dependence* of higher-level features on lower-level features. To say that phenomenal experience covaries with neurophysiological activity in the brain is to say that if one could create a perfect physical duplicate (Brain_2) of a fully functional living brain (Brain_1), then the Brain_2 and Brain_1 would also have to be mental copies of each other: if there is no physical difference between these two brains, then there cannot be any mental difference either. Conversely, if there is some mental difference (a different phenomenal experience) between two otherwise identical brains or between one and the same brain at two different times, then there must also be some physical difference between these two brains (or states of the same brain at the different times).

A difference at the level of consciousness thus necessarily implies a difference at the neurophysiological level. Incidentally, cognitive neuroscientists implicitly rely on this principle when they design experiments for discovering the neural correlates of consciousness. They try to create a well-defined difference between two states or two contents of consciousness in the same brain and then try to measure objectively what neural difference covaries with it.

To say that phenomenal experience *depends* on neurophysiological activity is to say that phenomenal experience can only come into existence in a system where there are neurophysiological entities and activities of the appropriate kind. Phenomenal consciousness cannot hang around all by itself. However, neurophysiological entities and activities are not dependent on phenomenal consciousness, but it is entirely possible to have some kind of neurophysiological activity going on even in a totally nonconscious system (say a person in deep coma). Neurophysiology per se does not depend on consciousness, but consciousness depends on neurophysiology.

The supervenience relationship is useful not only in the characterization of zombies but also in the context of another famous thought experiment in the philosophy of mind: *brains-in-a-vat* (BIV) (to be discussed in more detail in chapter 8). BIV invites us to imagine a fully functional, living brain that has been removed from the skull by skillful neurosurgeons and placed in a vat with all the essential nutritients, an artificial supply of oxygen and glucose, and the necessaries to satisfy the other physiological needs of the brain. The sensory input nerves are stimulated by a computer that carefully simulates real-life stimulation coming from sensory organs. Consequently the internal sensory state of the brain resembles that perceiving a multisensory environment. Now anyone who accepts the supervenience thesis that consciousness supervenes on the brain (and the brain alone) must accept that in this situation, more or less normal experiences are being produced inside the brain. The BIV necessarily enjoys primary, phenomenal consciousness if it is neurophysiologically in the same state as it would be when perceiving the external environment.

The BIV thought experiment carves off everything else but the constitutive neurophysiological basis on which phenomenal consciousness ontologically depends. The BIV possesses the minimal neural basis needed to support phenomenal consciousness. The experiment aims to isolate what is *minimally sufficient* for the existence of consciousness. By contrast, thought experiments involving zombies attempt to pinpoint those features in our mental and behavioral lives that, in the absence of the appropriate biological basis, are neither necessary nor sufficient by themselves to support consciousness: external behavior, complex organism-environment interaction, complex input-output transformations of information processing guiding flexible behavior, and so on. Thus, behavioral and functional zombies serve to show that consciousness does not supervene on purely behavioral or functional entities.

Summary

In science, meaningful research and discussion would be impossible without a clear conceptual basis shared by the researchers involved in the same domain of inquiry. In this chapter I have presented what I perceive to be the most fundamental concepts and distinctions that are necessary for the science of consciousness to get off the ground. The way in which I have framed them is not free of theoretical assumptions or philosophical commitments, and many will disagree with me about them. Nevertheless, a science of consciousness has to start from somewhere, and, as I see it, the biological research program aiming at the multilevel explanation of consciousness starts here.

Primary, phenomenal consciousness is the most fundamental concept for the science of consciousness. It refers to the immediate presence of qualitative experience (*qualia*) for a subject. Primary consciousness is organized as a unified sphere of subjective experiences, a sensory-perceptual world-for-me. A fundamental structural feature of this world is its *egocentricity,* also called the *first-person perspective.* The phenomenal contents of the world-for-me are spatially related to the center of the reference frame, where the self or the origin of the point of view of the world is located. Another fundamental structural feature is the dynamic *center-periphery organization* of the sphere of experience: at any given moment, some phenomenal contents form *the center of consciousness,* whereas the rest reside in the more vague *phenomenal background.*

Primary phenomenal consciousness should not be confused with *higher-order forms* of consciousness. The contents in the center of phenomenal consciousness are selected for further cognitive processing in *reflective consciousness.* The contents of the center of consciousness are within *the spotlight of attention.* Reflective consciousness takes the contents in the center of phenomenal consciousness as its object. Reflective consciousness is thus closely related to *selective attention* and *working memory. Self-awareness* and other types of "awareness-of-X" are special forms of reflective consciousness. *Introspection* is reflective consciousness coupled with the intention to report or communicate the contents of consciousness. Although introspection as a method has a bad reputation in psychology, introspective data are in fact commonly collected in psychological research, although the word "introspection" is rarely used anymore.

In different fields, several concepts of consciousness have been used that are to some extent in conflict with the current approach where phenomenality is taken as the most fundamental notion of consciousness. *Responsiveness* to external stimulation, the state of *wakefulness,* or the capability of *representing* or being *aware of* the surrounding world or *interacting with* it have been in some contexts defined as definitive criteria of "consciousness." However, all of these features may be dissociated from phenomenal consciousness. They bear no *necessary* relationship to the presence or absence of subjective experience. Thus, to avoid unnecessary confusion, they should not be regarded as the defining criteria for "consciousness" in theoretical contexts.

Phenomenal consciousness or the phenomenal level differentiates *conscious creatures* from *nonconscious creatures.* When considering the possibilities of *animal consciousness* or *machine consciousness,* the issue is whether the phenomenal level is present in an animal's brain or, respectively, whether it can be artificially reproduced in a machine. In conscious creatures, the temporary presence or absence of the phenomenal level constitutes the difference between the *conscious state* and *unconsciousness.* Conscious states can be divided into the *baseline state* of consciousness and various *altered states,* on the basis of the representational contents of consciousness. In altered states, consciousness temporarily misrepresents the world. However, the *representational contents of consciousness* should not be confused with the *phenomenal contents of consciousness.* Representational contents involve a reference to the world outside of consciousness, whereas the phenomenal contents of consciousness are just the internal patterns of subjective experience taken as such, without considering their external relations. *Dreaming* is the most important altered state of consciousness. Although in dream research the definition of dreaming remains unclear, one potentially fruitful way of defining dreaming considers it a spatiotemporally *organized form* of phenomenal consciousness during sleep: a *world simulation.*

In psychology, two concepts in particular have been used to characterize the absence of consciousness: *unconscious* and *nonconscious.* The distinction between them can be defined in terms of *accessibility* to consciousness: unconscious information in the brain can in principle modulate consciousness and thus exist in a phenomenal form, whereas nonconscious information in the brain cannot directly modulate phenomenal consciousness nor exist in a phenomenal form at all.

The concept of *zombie* has been used in philosophy and consciousness studies to describe something that constitutionally lacks consciousness. Many variations of zombies exist in the literature. In philosophy, they have been used as thought experiments to examine what is *not necessary* for consciousness. A creature can possess all of the non-necessary features (say intelligent behavior, or accurate representation of the world) but still remain a zombie. By contrast, the thought experiment involving a *brain-in-a-vat* has been used to examine what might be *minimally sufficient* for consciousness: an organism only needs the minimal basis to enjoy phenomenal consciousness. The relation between the minimal physical basis and consciousness has been described in terms of the *supervenience* relationship.

II The Dreaming Brain: A Model System for the Science and Philosophy of Consciousness

In part II, the theoretical and philosophical basis of biological realism will be put together. Productive research programs in biology often rely on fruitful model systems. In a good model system the nature of the explanandum can be exposed and efficiently investigated. We will examine the idea that the dreaming brain might be a particularly valuable model system for the science and philosophy of consciousness. First, we will establish, by exploring the results of empirical dream research, that phenomenal consciousness truly blooms in the dreaming brain. This observation gives us an adequate basis for treating the dreaming brain as a model system for consciousness (chapter 3). Then we examine the implications of this for the location of consciousness in the physical world (chapter 4). The data about the nature and location of phenomenal consciousness in the dreaming brain subsequently lead us toward a new metaphor of consciousness: the world simulation metaphor (chapters 5 and 6). That metaphor accurately conveys the essence of phenomenal consciousness. Furthermore, it suggests that the metaphysical core of phenomenality is to be found in the *inner presence* of consciousness. The philosophical nature of "presence" is consequently analyzed in detail, building the epistemological and metaphysical basis of the science of consciousness on the philosophy of presence (chapter 7). Finally, the most prominent alternative philosophical approaches to consciousness are reviewed: we try to understand how and why exactly they differ from biological realism and from the philosophy of presence (chapter 8).

3 The Dreaming Brain as a Model System

This chapter brings up the idea that *model systems* are useful tools in biological science. A model system is a particularly fruitful object of study, because it shows the phenomena under investigation in an exceptionally prominent form. A good model system allows focused and efficient experimental research to be performed on the most interesting phenomena. Furthermore, the model system may lead to theoretically significant observations and insights that would be difficult to reach otherwise. In consciousness research, visual awareness has become a popular model system. Another helpful model system is the dreaming brain, because it brings about phenomenal consciousness in a theoretically interesting form. The evidence from dream research is surveyed, showing that the dreaming brain indeed does bring about the entire sphere of subjective experience in a form closely mirroring waking reality. Thus the dreaming brain is a unique model system for the science of consciousness.

Model Systems in Biological Science

The first task for any new branch of science is to provide an initial identification of the phenomenon it is supposed to explain. For consciousness research, the task is to clarify what kind of system consciousness is and where it is located in the physical world. In this task, the history of biological science may be a valuable guide. It reveals the research strategies that have proved to be successful and thus should be utilized by consciousness research as well. There are several points in history where biologists had to face entirely novel phenomena. At first little was known about them and no theories to explain them were readily available. One strategy that seems to have worked well in biology when dealing with such unknown phenomena is the identification of a *model system.*

In a model system the explanandum manifests itself in a crystal clear form. In the ideal case the most interesting phenomenon can be sharply demarcated from other entities with which it might otherwise be confused. Furthermore, the model system usually allows easy observation and manipulation of the phenomenon, so that experimental research may proceed rapidly. The model system may not be prominent otherwise; consider the significance of the lowly fruit fly *Drosophila melanogaster* for the development of genetics. It hardly strikes anyone as a particularly significant organism—surely, for the layperson, all species of mammals and birds seem much more important forms of life—but still, the fruit fly proved to be crucial to theoretical and experimental progress in genetics.

In a new branch of biological science, if suitable model systems can be identified, then it is practical first to concentrate on the description and explanation of the model system. Exploring the novel phenomena in the limited but maximally clear cases provided by model systems may lead to rapid progress in the field. Model systems may quickly reveal the fundamental theoretical principles needed in the explanation of the phenomenon.

The idea of identifying a proper model system for consciousness research seems to be what Francis Crick (1994) was getting at when he wrote about the prospects for the scientific study of consciousness:

> Rather, one tries to select the most favourable system for the study of consciousness, as it appears at this time, and study it from as many aspects as possible. In a battle, you do not usually attack on all fronts. You probe for the weakest place and then concentrate your efforts there. (Crick, p. 19)

Crick and Koch (1990) proposed that *visual awareness* is the most favorable phenomenon for an initial experimental approach in consciousness research. They provided us with several weighty reasons for choosing visual awareness as the model system. We humans are very visual animals and our visual awareness is especially vivid and rich in information. There is no doubt that visual consciousness and visual qualities have an almost dominating role in human phenomenology. The visual system also has played a dominating role in research: of all our sensory-perceptual systems, vision is the one most intensively studied both in neuroscience and experimental psychology. Furthermore, the input to the visual system is highly structured and yet easy to control experimentally. Thus, visual awareness is open to relatively easy experimental manipulation in the laboratory—surely an important feature for a model system. Other higher primates have visual systems closely similar to that of humans, and therefore many experiments impossible for human subjects can be done in those animals.

In effect, visual awareness has turned out to be the fruit fly of consciousness research. Most of the groundbreaking experiments on the neural correlates of consciousness (NCC) have concentrated on various aspects of visual awareness: say blindsight, binocular rivalry, or change blindness. The intensive study of visual awareness has led to rapid progress in the neuroscience of consciousness. We know now much more about the relationship between visual awareness and various cortical areas than we did in 1990, when Crick and Koch first announced that the time is ripe for cognitive neuroscience to take subjective visual awareness into serious consideration. (I return to those findings in Chapters 18 and19 when discussing the NCC.)

I believe, however, that in addition to visual awareness, there is another immensely fruitful model system for consciousness research: the dreaming brain. It should be utilized, along with visual awareness, in the biological research program on consciousness. The dreaming brain brings out the phenomenal level of organization in a clear and distinct form. Dreaming is phenomenality pure and simple, untouched by external physical stimulation or behavioral activity. Furthermore, dreaming depicts consciousness first and foremost as a subjective world-*for-me.* Hence, the dreaming brain as a model system leads up to a particular conception of consciousness which I call the world-simulation metaphor of consciousness (chapter 6 is devoted to a closer examination of this metaphor).

The dreaming brain is a proper model system also because it is an excellent reminder of the *subjectivity* of conscious phenomena. A dream is a sequence of subjective experiences that takes place in a hallucinatory world. There is no way we could directly "see" or "observe" another person's dream world as it unfolds in the sleeping brain, and it is questionable whether this could ever be done even indirectly by using some fancy research instruments (but I shall have more to say about this in chapter 21). The dream world cannot be observed by using "objective" measurements, or described in "behavioral" terms, nor can its experiential content be characterized by purely neurophysiological concepts.

In spite of the fundamental subjectivity of dream experience, there is a large body of systematic empirical data on the phenomenal content of dreaming, thanks to the development of quantitative methods in dream content analysis (Domhoff, 1996; Foulkes, 1985; Strauch & Meier, 1996). This shows that the model system is viable for systematic empirical inquiry.

The Dreaming Brain

I suggest that the dreaming brain is a unique model system for the science of consciousness because it reveals consciousness in a very special, pure, and isolated form. This special form preserves the subjectivity and the first-person perspective of the explanandum, yet allows empirical investigations and leads to significant theoretical insights and implications.

To establish that the dreaming brain is a viable model system for consciousness science we should show that the following statements are accurate:

- The dreaming brain generates (or supports) phenomenal consciousness.
- Phenomenal consciousness generated by the dreaming brain includes the full range of phenomenal contents.

• Phenomenal consciousness generated by the dreaming brain has similar overall form as phenomenal consciousness during wakefulness.

I consider each of these points in the light of empirical evidence from dream research.

The Dreaming Brain Generates Phenomenal Consciousness

Personal Experience and Familiarity

There are two sources of evidence supporting the claim that phenomenal consciousness comes about during dreaming. The first is our own personal experience. Most people simply remember that they have enjoyed vivid subjective experiences during sleep, and require no further evidence that such things are possible.

In one study, 1000 people in Switzerland were asked the question "How often do you dream?" The results showed that 37% of the subjects remembered dreaming either every night or frequently. A further 33% reported dreaming every now and then and 24% answered that they dream only rarely. Only 6% of the study group responded "never" (Borbély, 1984, cited in Strauch & Meier, 1996). The results suggest that about 95% of people have personal experiences of dreaming, and for most people dreams are a familiar feature of their everyday lives.

When we appeal to personal experiences of dreams as evidence we are not appealing to some newly discovered, improbable fringe phenomenon that would only occasionally reveal itself in complex experimental settings, and whose significance or even existence could be seriously doubted. Unlike blindsight or phantom limbs, which very few people have ever experienced, dreaming hardly is an exotic abnormality or a rare pathological syndrome. On the contrary, dreaming is a perfectly normal biological process universally realized in the human brain in all cultures of the world and throughout the history of the human species. Dreaming is a phenomenon of consciousness familiar to just about everyone, revealing itself for most of us several times every night.

Laboratory Studies of Dream Recall

The second source of evidence comes from formal studies of dreaming in which people are systematically awakened from different stages of sleep. Dream recall strongly depends on the stage of sleep (see chapter 2). Vivid dreaming may be remembered in nine out of ten awakenings from REM sleep, but only one or two out of ten awakenings from NREM sleep lead to reports of vivid dreming. Most subjects who do not spontaneously remember any dreams are able to reach high rates of recall under laboratory conditions when awakened directly from REM sleep. However, a small proportion of infrequent dream recallers do not remember their dreams well even under laboratory conditions. In one study, seven out of ten poor dream recallers remembered their dreams significantly more often when awakened directly from REM sleep, but for three poor recallers the rate of recall remained low: for them, only 10 to 20% of awakenings from REM sleep produced dream reports (Strauch & Meier, 1996). It is unclear, however, whether the problem was their poor memory for dreams, or the infrequent appearance of dream experiences.

All in all, the evidence supports the view that most people experience dreams several times every night. Not all people, however, remember their dreams very well. A small proportion of people do not remember their dreams at all, or only very rarely. Futhermore, focal brain damage (especially bilateral damage of the parietal lobes) may wipe out dreaming altogether (Solms, 1997).

Skeptical Challenges to the Existence of Dreams

Despite these sources of evidence, the experiential reality of dreams has been flatly denied by some behavioristically oriented philosophers. They have argued that we should not accept introspective dream reports, composed during wakefulness, as valid evidence of subjective experiences that supposedly took place during sleep (see especially Norman Malcolm [1959] and Daniel Dennett [1976]; for critical analyses of their arguments, see Revonsuo [1995b] and Karlsson [2001])

Dennett (1976) considers the following possibility as an alternative explanation of dreams (or rather as an explanation of dream-reporting behavior): There may be a library of undreamed dreams somewhere in the brain. When the dreamer wakes up, one of the dream cassettes which has an ending consistent with the events at the time of waking up (say, hearing the alarm clock ring and merge with the dream events) is fetched and loaded into memory. Consequently, the contents of this dream cassette are recalled as a false memory of experiences supposedly happening during sleep. There were no conscious experiences going on during sleep as a matter of fact, just the unconscious insertion of a dream recollection into memory.

Dennett further develops his theory into the hypothesis that the unconscious dreams are recorded to the library during REM sleep, and upon waking, the unconscious dream just composed will be inserted into memory. This would explain the strong correlation between the duration of the REM stage before awakening and the length of subsequent dream reports. In a nutshell, Dennett's cassette theory of dreams suggests that dreams could be false memories, unconsciously composed during REM sleep, and unconsciously implanted to short-term memory just before awakening.

Although Dennett's theory is a *logically* possible explanation of dream-reporting behavior and recollections of dreams, it has turned out to be an *empirically invalid* idea. The force of Dennett's argument rests largely on the assumption that all the evidence that we will *ever* have about dreams consists of retrospective reports given during wakefulness, after the conjectured experience is already long gone. But since Dennett published his theory in the 1970s, new lines of evidence have turned up that support the view of dreams as subjective experiences during sleep. Skilled lucid dreamers are capable of becoming aware (in their reflective consciousness) of the fact that they are dreaming while they continue to dream. When lucid they are capable of controlling their movements at will within the dream. Although voluntary muscles are paralyzed during REM sleep and the movements they perform in the dream thus have little effect on the physical body, eye movement muscles work normally (otherwise the rapid eye movements characteristic of REM sleep would not be possible!). Voluntary eye movements are consequently employed to establish a channel of communication from the dream world to the world outside (LaBerge, Nagel, Dement, & Zarcone, 1981). The lucid dreamer can in principle report in real time to external observers in a sleep laboratory that he is just *now* enjoying dream experiences. The physiological recordings confirm that his body and brain remain in REM sleep when the communication occurs.

These messages from the dreamer in REM sleep constitute fairly strong evidence against Dennett's cassette view of dreams, although the really stubborn critic might reply that the evidence merely shows that *lucid* dreams are experiences, not that ordinary dreams are.

Fair enough, but there is another source of evidence against Dennett's theory that comes from ordinary dreams. In REM sleep behavior disorder (see chapter 23) the dreamer starts to show complex behaviors during REM sleep (Schenck, 1993; Schenck, Bundlie, Ettiger & Mahowald, 1986). He may show movements of the extremities or even whole-body locomotion: walking, jumping, running. When he wakes up, he is unaware of the behaviors he has just displayed, but he will report a dream in which he underwent exactly the same actions. Thus, the complex behavior that was objectively observed while the sleeper was still in REM sleep can only be explained by referring to the sequence of dream events and dream actions that the dreamer experienced during REM sleep without atonia. There is no reason to suppose that the removal of atonia as such should somehow cause dream experiences; thus, the most reasonable hypothesis is that dream experiences are brought about in the brain whether or not muscular atonia is present. Muscular atonia normally hides the behavioral consequences of dreamed behaviors, but removal of the atonia allows them to surface.

To briefly summarize: Careful consideration of the empirical data and the possible philosophical counterarguments lead me to conclude that the statement under examination is true—the dreaming brain indeed generates phenomenal consciousness. The burden of proof is on anyone who wants to deny this proposition. We are thus entitled to proceed to the closer examination of the phenomenal contents of consciousness during dreaming.

Phenomenal Consciousness Generated by the Dreaming Brain Includes the Full Range of Phenomenal Contents

If the phenomenal level is fully realized inside the brain during dreaming, then we should be able to enjoy the *full range* of subjective experiences during dreaming. As we shall see, this claim is well backed up by evidence from empirical dream research. The phenomenal level is put together from the same ingredients during dreaming as during wakefulness.

Perceptual Contents in Dreams

In one laboratory study of REM dreams (Strauch & Meier, 1996), dreamers were asked to describe in detail how they perceived their dreams, and what they had thought or felt. A total of 778 codes were assigned to the dreamers' descriptions. The results revealed that descriptions of perceptual content dominate dream experience (48.5% of the codes), thoughtlike contents (thinking, knowledge, memories) come next (42.7%), and emotional contents occupy a lesser role, about 10% of the information in the dream reports. When the perceptual contents are further subdivided into different sensory modalities, visual experience accounts for the lion's share, almost 60% of the codes assigned to the descriptions. Auditory impressions (nearly 25%) and bodily sensations (nearly 20%) are frequent, too, but smell and taste rarely occur, accounting for less than 1% of perceptual content in dreams (Strauch & Meier, 1996).

What makes the above study special is that the dreamers were closely questioned about their phenomenal experiences immediately after awakening, which yielded a great deal of additional information, not explicit in the original dream report. The researchers summarized the results in this way:

> Our dreamers had seen something in every dream and heard something in most dreams. Furthermore, they also recalled that they felt and thought something in many of the dreams. Impressions of smell and taste were, however, only rarely reported during such intensive inquiry. (Strauch & Meier, 1996, pp. 78–79)

In many earlier studies, the sensory content of dreams has been calculated in a different manner, as the percentage of dream reports that contain at least one instance of a particular sensory experience. When calculated in this manner, a review of seven studies showed that visual experiences occur in 100% of dreams, auditory in 69%, kinesthetic in 11.5%, touch in 10%, taste in 1%, and smell in less than 1% of dream reports (F. Snyder, 1970). In a recent, extremely detailed study of over three thousand dream reports, A. L. Zadra, Nielsen, and Donderi (1998a) found that 53% of dreams contained auditory, 1% olfactory (smell), and 0.9% gustatory (taste) experiences.

It is thus a well-established fact of dream research that experiences in all our sensory modalities appear during dreaming. Furthermore, different sensory modalities are involved approximately in proportion to their frequency in the waking state, as also during wakefulness smell and taste experiences occur much more rarely than visual or auditory ones.

Even if all our sensory modalities are engaged, this still leaves open whether all of our sensory *qualities* are present during dreaming. Two types of qualities are perhaps of most significance: visual qualities of color and bodily sensations of pain. They are the favorite paradigm cases of qualia in philosophical discussions as well, and their occurrence in dreams has been discussed in dream research, too.

Color Qualities in Dreams

Let us first consider the qualities of color vision. Do we dream in chromatic colors or in shades of gray and in black and white?

In a review of five studies, the percentage of dream reports including explicit color sensations varied from 50 to 83% (Rechtschaffen & Buchignani 1992). Thus we can safely say that most but not all dreams contain at least some qualities of color. Moreover, these figures are likely to be an underestimation of the occurrence of colors in dreams. Unless the subjects are explicitly inquired about the colors in their dreams, they might not mention them in the dream report. Consider the following report (from Strauch & Meier, 1996):

> I am on the road, in a car, and I get to a big intersection, in fact it is a traffic circle. And a car in front of me explodes, a truck, which blocks the road. Now I have to wait and I am on the side, over on the shoulder. And Roger comes along and does some controlling (24-year-old male). (p. 81)

In the original report, no colors are mentioned. Yet, when inquired, the subject reported that the truck was sheer white, the explosion created lightning yellow, and Roger wore a dark blue suit, a white shirt, and a tie that was diagonally striped in either red and black or red and blue.

In one extremely detailed and methodologically ingenious study, the visual qualities of dream experience were explored in detail. Rechtschaffen and Buchignani (1992) had their subjects match the visual sensory quality of their best remembered or most recent dream scene, immediately after waking up, with a selection of over 100 photographs with variations on different basic visual features (chromaticity, saturation, diffusion, illumination, etc.).

The single most selected category of photographs was one with entirely normal visual characteristics or only slight deviation from them. Thus a little over 40% of the dream scenes were visually normal and experienced just the same as external reality. The category of achromatic pictures came next; about 20% of the visual scenes in dreams were matched with black-and-white photographs.

There were notable interindividual differences, however, as to the chromaticity of dream experience. Thirty-three percent of the subjects chose only color photos whereas 29% chose only achromatic photos. The rest (37.5%) of the subjects reported both chromatic and achromatic dreams. We should remember, though, that achromatic vision is not unnatural, even in the waking state, because in low levels of illumination we still see shapes and recognize objects but we do not see chromatic colors.

Deviations from normal visual perception were quite rare. The most common type was a moderate "bleaching" effect, where the colors were moderately desaturated, illumination was high, and background detail was to some extent lost. This kind of dream scene constituted 11% of the reported scenes. In about 8% of dream scenes, the central objects were seen vividly and normally, but the background detail was almost completely lost. Soft haze characterized dream scenes in only about 6% of reports. When different types of deviations were combined, 22.4% of scenes suffered from loss of background detail. This might not be a sign of any serious deviation from normal waking perception, however, but simply a reflection of the center-periphery structure of visual consciousness, and the effect of selective attention. No dream images in this study were reported to be severely visually disorganized. The first REM period of the night was correlated with a loss of color saturation and figure and background clarity, as compared with later REM periods. The results were summarized as follows:

These departures from reality notwithstanding, it must be recognized that dreams only very rarely have the dark, murky, confused qualities that are frequently attributed to them in myths and movies. From what subjects have conveyed to us by their matches of photographs to dream images, the dream is most frequently a highly organized, coherent perceptual production that is usually not drastically different from the way we see the outside world while we are awake. (Rechtschaffen and Buchignani, 1992, p. 155)

Pain in Dreams

Some classic sources in dream research (e.g., see de Saint-Denys, [1867] 1982) suggest that the phenomenology of dreams is inconsistent with the experience of pain. However, recent research has overthrown this idea and shown that it is possible to feel pain in a dream even when absolutely nothing is physically wrong with the body part where an intense dream pain is clearly felt to be located. Nearly 50% of participants report that they remember experiencing pain in dreams at least once. During a period of 2 weeks of home-based dream reporting, 16 participants out of 185 (9%) reported dreams with experiences of pain. The pain sensations reported in dreams were realistic, were localized in a specific area of the body, and typically resulted from violent encounters with other dream characters (A. L. Zadra, Nielsen, & Donderi 1998a).

Cases of pain in dreams reported in the study by A. L. Zadra, Nielsen, Germain, Lavigne, & Donderi et al. (1998b) also show how remarkably realistic dream sensations can be. Here are a couple of examples from the home dream logs of their subjects:

I'm listening to a colleague and I begin to scratch my left forearm. It's itchy and it burns. I look at my left arm and I see that I have many "pimples." I try not to scratch my arm but it's really burning. I think that maybe it's not poison ivy but a really bad allergic reaction. When I woke up I turned on the light to look at my arm [pain dream reported by a 41-year-old women]. (p. 158)

. . . I try to close my hand but they just pry my hands open. Then they put a hot coal in the palm of my hand. It really burns and I yell "No, Stop! Stop!" To my surprise they stop and remove the coal. My hand still hurts and I can see that my skin is burned. The man holding the coals starts looking straight into my eyes and then I woke up. The pain was so intense that I was amazed when

I awoke that it existed only in the dream [excerpt from a pain dream reported by a 34-year-old man]. (p. 158)

In conclusion, dream research confirms that we can see, hear, touch, taste, smell, and feel in dreams. We even enjoy vivid color vision and suffer from unpleasant, sharply localized pain sensations. We also think, have emotional experiences, and feel our own body image in dreams. Not all of these experiences occur in every dream, but all of them may occur and do occur in our dreams at least once in a while. The evidence from dream research thus shows that there is nothing in the experience itself, in the actual qualitative character of the experience, that necessarily distinguishes the dream experience from a corresponding perceptual experience in the waking state.

The statement, "Phenomenal consciousness generated by the dreaming brain includes the full range of qualitative phenomenal content," receives considerable empirical support and can be regarded as accurate.

Phenomenal Consciousness Generated by the Dreaming Brain Has Similar Overall Form and Contents as Phenomenal Consciousness during Wakefulness

Granted that the sensory elements of dreams are the same as those of waking phenomenal experience, what is the overall *form* and *organization* of consciousness during dreaming? Is it in some sense equivalent to the organization of perceptual experience during wakefulness?

Dream Experience Presents a Sensory-Perceptual World

F. Snyder (1970), who conducted the first systematic laboratory study of the content of REM dreams, described the equivalence between dream experience and waking experience with the words that the dreaming consciousness is a *remarkably faithful replica* of waking life. On the basis of the data collected in his study, he commented that the progression of complex visual imagery was in almost every instance *a realistic facsimile* of the perception of external reality. Dream experiences are carefully organized: dreaming involves highly structured rather than random or chaotic experiences. Therefore, the global organization of the phenomenal level during dreaming can be characterized as a "world" or a "reality."

The Dream Self in the Center of the Dream World

In F. Snyder's (1970) study the dreamer was present and the central character in 95% of the 285 REM reports that were over 150 words long. In another laboratory study of REM dreams, the dream self was present in 90% of the dream reports, and active in over 70% of the reports (Strauch & Meier, 1996). Hence, the dream world seems to have at least one permanent inhabitant: the dreamer herself. In most dreams the dreamer appears in the center of the dream world and interacts with the surrounding dream environment. The overall form and content of phenomenal consciousness during dreaming appears to closely resemble the form and content of our everyday experiences. There is an entire *sphere* of phenomenal experience surrounding us. We ourselves are posited in the center of events and see the surrounding world from our first-person perspective.

The Dream World Is Taken as the Real World

The phenomenal level during dreaming is experienced as a reality, not as a dream or as a hallucination. Only rarely do we realize during the dream that it is only a dream. The estimated frequency of lucid dreams varies in different studies. Approximately 1 to 10% of dream reports include lucidity and about 60% of the population have experienced a lucid dream at least once in their lifetime (Farthing, 1992; T. V. Snyder & Gackenbach, 1988).Thus, as many as 90 to 99% of dreams are completely nonlucid, so that the dream world is taken for real by the dreamer.

The dream world hence constitutes the dreamer's actual "reality-now"—the only reality that exists at that very moment for the dreamer. Any past or future realities are at best distant echoes around the periphery of awareness. Access to autobiographical memory or future plans is diminished during dreaming. We are not able to conduct "mental time travel" in the same way as during wakefulness. We are not aware what happened before the dream commenced (that we went to sleep), nor are we aware what we are supposed to do in the morning after the dreaming is over. Awareness of the temporal continuity of our lives, a variety of self-awareness, is diminished in dreams.

From the point of view of the dreamer the waking world is as unreal as the dream world is from the point of view of a person awake. Dreams become labeled as dreams only in retrospect, and subsequently regarded as unreal.

Even in a lucid dream, where one realizes that it is all a dream while the dream still lasts, the dream world does not suddenly begin to look like an old Hollywood B movie with cardboard scenery, plastic monsters, or strings attached to flying saucers. On the contrary, lucid dreaming is, paradoxically perhaps, often accompanied by a *heightened* sense of reality. In a lucid dream, one readily becomes very attentive to the surroundings, which may make the dream world seem almost supernaturally clear and brilliant. Though the dreamer knows for a fact that it is only a dream, she may find it ever harder to believe that the spatially extended world all around her is actually somewhere in her own mind (or brain).

In conclusion, phenomenal consciousness generated by the dreaming brain has the same overall quality and form as phenomenal consciousness during wakefulness. The statistical properties of dreams, appearing over and over again in thousands of dream reports from different studies and laboratories, confirm the following general features of dreams (for reviews of the evidence, see Foulkes [1985], Domhoff [1996], Strauch & Meier [1996], Farthing [1992], Hobson [1988]). The dreamer typically experiences being personally present in the center of a spatially extended world surrounding her. The dreamer has perceptual experiences of objects, people, and other living creatures inhabiting the dream world all around. The dream is not a static image, but an animated world with temporally progressing events going on. All sensory modalities may be involved in dream experience, but vision is dominant (as it is during wakefulness). The dreamer usually posseses a body image much like the one experienced during waking; the dreamer is embodied in most dreams as a dream self. The dreamer seems to be able to control the actions of the body image and can sense her own movements through dreamed space.

Summary

The available evidence from the phenomenology of dream experience was summarized to show that the dreaming brain brings about a phenomenal *world-for-me* during sleep. For most people, this is a familiar experience. Laboratory research confirms that most people experience dreaming several times every night.

Philosophical skepticism about the reality of subjective experiences during sleep was demonstrated to be baseless, especially in the light of new evidence from lucid dreaming and REM sleep behavior disorder. In lucid dreams, the dreamer may communicate to outsiders the fact that he is dreaming while he is dreaming and while there is objective evidence that his brain remains in REM sleep. In REM sleep behavior disorder, the dreamer shows patterns of external behavior isomorphic with patterns of dreamed behavior. Both facts speak for the reality of phenomenal consciousness during sleep.

Systematic sampling of people's dream life has furthermore shown that the qualities of dream experience are identical with the qualities of waking experience. Dreams contain the full range of sensory qualities. Visual dream experiences are in color most of the time. Even realistic pain experiences come about during dreaming every now and then. The qualities of experience are carefully organized to form a dream world and a representation of the dreamer in the center of that world. The dreamer takes the dream world as a real world, hardly ever realizing that it is not the real world.

These facts establish that phenomenal consciousness in all its glory comes about in the sleeping brain. It is a normal, typical feature of the sleeping brain, especially in the REM stage. The form and content of phenomenal consciousness during dreaming closely resemble the form and content of phenomenal consciousness during wakefulness. Hence, the dreaming brain can be regarded as an incomparable model system for the science of consciousness.

4 The Dreaming Brain and the Location of Consciousness

The question about the location of consciousness is central to any research program on consciousness. The question is also highly controversial in philosophy, where several lines of thought resist the conclusion that consciousness is located in the brain. The evidence from the dreaming brain nonetheless establishes that the phenomenal level resides somewhere inside the brain, and that consciousness is ontologically independent of sensorimotor mechanisms.

The Localization Problem

The dreaming brain isolates the phenomenal level from many other systems with which it normally is in interaction. Therefore this model system of consciousness research might provide us with an answer to the *localization problem:* Where is the phenomenal realm to be found in the physical world? A scientific research program on consciousness must have a clear and empirically plausible answer to the location question. After all, the research efforts have to be targeted *somewhere.*

Biological realism is committed to the thesis that consciousness is located within the confines of the brain. We should not accept any such thesis purely on faith, though. Many philosophical approaches to consciousness in fact deny this thesis (see chapter 8). In this chapter we inspect some compelling empirical evidence that serves to defend the idea that consciousness literally resides in the brain. Most of this evidence comes from the two model systems of the research program: the dreaming brain and visual awareness.

The question about the location of a natural phenomenon can be formulated in terms of finding or isolating *the locus of control* for that phenomenon (Bechtel & Richardson, 1993). The locus of control for a given phenomenon is simply the system that exercises significant autonomy or internal control over its occurrence. For example, the locus of control in the living cell for storing information about the constitution of proteins is encoded in DNA genes: the proteins themselves do not possess the information needed for their own synthesis in the cell. The information encoded in DNA dictates (by way of RNA transcriptions) the assembly of practically all known proteins (DeDuve, 1991). Although DNA cannot bring about proteins in isolation all by itself without the surrounding biological machinery being involved, the machinery of the cell will bring about just those proteins dictated by the information encoded in DNA (regardless of how the DNA ended up in the nucleus; even artificially inserted DNA will handle the job). DNA is the locus of control for the information expressed in the cell's protein synthesis. The cell nucleus (DNA and messenger RNA interaction) is the locus of control for the transcription of the information.

To isolate the locus of control for a phenomenon does not mean that the phenomenon would be normally isolated from everything else. On the contrary, most biological mechanisms are open systems in constant causal interaction with other systems surrounding them. The locus of control for a phenomenon merely points to those systems on which the phenomenon is ontologically dependent, without which it could not exist. For example, protein synthesis could not exist without DNA, RNA, and their complex interaction inside individual cells.

The phenomenon itself, as well as its microlevel mechanisms, is presumed to rest somewhere inside the locus of control. The choice of a particular locus determines the course of subsequent research, because most of the further research efforts will then be targeted to the chosen locus of control. If a particular locus of control is, however, rejected, then an alternative and more appropriate source of control should be identified. Without any clear locus of control identified for a phenomenon, research concerning the phenomenon would not be targeted anywhere in particular. In that case the whole research progam would be adrift like a ship that has lost its rudder.

The Dreaming Brain: Constraints on the Locus of Control

Whenever the sphere of phenomenal experience comes about, then the physical basis of consciousness must be responsible for this. There is overwhelming evidence that the whole range of subjective conscious experiences—the entire phenomenal level of organization—does come into existence during dreaming (see chapter 3). From this simple, well-attested fact it follows that the same physical or neural realizing basis of consciousness must be responsible for the sphere of subjective experiences both during wakefulness as well as during dreaming. The mechanisms of consciousness must be active in both states and furthermore organized in a closely similar way—otherwise dream experience would not amount to a faithful simulation of the perceptual world.

Knowledge of the physiological activity in the brain during dreaming could be utilized to constrain hypotheses about the locus of control for consciousness. Many of the sensory and motor systems that normally during wakefulness are in causal interaction with the phenomenal level, are no longer so in REM sleep. As the phenomenal level is fully realized all the same, the sensorimotor systems disengaged from phenomenal consciousness during dreaming can be excluded from the locus of control of the phenomenal level. Phenomenal consciousness cannot be ontologically dependent on any bodily or physiological state that is missing during dreaming. No state missing during dreaming can be absolutely necessary for the existence of the phenomenal level. Therefore, physiological states or activities missing during dreaming cannot be constitutive of phenomenal consciousness. We can consequently rule them out from the locus of control of phenomenal consciousness.

During REM sleep in the brain there is a *sensory input blockade* (preventing stimuli from reaching consciousness), a *motor output blockade* (preventing motor commands from reaching the muscles), and a *highly active brain in between* them. As a result of all this, the phenomenal level of subjective experience is brought about inside the brain. Yet, for an external observer the dreaming person's body appears to be paralyzed and unresponsive, revealing no behavioral signs of the vivid phenomenal world wherein the dreaming subject is immersed in all sorts of colorful adventures.

Even so, physical stimuli are received and processed by our sensory systems, but only at levels not involving consciousness. To find out more about the location of consciousness in the sleeping person, we should figure out which physiological processes are totally dissociated from dream experience.

Sensory Organs Never Sleep

When the brain is asleep and REM dreaming, the sensory arousal thresholds are high—an external stimulus has to be quite strong (or highly meaningful) in order to modulate the contents of the phenomenal level, or to awaken the dreamer. Sensory transmission in the periphery is, however, largely preserved (Wu, 1993). In the auditory modality, the cochlear evoked potentials show that vibrations of air continue to be transformed into neural impulses in the inner ear. Evoked responses in the auditory relay nuclei in the thalamus are either unchanged or only slightly reduced during sleep. Cortical auditory evoked potentials are amplified in slow-wave sleep and reduced in REM sleep, but auditory stimuli are not experienced in either condition. In the visual modality, responses to stimulation are not altered at the peripheral stage; the retina responds to the visual stimulus field all the same, no matter whether the subject is awake or asleep—*the retina never sleeps!* Higher levels of visual stimulus processing (thalamic and cortical) are, however, reduced. Peripheral transmission of somatic information is unchanged during sleep, but thalamic and cortical responses to somatic stimulation are reduced.

Our sensory receptors themselves are thus quite oblivious to the stage of sleep, as is the ensuing neural activity up to the thalamocortical level. In this way the brain assures prompt processing of important or threatening information, but at the same time preserves sleep continuity if the stimuli prove to be insignificant (for a review, see Wu, 1993). Hobson (1988) calls this barrier between the external stimulus inputs and consciousness *the sensory input blockade.* The blockade results from both *active inhibition* of messages arriving from the outside world and *occlusion* or *competition* between externally originated and internally generated stimulation.

What Would We Dream about if We Slept with Our Eyes Open?

An ancient conception of seeing postulates a vision beam that projects from the eye outward to external objects. During dreaming the beam cannot get out because our eyes are closed, so it has to bounce back from the closed eyelids and thus are dream images created. Plato believed that dreams are created in this way. This theory is empirically testable: the hypothesis predicts that if one could somehow sleep with the eyelids open, the vision beam could scan the external world and, consequently, dreams should contain images of the actual physical surroundings. In fact, modern dream research has conducted some fascinating experiments that reveal what happens when a person sleeps with the eyes fully open.

Well, what happens? Did the persons falling asleep with their eyes open report dreams of the objects and persons surrounding their bed? Why not? After all, the retina could not have been asleep. Nonetheless, that does not seem to be the case. Instead, when we fall asleep, we become functionally blind, no matter whether our eyes are open or closed. That is, the phenomenal level suddenly loses its contact with external sensory events. We do not notice the sudden onset of blindness, for normally we lie in darkness with our eyes closed so there is not much to see anyway. But the dramatic emergence of blindness can be shown experimentally. It is possible to tape a subject's eyes open and let him fall asleep.

Dement (1972) described one such experiment, in which a very bright light is flashed 6 inches in front of the subject's eyes every few seconds. The subject's eyes are taped open, and so there is no way his eyes could avoid receiving the strong input. The subject is instructed to respond every time he sees the light flash by pressing a switch taped to his finger. The subject presses and presses, but sooner or later he suddenly stops. The light keeps on exploding right into his widely open eyes, but he has become totally blind and unaware of it: he has fallen asleep. And yet we know that the sensory receptors, the retina, the visual pathway, at least up to the thalamus, obediently continues transmitting the neural impulses and signaling the presence of a bright flash right before the eyes—it is just that the level at which subjective visual awareness is generated in the brain has shut itself off from all that.

Another dramatic illustration of functional blindness during sleep was reported by Rechtschaffen and Foulkes (1965). They taped the eyes of their subjects wide-open and made arrangements to keep the cornea moist and the pupils chemically dilated. While the subjects slept and entered REM sleep, various brightly illuminated objects were placed right in front of their eyes: a white card with a large black *X* printed on it, a red-covered book, a white handkerchief (which was waved in front of the subject's eyes), and an aluminum coffee pot.

The results showed, however, that the sleepers could neither see those objects nor dream about them: not a single clear instance of stimulus incorporation into the dreams could be detected. In other words, the external sensory input that the visual system received during REM sleep did not modulate the phenomenal level of organization in any detectable way. The subjects were, apparently, staring at the objects all the time, but they had become as blind as bats. One subject was shown the coffee pot, and at that time there was so much light coming from the window that, if awake, he would have had no difficulty in seeing the entire room. When the REM period started, his eyes opened very wide and the rapid eye movements made it appear that he was looking all about the room and was awake but motionless. The coffee pot was presented to him and after awakening he remembered a dream where he was bowling with two friends. None of the objects or colors he reported having experienced in the dream bore any resemblance to the objects and colors that were before his wide-open, actively scanning eyes during the REM episode.

These experiments demonstrate unequivocally that patterns of retinal excitation are not by themselves sufficient for the phenomenal level to be realized. Our sensory apparatus and input mechanisms below the thalamic level can be as active during sleep as during wakefulness, but no consciousness whatsoever results from this activity. Those levels of organization do not constitute the locus of control for producing the phenomenal level. The external sensory environment may exert its influence on the sensory organs and peripheral sensory systems quite normally, but those events have nothing directly or necessarily to do with the phenomenal level of organization. Therefore, the physiological events in the peripheral sensory organs and pathways must be excluded once and for all from the list of potential candidates for the locus of control of the phenomenal level. They are not by themselves capable of realizing or supporting the phenomenal level, or any phenomenal features whatsoever, nor is their contribution necessary for the phenomenal level to come about inside the brain.

Where the Blind Can See Again

Furthermore, activation at those levels is not even a necessary condition for bringing about the phenomenal level. People who have become adventitiously blind after the age of 7 years can continue to have clear and vivid visual experiences in their dreams all their lives, although their visual sensory apparatus may be completely destroyed and they may not have had a single episode of visual perception for years or even decades. Adventitiously blind people can have visual dreams about both familiar and new contents (Kerr, 1993); they can actually *see* (in the sense of *visually experience*) new places and faces of people they have never seen in their lives, although they cannot see anything at all while awake. During dreaming they enjoy the subjective experience of sight; still, they lack all visual perception. The content of their visual awareness can never be modulated by sensory input from the eyes anymore. They may be totally blind when it comes to visual perception, but, amazing as it is, that sort of blindness by no means entails the total absence of visual phenomenology. On the contrary, in dreams the adventitiously blind person can see again: she may enjoy highly organized visual sensations and she experiences being fully immersed in a visual environment.

Visual dream phenomenology has great emotional and personal significance for blind people (Rainville, 1994): the dream world is the only place in the universe where sight can still be restored to them; where it is still possible to genuinely see—to have the visual experience of—the face of a loved one, beautiful scenery, or the color of the sky. When the blind person awakes from a dream, he is cruelly returned to the world of absolute blindness from the momentary, almost miraculous relief offered by the dream world.

Dreams are not only isolated from the sensory input information coming from the outside world, they are isolated overall from the organismic condition of the physical body of the dreamer as well (Rechtschaffen, 1978). Dream content correlates poorly with the physiological states of the body or its autonomic regulatory systems. For example, subjects who were deprived of water for 24 hours had few if any dreams related to thirst. Erections occur in the absence of sexual content in dreams and vice versa. Quadriplegic patients without any sensations arising from their genital areas were capable of having dreams with orgasms (or "phantom orgasms" as they were called in the original study of Money [1960], cited in Rechtschaffen [1978]).

When the Physical Body Is Fully Paralyzed

Dreaming occurs behind a sensory barricade, isolated from both the external world and the physical body. The story concerning motor output is no less dramatic. During REM sleep, the final common-path motor neurons of the spinal cord are actively inhibited by postsynaptic inhibition arising in the brain stem (Hobson, 1988). This means that all the motor commands originating in the motor cortex are stopped long before they ever reach the muscles. During REM sleep there is a complete lack of muscle tone, or complete atonia, of all voluntary muscles (apart from those concerned with eye movements and breathing)—even those muscles that maintain posture in waking. People suffering from *narcolepsy,* a sleep disorder with sudden REM attacks, may experience cataplexia or sudden loss of muscle tone, and abruptly fall down like a wet rug.

Subjectively, however, we do not have the slightest idea that our physical body is in a state of complete paralysis while we dream: our dreams are full of vivid bodily movement. Sometimes it is possible, though, to experience a curious state called *sleep paralysis* in which the person is at least partially awake, but the muscle atonia of REM sleep is still present, and the content of consciousness at the phenomenal level is modulated by this condition. It is usually a rather frightening experience, for one finds oneself unable to move even a finger, unable to speak or call for help, and unable to open one's eyes. This experience of absolute paralysis may be accompanied by intense fear or by dream imagery of an approaching threat of some kind, and by a struggle to escape the paralysis or to wake up. To outside observers, the subject appears to be sleeping quietly with eyes closed (see also chapter 10).

Where the Crippled Can Walk Again

During REM sleep, muscular atonia is brought about by the inhibition of spinal motor neurons. Voluntary muscles are thus virtually paralyzed during REM sleep. Yet, at the same time motor commands are being actively produced in the brain. Converging evidence for the existence of motor commands during REM sleep come from a number of sources. First, observations of humans and animals in REM sleep confirm that small muscle twitches, sometimes even small movements of the extremities, occur during REM sleep. Second, if the inhibitory mechanisms in the reticular formation in the pons are experimentally lesioned in the cat, the animal will show complex behaviors, movements, and locomotion while in REM sleep (Morrison, 1983). Third, if the same mechanism is damaged in humans, a syndrome called REM sleep behavior disorder (RBD) follows (Schenck, 1993). Patients suffering from it act out the movements that they are dreaming about. Fourth, microelectrode studies in animals have shown that motor cortex and subcortical motor areas are activated during REM sleep. In functional brain imaging of humans during REM sleep, activation of motor and supplementary motor areas has been observed (Schwartz & Maquet, 2002).

Even a physically injured or severely disabled physical body does not necessarily enter the dream world. The famous philosopher of science, Paul Feyerabend, was wounded during World War II and remained crippled, but related that all his life he had recurrent dreams of restored ability to walk:

> The situation is always the same. I get the draft notice. "Ah," I say, "I don't have to go, I'm a cripple" (which I am—I have been on crutches since 1946). I enter the barracks, get into line, and then—lo and behold!— I can walk. "What a lousy joke," I think. "There I was, dragging myself around for years, but now that I don't need it my legs suddenly work." (Feyerabend, 1995, p. 52)

Even quadriplegic patients (e.g., Christopher Reeve, the actor best known for playing Superman, who became paralyzed after a riding accident damaged his spinal cord) sometimes report that in their dreams they have a fully functional body. Despite the severe, irreversible paralysis that prevents almost all voluntary movements of the physical body, miraculously, in the dream world, the patient can still sense his limbs and control their movements perfectly. In his dreams the quadriplegic patient may be able to move freely and powerfully.

The Phenomenal Reality in the Brain

As the above discussion shows, dreaming is a very peculiar state indeed. On the one hand, normal healthy people suddenly become functionally blind and completely paralyzed. On the other hand, subjectively, dreaming is a state in which even the blind may have their sight restored, and the crippled and truly paralyzed may experience their fully functional bodies walking and running once more, and may sense the parts of their body they cannot sense when awake. No wonder people have believed that while dreaming, the soul enters another reality altogether.

The facts that we have now collected about dreaming lead us to the following conclusions:

1. The external stimulus environment or the peripheral parts of the sensory input systems are not the locus of control for consciousness; they are no part of the necessary realizing ground of the phenomenal level of organization.
2. The *external stimulus fields* (the *distal* visual field of physical objects reflecting electromagnetic radiation at the visible wavelengths and the *proximal* stimulus field falling on the retinas) have to be clearly separated from the *subjective visual field* (J. Smythies, 1996). The external stimulus fields can modulate the contents of the phenomenal visual field when we are awake, but the latter is ontologically separate from and independent of the former.
3. The lived body, or the *phenomenal body image,* is not identical with the organism's physical body of flesh and bones. The body we have in our dreams, the body in which phenomenal embodiment is experienced, could not be literally identical with the physical body with muscles and bones and all the rest, for during dreaming that body is in a completely different state from the body image that we vividly experience. If the content of bodily awareness were identical with the state of the physical body, we should, during REM sleep, be constantly aware of our real surroundings (because the peripheral sensory systems work just like they do when we are awake) and we should experience a complete bodily paralysis during REM sleep (because all of our voluntary muscles are truly paralyzed). As we all know, nothing could be further from the truth: the contents of both perceptual and bodily awareness are, during REM dreaming, totally dissociated from the corresponding states of the physical body. This full-scale dissociation is what Allan Rechtschaffen (1978) calls the "isolation" of dreams. Furthermore, if the phenomenal body were identical with the physical body, the crippled would never possess an intact body in their dreams; nor would phantom limbs be possible in patients whose real flesh-and-bones limb has been amputated.

The phenomenal body image is a construction at the phenomenal level of organization in the brain, whereas the physical body of flesh and bones surrounds the brain and is in tight causal contact with it. When awake, the state of the physical body of course modulates the state of the lived body at the level of phenomenal organization, just as the external visual stimulus fields modulate the states of the subjective visual field at the phenomenal level, but in no way are the two ever identical. When awake, the states of the physical body figure as causes of the states of the phenomenal body image, but when dreaming, that causal relation is broken.

The thoroughgoing distinction between the physical body and the phenomenal body image (or virtual body) is one of the most difficult facts to take in. In our everyday thinking we seem to be in such a close and intimate contact with our own physical body that absolutely nothing would seem to be able to separate us from it. Yet, this amazing fact has been clearly appreciated 75 years ago by the Gestalt psychologist Wolfgang Köhler ([1929] 1947). Let me quote some insightful passages from his writings on the matter:

> The only consideration required for the solution of our curious problem now consists in the fact that "my body," before which and outside of which the phenomenal objects are perceived, is itself such a phenomenal object along with others, in the same phenomenal space, and that under no circumstances may it be identified with the organism as the physical object which is investigated by the natural sciences, anatomy and physiology. (p. 130)

> If Schopenhauer and many natural scientists after him were astonished by the "external localization" of phenomenal objects, the reason was only that they failed to apply to their own body an assumption which had become natural to them in considering other objects. For the body they retained the naive identification or confusion of physical and phenomenal object. But if we say some object is in front of "us," then what we mean by "us" is not the organism in the physical, physiological sense. (p. 131)

More recently, John Smythies has repeatedly emphasized that this distinction is absolutely critical for formulating the mind-body problem in a clear way: "The fact is that we never experience any event in the physical body outside the brain at all. The body-image is a construct of the parietal lobe in the brain. It is in no way identical with the physical body that it represents. Most philosophers continue to confuse the body-image and the physical body" (J. Smythies, 1994a, p. 315). "No-one can even begin to understand the nature of the brain-consciousness problem without thoroughly grasping this point—extremely counter-intuitive and contrary to 'common sense' (folk psychology) though it is" (J. Smythies, 1994b, p. 87). [1]

The evidence from dreaming now establishes, perhaps more clearly and compellingly than any other piece of evidence, that the phenomenal body and the physical body must be categorically distinguished from each other.

Frederick van Eeden ([1913] 1990) was an early dream researcher who experimented with lucid dreaming. When he was dreaming lucidly, he was totally aware of his condition and decided to perform various experiments, just out of curiosity, to see what would happen. Some of his experiments are perfect demonstrations of the differentiation of the phenomenal body image from the physical body:

> In the night of January 19–20 [1898], I dreamt that I was lying in the garden before the windows of my study and saw the eyes of my dog through the glass. I was lying on my chest and observing the dog very keenly. At the same time, however, I knew with perfect certainty that I was dreaming and lying on my back in my bed. And then I resolved to wake up slowly and carefully and observe how my sensation of lying on my chest would change into the sensation of lying on my back. And so I did, slowly and deliberately, and the transition—which I have since undergone many times—is most wonderful. It is like the feeling of slipping from one body into another, and there is distinctly a double recollection of the two bodies. . . . This observation of a double memory I have had many times since. It is so indubitable that it leads almost unavoidably to the conception of a dream-body. . . . In a lucid dream the sensation of having a body—having eyes, hands, a mouth that speaks, and so on—is perfectly distinct; yet I know at the same time that the physical body is sleeping and has quite a different position. In waking up the two sensations blend together, so to speak. (pp. 181–182)

Van Eeden's experiment shows how the information sources that modulate the phenomenal body switched from internal ("dream-body") to external ("physical body"), and for a fleeting moment he could experience both at the same time, the former gradually transforming into the latter.

The Neural Basis of the Phenomenal Level in the Dreaming Brain

The phenomenal level is realized both during REM sleep and in the awake state. In REM sleep it is easy to observe its isolation from the various stimulus fields which modulate it when awake. What can be learned about the lower-level constitutive mechanisms or the neural realizing ground of consciousness by looking at REM sleep physiology? If what goes on in the body and the peripheral nervous system is completely isolated from consciousness, what kind of activity in the brain then generates the contents of consciousness that closely simulate waking reality?

There are two factors involved: first, *the general activation in the brain* must reach a certain level to be in a conscious state (as opposed to an unconscious state). Second, there must be *specific internal activation patterns* that generate specific sensations and images as the content of dream consciousness. The dreaming brain fulfills both of these requirements.

The level of general activation in the forebrain is controlled by ascending arousal systems in the brain stem reticular activating system. One way of measuring the activation level is to look at the firing levels of reticular activating neurons in the midbrain. Such experiments, however, require invasive microelectrodes and can only be conducted in animals. The rate of firing has been found to be as high in REM sleep as it is during wakefulness; in this respect there is no difference between these two states (Hobson,

1988). In humans, EEG activity as measured by scalp electrodes reflects the activity of the intrinsic arousal systems. During REM sleep, the scalp-recorded EEG becomes desynchronized: it shows a mixture of high frequencies (fast waves) with a low amplitude. This is unlike slow-wave sleep, but very much like wakefulness. In fact, to reliably differentiate REM sleep from wakefulness, one must look at phenomena other than the spontaneous electrical activity of the brain alone, namely eye movements and muscle tension. Brain activation levels can also be measured by looking at brain glucose metabolism, for active neurons use glucose as their fuel. In slow-wave sleep, glucose metabolism decreases in the brain, but during REM sleep the brain uses up at least as much energy as it does during wakefulness (Heiss, Pawlik, Herholtz, Wagner, & Wienhard, 1985; Jouvet, 1993).

Hobson (1992) points out that if the brain's activation level alone were involved in generating our overall mental state, then waking and REM sleep would be identical. Llinás and Paré (1991) emphasize that the overall functional states present during REM sleep and wakefulness are fundamentally equivalent and that they can be seen as almost identical intrinsic functional states in which subjective awareness is generated.

The wakefulness-like electrical activation of the cortex is accompanied by bursts of PGO waves (ponto-geniculo-occipital waves). They may be the causal key element in bringing about specific phenomenal contents during dreaming. PGO waves are bursts of neural activity originating in the pons, shortly afterward detectable in the lateral geniculate nucleus (LGN) of the thalamus, whence they travel to the occipital cortex. In fact, despite their name, which reflects the locations in which they were first detected, PGO waves are not restricted to the anatomical areas their name suggests. By contrast, they have been recorded in many other brain regions as well, including all types of thalamic relay nuclei and cortical areas outside the occipital cortex (G. A. Marks, 1993).

When it comes to the experience of dreaming, one of the most significant features of the PGO waves is that when they pass from the thalamus to the cortex, they *use exactly the same pathways that are used by our external senses* in waking perception when sensory input passes from the sense organs through the thalamus to the cortex. The main pathway from the retina to the primary visual cortex goes through the LGN in the thalamus. During REM sleep, we are functionally blind to external stimulation, but PGO waves keep bombarding V1 and other cortical areas. Also, the limbic lobe and amygdala are activated by PGO waves; their activation probably mediates dream emotion (Hobson, 1999). The realizing ground of the phenomenal level is modulated by this internal stimulation, but the phenomenal level itself has no way of knowing where the causal chain originated: in the external sensory fields or in the internal dream stimulation mechanism. The dream stimulation bears no labels that reveal its original source.

Further evidence supporting the view that the neural basis of consciousness is realized during REM sleep comes from studies of synchronous gamma-band oscillations, which have been shown to correlate with consciousness in humans and animals (Sauve, 1999). High-frequency gamma activity is prominent both in active waking episodes and in REM sleep in rats (Maloney, Cape, Gotman, & Jones, 1997) and PGO potentials during REM sleep are consistently followed by synchronized cortical oscillations within the gamma frequency range of 30 to 40 Hz (Amzica & Steriade, 1996). In human subjects, synchronized gamma rhythyms have been recorded over the neocortex during waking and REM sleep by using magnetoencephalography (Llinás & Ribary, 1993). The subjective perception of visual objects also seems to elicit cortical gamma synchronization. Gamma-band responses have been found to be closely correlated with visual awareness and binding of coherent visual stimuli (Crick & Koch, 1990; Tallon-Baudry & Bertrand, 1999; Engel, Fries, König, Brecht, & Singer, 1999; Revonsuo, Wilenius-Emet, Kuusela, & Lehto, 1997).

Taken together, this evidence reveals that gamma-band synchronous oscillations are associated with the realization of the phenomenal level in the awake state; therefore, similar neural activity detected during REM sleep is probably related to the realization of the phenomenal level that constitutes dreaming. Functional brain imaging with positron emission tomography (PET) further supports the idea of large-scale activation in the brain during REM sleep (Maquet et al., 1996; Braun et al., 1998); in particular, the occipitotemporal visual cortex and the amygdala are strongly activated, which is well in harmony with the abundant visual and emotional experiences during dreaming.

The evidence is now all in for the view that during REM sleep the neural basis of the phenomenal level is effectively isolated from external reality and from the physical body but at the same time internally activated in a way that closely simulates the activation originating in the external sensory fields during wakefulness. Consequently, the phenomenal level of organization is brought about in a way almost identical to that of wakefulness.

This is not to say that there are *no* differences between these two states as to the content of experience, neurochemical balance, or forebrain activation. There surely are quite radical differences in all these respects (for reviews, see Hobson et al. [2000] and Schwartz & Maquet [2002]). Recent PET studies have revealed that fairly large parts of the prefrontal cortex are less active in REM sleep than in the waking state. This deactivation is probably connected to the fact that in dreams it is difficult (though not impossible) to make deliberate plans, or to take a critical and reflective stance toward even highly bizarre dream events, or to deliberately make decisions and control the dream events. Such cognitive functions are subserved by the prefrontal areas deactivated during REM sleep. Their relative deactivation probably contributes to our utter gullibility during dreaming: we take the dream world with all its peculiarities for real, because our skeptical and critical attitude, as well as our powers of ratiocination, are greatly (but not totally) suppressed.

This state of affairs serves to make the world simulation in dreams seem even more realistic, for we tend to take the dream reality altogether seriously, no matter how unlikely the events are that we there encounter.

Summary

The significance of the dreaming brain for the theoretical description and explanation of consciousness lies in the fact that dreaming effectively *isolates* the explanandum from the surrounding nonconscious biological mechanisms. When considering the dreaming brain we acquire a crystal clear distinction between the phenomenal level itself and what lies just beyond its borderlines: the preceding causes and the underlying microlevel mechanisms of consciousness, tightly surrounding the phenomenal level, but fundamentally distinct from it nonetheless.

The isolation of consciousness consists of the following elements: Sensory input is received normally by peripheral sensory organs during sleep, but blocked from consciousness at higher thalamocortical processing levels. Sensory input thus does not modulate phenomenal consciousness in any way. This is the *sensory input blockade.* Bodily action is experienced in dreams and related motor output is being produced by cortical motor areas during REM sleep. The motor output is blocked from reaching the muscles. This is the *motor output blockade.*

The isolation of consciousness in the dreaming brain establishes that sensory input and motor output (and the mechanisms involved in dealing with them) are *not necessary* for producing phenomenal consciousness. The dreaming brain furthermore provides us with insights into the internal biological mechanisms that are entirely *sufficient* by themselves for supporting the phenomenal level. During REM sleep, the level of *general activation* in the brain is similar to that during wakefulness. Furthermore, specific internal activation patterns are being produced that mimic the neurophysiological events during perception (PGO waves and gamma-band activity in the EEG). Recent brain-imaging results show that emotional, visual, and motor areas in the brain are particularly activated during REM sleep. The internal activation appears to be sufficient for producing the full range of phenomenal experience. People who have lost peripheral sensorimotor capacities still experience the phenomenal contents that were once connected with those capacities. Blind people still have visual experiences in their dreams. Crippled or paralyzed people continue to have experiences of bodily movement in their dreams.

The evidence gathered concerning the location of consciousness in the physical world now seems definite: *the entire sphere of phenomenal consciousness resides within the confines of the brain.* It is ontologically dependent neither on the sensory input mechanisms leading to the brain, nor on the motor output mechanisms reaching out from the brain.

Our sensory-perceptual and bodily presence in the world is brought about by wholly internal neural mechanisms that work in a similar manner during wakefulness and dreaming. The experience of a seemingly external perceptual world and the experience of being personally embodied and situated in the center of the world are grand illusions brought about by the internal workings of the brain.

The above conclusion about the place of consciousness in the world is highly controversial in philosophy, where several lines of thought resist the idea that consciousness resides in the brain (see chapter 8). Now the burden of proof is on the advocates of those views. Anyone who denies that consciousness is in the brain should come up with an alternative interpretation of the evidence provided by the dreaming brain. Furthermore, he should come up with a clear answer to the question, If consciousness is *not* located in the brain, *where then is it to be found*?

5 Metaphors of Consciousness

In this chapter, the role of metaphors in science is first elucidated by presenting some illuminating examples from the history of biology. Then the most prominent traditional metaphors of consciousness are briefly described. A more detailed analysis is provided about two particular metaphors of consciousness that play a major role in current theories of consciousness: the multiple drafts metaphor and the theater-spotlight metaphor. Neither of them is found adequate as they seem to misconstrue phenomenal consciousness, the most important explanandum for the science of consciousness. Therefore, a new metaphor is needed that is above all faithful to the phenomenology of consciousness from the first-person perspective. The chapter concludes by showing how a promising theoretical metaphor may be derived from the model system of consciousness science, the dreaming brain.

Metaphors as Tools of Thought in Science

At a stage in scientific research when there is no well-developed theory available of the phenomenon to be explained, the explanandum is often described in terms of a suitable *metaphor.* A fruitful metaphor captures the essential features of the phenomenon in a single, captivating picture. For example, at the time when biologists had virtually no idea about the internal microstructure or constitution of genetic material, extremely useful models of genes were constructed by treating them as distinct units that are arranged linearly in the chromosome *like beads on a string.* This was a simple, powerful visuospatial metaphor that guided theoretical thinking in classical genetics for years.

To take another example, in the 1920s cell cleavage patterns were represented in what were called *soap bubble models.* This analogy between complex microscopic biological events and relatively simple macroscopic physical events allowed researchers to suggest theoretical explanations about cells, based on knowledge about soap bubbles (Maienschein, 1991). A famous metaphor in physics is Bohr's model of the internal structure of the atom. The atom was compared to the solar system where several planets (electrons) orbit around the sun (the nucleus).

An illuminating or helpful metaphor hence captures some key features of the phenomenon in a clear and simple image. Several different metaphors of consciousness have been proposed in consciousness research. William James proposed that consciousness is like a flowing *stream.* This famous *stream of consciousness* metaphor emphasizes the temporal dynamics of consciousness: that it consists of ever-changing patterns of thought and experience. Although temporal flow is an important feature of consciousness, the stream metaphor alone hardly offers a sufficient basis for a full theory and philosophy of consciousness.

Another popular metaphor of consciousness is to say that it is "like the tip of the iceberg." The (perhaps rather Freudian) idea behind this metaphor is to stress the fact that consciousness occupies only a small (and insignificant?) corner of the mind-brain, surrounded by a vast and powerful (but mostly invisible) machinery of nonconscious neurophysiological (and psychodynamic) mechanisms. Again, although this observation is probably true and should be taken seriously by any theory of consciousness, it falls short of guiding us toward the science of consciousness in any detail.

Why, then, does the biological research program need yet another metaphor of consciousness? Are there not plenty of them around already? I am afraid that most of the currently popular metaphors suffer from one crucial weakness: they do not manage to capture the explanandum—the phenomenal level of organization—but either totally eliminate it or at least ignore its fundamental features. Two recently popular metaphors, the multiple drafts metaphor (Dennett, 1991) and the theater-spotlight metaphor, are cases in point.

The Multiple Drafts Metaphor

The multiple drafts metaphor, presented in the context of Daniel Dennett's (1991) theory of consciousness, is not a metaphor of consciousness in the sense in which the concept is defined in biological realism, the phenomenal level in the brain (Revonsuo, 1993, 1994b). In Dennett's philosophy the reality of both phenomenal consciousness and qualia is denied (chapter 8). In Dennett's view of the mind, multiple drafts of objective information processing in the brain replace our everyday ideas of what consciousness is. The idea of a single, subjective stream of consciousness that posesses determinate contents is, according to Dennett, only an illusion. In the brain, there is no such thing as a *single* internal stream of consciousness that would constitute the *actual* stream of consciousness of the subject and hold the determinate contents of the subject's consciousness. There are only multiple streams of processing, but no line can be drawn that would separate the conscious from the nonconscious streams. The property of "consciousness" is not something that can be ascribed to internal brain processes. In Dennett's theory, consciousness is to be found in the objective patterns of behavior and organism-environment interaction that are attributes of the *whole* organism rather than any of its parts. The contents of consciousness ascribed to the system are always open to revision and further interpretation by external observers (and even by the person who has the conscious states). There is no single "right" answer to the question, What exactly are the contents of my consciousness right now?

Dennett denies that there is any "center" in the brain where it all comes together in a unified sphere of consciousness. He argues that nothing in neuroanatomy suggests that such a center exists. Postulating a center of consciousness in the brain is a category mistake for him, as it ascribes what he believes is a system-level property to a part of the system. In his view, it is the person as a whole who possesses consciousness, not any of the person's parts (nor any parts of his brain). Assuming a system-level property to a subsystem only duplicates the problem at the lower level. Therefore, Dennett does not believe that any phenomenal *world-for-me* even exists in the brain. On the contrary, he tries to discredit the whole idea with the concept of a Cartesian theater—a philosophical caricature of all theories that posit a phenomenal world-for-me in the brain.

The multiple drafts metaphor is hardly a satisfactory metaphor for the purposes of a biological science of consciousness, because it eliminates from serious discussion the phenomenal level of organization in the brain.

The Theater-Spotlight Metaphor

In the theater metaphor (or spotlight metaphor) consciousness resembles a bright searchlight beam in an otherwise dark theater. The spotlight moves around the stage, and inside of its beam appear, one by one, various persons and objects, which then disappear again into the darkness. The darkness where the audience sits resembles the nonconscious processing mechanisms in the brain that surround consciousness. They observe the contents of the stage, they compete for access to the stage in trying to send their own informational contributions to the spotlight, and they receive globally distributed information from the stage—the information that won the competition. Bernie Baars has used the theater metaphor as the basis for his global workspace theory, one of the leading empirically based theories of consciousness. The theater metaphor thus seems to be useful in guiding further theory-building in the science of consciousness.

The global workspace theory is closely related to cognitive models of attention and working memory. Baars (1998) describes working memory as resembling a theater stage, and the spotlight of attention as resembling the limited capacity of working memory, whereas the serially shifting contents in the spotlight resemble the stream of consciousness. The audience in the darkness resembles unconscious processors and contexts in the brain to whom the information in the spotlight is disseminated.

The theater-spotlight metaphor seems to be erected on the following background assumption: consciousness is ontologically dependent on attention, or, conversely, attention is necessary for consciousness. According to the theater metaphor, contents of consciousness only come into existence when the bright searchlight beam of selective attention touches on them. When the spotlight departs, the phenomenal contents disappear into the nonconscious darkness again, as quickly as they came into existence. While they persist within the spotlight, they form the contents of consciousness and the contents of the spotlight of selective attention: "Thus, attention involves the selection of the targets for the searchlight to shine on, while consciousness results from the illumination of the target" (Baars, 1998, p. 59).

The theory of consciousness that more or less naturally follows from this metaphor seems to reduce consciousness to the cognitive concepts of attention and working memory. Consciousness is really nothing over and above the cognitive and neural mechanisms underlying the spotlight of selective attention and the global workspace of working memory. Such a view appears to be surprisingly popular in cognitive psychology and cognitive neuroscience. Recently, Dehaene and Naccache (2001) proposed that one of the cornerstones of the cognitive neuroscience of consciousness should be the fact that attention is a necessary prerequisite of consciousness; according to them there is no doubt that attention serves as a filter prior to conscious perception.

If the theater-spotlight metaphor is accepted, then consciousness science does not really need any fundamentally new concepts or novel levels of description: traditional cognitive concepts and their neurophysiological mechanisms can do all the work that is required. Hence, in Baars's global workspace theory (Baars, 1988, 1997), the cognitive level of description is worked out in much detail, and then an attempt to map it to brain function is carried out. After all this standard cognitive neuroscience theorizing it remains a bit unclear whether the theory simply describes the cognitive and neural mechanisms of attention and working memory rather than the phenomenal level of subjective experience.

The main problems with the theater metaphor are its commitment to a kind of "cognitive reduction" of consciousness and its phenomenological inadequacy. Phenomenal consciousness does *not* feel like sitting in a dark theater looking at characters or events appearing one by one on a faraway stage. Phenomenal consciousness is not just a narrow spotlight jumping around in total darkness. The contents of phenomenal consciousness are not necessarily first selected or filtered by a beam of attention and only subsequently to become the contents of experience.

Rather, moment-to-moment phenomenal consciousness feels like being bodily immersed in the center of a temporally progressing, multimodal *phenomenal world* which is present for the subject all at once (though perhaps not in full detail, apart from the objects in focal consciousness). The phenomenal level includes the externalized sensory-perceptual events, the subject's own body-image, and those events that are felt to be going on within the confines of the body or the mind, say emotions or inner speech (for a similar view, see Velmans, 2000). Phenomenal contents fill an entire sphere of subjective experience. The spotlight of attention selects particular experiences for more detailed processing within this field of already subjectively experienced contents. Thus, primary phenomenal consciousness is not dependent on selective attention; only reflective consciousness is (see chapters 2 and 15). The theater-spotlight metaphor seems to pass over primary phenomenal consciousness. It suggests that there is only reflective consciousness. All phenomenal experience is taken to be dependent on selective attention and working memory.

Hence, a new metaphor of consciousness is needed that first and foremost captures the structure and organization of the phenomenal level. The new metaphor should give a proper place to both primary and reflective consciousness and should not reduce consciousness to the cognitive concepts of attention and working memory (or to anything else either). It should faithfully describe the phenomenal level rather than reduce, eliminate, or distort it.

From the Dreaming Brain to a Novel Metaphor of Consciousness

As I argued above, the dreaming brain can be regarded as a theoretically fruitful model system for consciousness research. Furthermore, I believe that it could also serve as the basis for an appropriate metaphor of the phenomenal level: the world-simulation metaphor of consciousness.

The Phenomenal Level as a "World"

The concept of "world" has often been used to capture the nature of dreams. The pioneer in the study of lucid dreaming, Frederik van Eeden ([1913] 1990) once described dreaming as comparable to being in a "cleverly imitated fake-world." The pioneer of sleep-laboratory dream research, Frederic Snyder (1970) described dreaming as a "realistic facsimile" of the perception of external reality. A German dream researcher, Detlev von Uslar (1990), wrote a whole book devoted to the idea that the dream is a world of its own, *Der Traum als Welt.* Of contemporary dream researchers, David Foulkes (1985) holds that dreams are "simulations" of what life is like, or "multimodal world analogs."

Such characterizations are in harmony with our everyday understanding of dreams: most laypersons would be quite comfortable saying that their nocturnal experiences happen in a "dream world." But why exactly are both laypersons and dream researchers inclined to take the dream as a "world" or "reality?" Why don't they, instead, describe it as an unreal mental representation or image, or a sequence of delusional thought? Probably because of the following simple reason: dreaming does not consist of what we ordinarily call "mental images" or "thoughts." Mental images and thought processes are psychological events that a subject experiences taking place within her own head or within the mind and over which she has some voluntary control. By contrast, a subject experiences the dream as taking place all around her, certainly not somewhere within her mind or her head (which usually occupies only a small region located in the perspectival center of the dream world). Furthermore, the dreamer does not usually have any significant control over the dream world and its events.

It is therefore slightly misleading to characterize the dream as a "purely mental" event, for it is *not experienced as* a mental event, at least insofar as mental events refer to those inner psychological processes that we experience happening within our heads, in the mind, and under some degree of control. I would rather say that the dream, while it is going on, happens all around me, not within my mind. When I am dreaming, the phenomenological facts are that I simply find myself, as an embodied subject, in the middle of a perceptual world where I am surrounded by objects, people, and events. I do not find myself engaged in any particular inner "mental" process called "dreaming," although of course it is possible for me also to entertain inner thoughts and even mental images (in the ordinary sense of the word) while I am in the dream world. But the dream does not consist of those inner events; it would be perfectly possible to have a vivid dream without having a single inner thought or mental image.

It is also misleading to think about the dream as happening on the stage of a mental theater (or perhaps a Cartesian theater). The "mental stage" on which the dream events unfold is nothing like a theater stage. The stage in a real theater is a restricted area, decorated with fake scenery—a rather poor, make-believe imitation of actual places or settings. Nobody would be inclined to confuse the theater stage with an actual place in the world. By contrast, the dream "stage" is no stage at all, but a world that seems to have a potentially limitless spatial extension in all directions. If the dream events happen in an outside setting, the dreamer may have a view extending all the way to a distant horizon.

Did I have a dream or did the dream have me? When I am in a dream, there seem to be three-dimensional objects all around me, and other people, independent of myself, are going about their business. There are events going on; the dream is not like a still photograph, but like an animated world. Unless it is a lucid dream, I do not orchestrate the unfolding dream events at will; they happen to me—I do not voluntarily plan them, or even have an idea where they come from, or what is going to happen next. Other dream characters may speak to me but I have no idea what they are going to say, although this must be a world of my own creation (or at least of my own brain's creation). However, I can voluntarily move in relation to the objects around me. I have a sense of moving through a space. And the entity thus moving and voluntarily controlled by the dreamer, is the "self," usually attached to a phenomenal body image not unlike the one experienced when awake. Even in dreams, I am still *me;* I go around the dream world and the dream events happen to *me.* There is a continuity of the sense of self. There is a first-person perspective from which the dream world is apprehended. The dream indeed seems to *have me,* rather than the other way around.

The dream world is experienced as a spatially extended and animated world, containing objects, people, and events completely independent of myself and beyond my control. The representation of the world in dreams is so amazingly realistic that it is fully justified to call it a "reality." After all, we call the representation of the world delivered to us by our waking perception a "reality" and not a "representation" (of reality); why should we call a similar representation in another situation anything else but a "reality" too? Dreaming is not an unrealistic, faint, or poor imitation of the true waking reality we experience. The fact is that in both cases we have similar representations of a "world" or a "reality," but in everyday waking perception we take the representation for the real thing. We have the naive realist stance in everyday waking perception, for we regard the mere representation of reality as the external physical reality itself. Thus, when there is a similar representation created in the brain during dreaming, we cannot help but call it a "reality" as well, although we do realize (retrospectively, though) that the phenomenal reality in that case does not represent any external state of affairs.

That it is perfectly natural for us to describe the dream as a "reality" or a "world" reminds us of the important fact that for us as subjects, the reality we are *directly* in touch with is necessarily our inner phenomenal reality and could not possibly be anything else. The word "reality" as we understand it in everyday life refers to all the stuff that seems to be located out there in the extended space beyond ourselves (including the space itself and our own body in the center of that space), inhabited by objects and people seemingly independent of ourselves. And we do indeed find such a reality within our dreams; or rather, we find ourselves within such a reality when we dream. In contrast, we do not find it natural to call the reality all around us a representation (of reality). Why might that be the case? Typical representations are not perfectly realistic copies of the real thing. A painting of an apple, or the word "apple," stands for, or *only* represents, the real thing, and nobody would mistake a painting or a printed word for a real fruit. But when you can see the apple, touch it, pick it up, and even bite into it and taste it, it no longer seems like a representation at all—on the contrary it seems just like an apple. A statue or a photograph or a video of a person is an unmistakeable representation of her, but when you can see her, talk to her, even embrace her, you no longer think it is a representation: it is the person herself (or at least some person or other, possibly an impostor). A dream in which one eats an apple and meets a person is experienced and described as eating an apple and meeting a person, not as seeing a representation of oneself eating an apple and meeting a person, or oneself eating a representation of an apple and meeting a representation of a person.

The Dream as a Transparent Surrogate World

In the phenomenal realm, whether dreamed or not, the objects and persons encountered are never experienced as representations, although from an external point of view they can be regarded as such. The philosopher Thomas Metzinger (1995b, 2000) calls this the "transparency of phenomenal states": phenomenal content seems to bring us into direct contact with the world; conscious life always takes place in the world. Our brain is a biological system that does not recognize its own phenomenal representations as representations; by contrast, we just look through the representations as if they were the real world itself, somehow immediately present or directly perceived.

The notion of transparency may be slightly misleading as it suggests that consciousness is the invisible, featureless window through which we are in direct contact with an external physical world. But the "reaching out" through a transparent window is just an illusion, for consciousness does not in actual fact reach out into the external world. Instead, the phenomenal level is engaged in internal *world simulation* and *world presentation.* The objects we experience around us, the objects directly present for us, are not the real physical objects out there in physical space, but purely experiential phenomena, located entirely within the sphere of the phenomenal level.

The philosopher Ivan Fox (1994) makes a distinction between surrogates and representations of external objects, which seems relevant here. He points out that since the external physical objects themselves certainly cannot enter the mind, they must have some sorts of mental representatives, which come in two varieties. Ordinary mental representations represent external objects through an arbitrary but consistent input-output correspondence with them, just like words, images, or symbols do. In this case, there is a perfectly clear distinction between the thing and its representation; they do not necessarily resemble each other very much if at all. A surrogate, by contrast, acts in the system as if it were the thing itself that it is a representative of. The system cannot distinguish the surrogate of the thing from the thing itself. In dreams, all the objects and persons we encounter are only surrogates, but we describe them with the same concepts we would use to describe similar things during perception. We do not have separate concepts for the surrogate persons and objects that we encounter in our dreams and the "real" persons and objects we encounter during wakefulness, but we say, "*You* were in my dream last night"; "I saw *a snake* in my dream."

The phenomenal level of organization thus includes surrogates (or simulations) rather than representations. The concepts of "transparency" and "surrogate" characterize the phenomenal contents of consciousness both during wakefulness and dreaming, and thereby explain why it is natural for us to conceptualize dreaming as a world. Phenomenal contents are fully transparent: they give the impression of being actual things *out there* in the world rather than some sort of merely secondary representations of those things *in here,* in my mind or my brain. The phenomenal level of organization in the brain consists of transparent surrogates (or realistic simulations) of physical objects. The surrogates are (mis)taken by the subject (or, in fact, by the brain) for the external objects themselves rather than only as mediated representatives or mental images of those objects.

The dreaming brain dramatically exposes this grand illusion to us because even though the dream world is not in touch with any external sensory environment, it includes fully convincing transparent surrogates of objects and scenery. The transparent surrogates establish the dream world as a world (for the subject). The experience of dreaming is, at bottom, the experience of *being in the world* or *world-presenting* rather than the experience of inner thinking, or private mental imagery, or an inner experiential medium that intervenes between us and the external world.

The conception of the phenomenal level as a *transparent surrogate world* or *world simulation* paves the way for the world-simulation metaphor of consciousness, one of the fundamental cornerstones of the research program advanced in this book. The next chapter is devoted to a closer examination of the world-simulation metaphor.

Summary

Metaphors are useful, indeed necessary, for theoretical progress in science. The science of consciousness should discover its own metaphors that faithfully convey the intuitive theoretical ideas we have about the nature of phenomenal consciousness. Many previously proposed metaphors were found to be either misleading or inadequate for capturing phenomenal consciousness from the first person perspective. The multiple drafts metaphor disregards phenomenal consciousness altogether. The theater-spotlight metaphor perhaps adequately describes selective attention, working memory, and some aspects of reflective consciousness, but it sidesteps phenomenal consciousness. Therefore, a metaphor is needed that captures precisely the nature of the experiences that phenomenal consciousness is all about. An investigation of the dreaming brain suggests that the concept of "world simulation" might be on the right track. Dream experiences establish that the world simulation in consciousness has certain defining features that make it a fully convincing experience of "being in the real world." The simulation includes entities that we may call "transparent surrogates" of real things. That concept implies that we do not recognize the phenomenal simulations in our brain as simulations at all, but instead treat them as the real external physical objects themselves. An adequate theoretical metaphor of consciousness should thus convey the fact that phenomenal consciousness is a transparent surrogate world in the brain.

6 The World-Simulation Metaphor of Consciousness

The dreaming brain as the model system for consciousness science has now led us to the world-simulation metaphor of consciousness. This metaphor takes into account what phenomenal consciousness feels like from the first-person perspective: It feels like being directly present or bodily immersed in the center of a world—the *world-for-me*—and being there surrounded by meaningful objects. The concepts *immersion* and *presence* have been introduced in the context of technologically produced world simulations: virtual reality technology. Thus, we might learn something about consciousness by examining that field. This exploration leads us toward an internalist conception of experience: the world simulation in our phenomenal consciousness takes place inside the brain, yet we never experience actually *being* inside the brain. This paradox can be solved if we realize that in world simulation, the brain creates for us only virtual presence or telepresence in the surrounding world, but we ourselves, and our consciousness, never in actual fact escape the confines of the brain.

World Simulation

The world-simulation metaphor captures consciousness from the first-person point of view—the way we subjectively experience it—rather than from an external or third-person point of view. It also depicts the relations between consciousness, brain, and external physical reality in the correct way.[1]

Let us take a look at the core features of phenomenal organization and see how the concept of world simulation helps us to think about them. As I argued above, the phenomenal level of organization as a whole is a momentary reality or world. I pointed out several reasons why it is natural to call the dream a "reality" or a "world"; why dreaming is "being-in-the-world" or "world-presenting." To dream is to have a multimodal realistic simulation of objects and events in a three-dimensional experiential space within which the subject finds herself and where she can move about and interact with the environment. The objects and events in a dream are transparent surrogates of the real thing, closely similar to those transparent surrogates constructed in the brain during waking perception. The only difference between them is that the surrogates we experience during dreaming do not involve an immediate causal chain reaching backward to the external world.

For exactly the same reasons, computer-generated simulations of objects and events in a 3D space are called "virtual realities" or "virtual worlds" (or sometimes "cyberspace" or "synthetic environments"). They are also transparent surrogates of coherently organized objects and events. A virtual reality (VR) is a computer-generated world simulation, a sensory environment which can be manipulated in real time and through which it is possible to move. The simulated worlds do not exist, as worlds, anywhere inside the computer or the program, only inside the consciousness of the subject whose brain is confronted with coherent information through several sensory channels and whose actions (say moving the head and gazing around) are tracked by the computer and used in updating the images in a way corresponding to the movements.

There are several types of VR systems. The simplest ones are called "desktop VR" or "window-on-world" systems. They use the conventional computer monitor to display a visual world as if one were looking through a window and seeing a real world out there. This sort of system, however, is not a good metaphor of consciousness, because the phenomenal level is not organized as a window-on-world system. What is the crucial difference? Consider the structure of the phenomenal level in most dreams. Empirical dream research has confirmed that almost all dreams (90 to 95%) have a dream self: a character with whom the dreamer identifies himself or herself and who is taken to be continuous with the waking self (Strauch & Meier, 1996; F. Snyder, 1970): it is *me* within the dream, not somebody else, or nobody at all. The dream self is not usually described in great detail in the dream reports; in most cases its existence is merely implied in the manner in which the dream is reported using first-person expressions: *I* was there and *I* did this or that. Only rarely is the dream self reported to depart from the waking self in its appearance, sex, age or identity (Revonsuo & Salmivalli, 1995). In most dreams the dream self is an active participant in the dream events (Strauch & Meier, 1996), and practically all dreams with animated (as opposed to static) visual imagery are experienced from the point of view of the dream self, that is, from an own-eyes', first-person perspective (Foulkes & Kerr, 1994).

The most universal form of the phenomenal level of organization in fully animated dreams therefore is that the dream self resides in the center of the dream world and dynamically interacts with whatever objects, persons, and events are to be found in the surrounding dream environment. This overall structure of the phenomenal level can be characterized as "self-in-world": immersion of the dreamer's perspective in the center of the dream world. It cannot be accurately characterized as a window-on-world system, where the self is an external observer looking at the world through a window but not being a part of the very same world. The phenomenal level does not separate the self from the world in that way.[2]

The overall "self-in-world" organization of the phenomenal level has not gone unnoticed in the VR circles where a vocabulary has been introduced that attempts to describe the effects of the VR system on the user's consciousness. These concepts actually manage to capture the global features of the phenomenal level itself. This is because they essentially describe the *effects* of VR technology on *human consciousness,* and those effects are realized at the phenomenal level of organization.

The Sense of Presence

In connection with dreaming, the overall organization of the phenomenal level is described as "self-in-world" and "transparent surrogate reality," while in the context of VR technology it is discussed in terms of "immersion," the sense of "presence," and the sense of "being there." Full immersion or presence is the *you-are-there* experience. A VR system is capable of creating full immersion when no efforts are required on the user's part to create the sense of presence in the virtual environment, or conversely, special efforts are required to avoid it (Heim, 1998). The "sense of presence" seems to be just another way to capture the fact that a perceptual object or scene ceases to be a representation of the real thing and becomes a fully transparent surrogate of it.

The ultimate VR systems are those that completely immerse the user's viewpoint in the virtual world (and in that way achieve transparency and the sense of presence). Currently, there are two different ways of achieving full immersion: head-mounted displays and projection-based virtual environments. A head-mounted display is a helmet or face mask holding the visual and auditory displays. The displayed information is adjusted according to the position of the head, thereby creating the illusion of being physically present within the virtual environment.

In projection-based virtual environments, no helmets or gloves are required. The images are projected onto the inside of a large hemispherical surface, as in a planetarium, or back-projected onto the walls and floor of a room within which the observer views and interacts with the virtual environment. A science-fiction example of an immensely advanced projection-based virtual environment is the holodeck in *Star Trek: The Next Generation.*

The best-known actually functioning projection based VR is called the CAVE system (incidentally, the name refers to the famous myth of the cave in Plato's *Republic*) (Heim, 1998). An even more advanced projection-based VR system is the Fully Immersive Spherical Projection System or Cybersphere: a large , hollow, translucent sphere, several meters in diameter, provided with a means of entry for an observer, and supported by a ring of bearings. The walking motion of the observer causes the sphere to rotate. Computer-generated images, updated in response to the subject's movement, are projected onto the outer surface of the sphere. These images are viewed by the observer from within the sphere. The observer is able to walk, run, jump, or crawl in any direction, while at the same time being able to observe an all-encompassing virtual environment. The Cybersphere allows completely free and limitless movement within the virtual world.[3]

A VR system must fulfill several requirements to be fully immersive. These requirements might, in fact, reveal some basic features of the phenomenal level or its underlying mechanisms, because for a VR system to produce "full immersion" is for it to modulate the phenomenal level in a way that produces a fully convincing "self-in-world" experience. Satisfaction of those requirements, or creating full immersion, reveals how much and what kind of information must be fed into the brain through the sensory systems to create a flawless, gapless world simulation at the phenomenal level. The most important modalities for immersion are vision, movement, and touch, and their coherent interplay. In the following I consider especially the prerequisites of visual immersion.

One essential requirement of visual immersion concerns the field of view. Its scope must be wide enough to create the sense of full immersion and subjective presence-in-a-world. If the field of view is too narrow, the observer will get the impression of looking out from a small window that opens into a world, but he will not acquire the sense of actually *being* there, inside the world. The horizontal scope of the normal field of view is about 200 degrees of visual angle. However, this very wide field need not be wholly covered by the VR display to create immersion. Estimations vary between 90 and 120 degrees of visual angle as to how large a field should be covered at the very least to create an immersible visual world (Reitmaa, Vanhala, Kauttu, & Antila, 1995). The range of binocular overlap (the area seen by both eyes simultaneously) should be about 30 degrees. Although in natural vision the field of binocular overlap is about 120 degrees, only about 30 degrees of this is significant for stereo vision. Thus, to achieve full visual immersion it is necessary to cover the area important for stereo vision completely, and in addition, a fairly large range of the monocular fields as well.

The fact that information must be fed into the visual system as a fairly large *field* to create immersion shows that visual consciousness is not some sort of narrow spotlight, only the center of which enters the phenomenal level of organization. If that were the case, the field of view required to create a convincing VR would be relatively narrow, for the foveal area where humans have high resolution and high-acuity vision is very small, encompassing only about 2 degrees of visual angle. The sense of "being there" requires the sense of a wide field surrounding the observer, although it does not require that all objects outside the current focus be represented in fine detail. The theater-spotlight metaphor of consciousness and theories that identify visual consciousness with the focus of selective attention (e.g., O'Regan & Noë, 2001) disregard the fact that the experience of sight has a fieldlike phenomenal structure.

The resolution of the display or projection must be relatively high, both in the spatial and in the temporal domain. In ordinary perception, our phenomenal field of vision does not have a subjectively observable grain; it does not seem to be composed of any basic pixels or voxels with an observable minimum size. On the contrary, regions of uniformly colored surfaces, for example, seem to have no grain at all, as phenomenally experienced. Therefore, if a VR display or projection does have elementary pixels of a relatively coarse grain, it immediately makes the world simulation look like an artificial image rather than a true world. A visible grain destroys the transparency of the environment; it will look like a mere representation, not like a reality in itself.[4]

The same principle applies to the grain, or refreshment rate, in the temporal domain. In everyday perception, we never notice how the phenomenal visual field is updated. We are capable of recognizing and understanding very briefly (~100 ms) flashed complex images of scenery. If we turn our eyes or head very rapidly, our phenomenal field is instantly updated to accommodate the new perspective. There is no perceptible delay. However, in VR systems, it is still very difficult to compute and update the visual stimulus field with sufficient temporal resolution. The temporal resolution of our internal phenomenal field surpasses that of our best VR technology. Thus, the neural mechanisms underlying the phenomenal field must be capable of extremely rapid reorganization of their informational content.

Furthermore, the phenomenal field tends to retain a coherent multisensory coordination and organization. A powerful factor in immersion is the coherence of the different perceptual cues. Shape, color, location, touch, and other sensory features defining a perceptual object should be perfectly coordinated to create a convincing experience of one coherent multisensory object. The coherence of the phenomenal level of organization would seem to reflect the fact that, behind our ordinary experience of the world, there are multiple binding mechanisms at work that create the sense of one unified perceptual world. If different perceptual cues are conflicting with each other, it is difficult to reach a coherent interpretation and experience of the perceptual world.

Other requirements for immersion are interactivity and autonomy. Interactivity means that the virtual environment must respond to the observer's actions in a natural manner. The relationship between the observer and the environment must change according to the observer's movements and actions toward the virtual objects. Autonomy refers to the freedom of will of the observer in the virtual world: she must be able to choose her path and course of action within the world; they must not be predetermined.

The Sense of Presence in Virtual Reality and Dream Consciousness

The world-simulation metaphor of consciousness states that "immersion" and the "sense of presence" are not only the most fundamental concepts in VR technology but also essential features of the phenomenal level of organization itself. Immersion and presence have nothing to do with computer technology per se. In actual fact they are *phenomenological* notions: they name basic features of subjective experience.

This point can be easily appreciated when considering the dreaming brain. When I dream during sleep, the phenomenal level is realized in all its glory inside my brain. That feels like being fully immersed in the center of a spatially extended, multimodal perceptual world. I have the sense of presence; the sense of really being there, inside that very reality. Furthermore, dream experience includes all sensory modalities in a full-scale, well-organized world simulation.

But why should we call the reality of consciousness a *virtual* reality? Again, the dreaming brain makes this point crystal clear. As far as we know anything at all about dreaming and its neurophysiological basis, we know that all the biological processes that somehow generate the dream experience are occurring inside the brain. Hence, the dream world can be regarded as "virtual" for the following reasons. The dream world, though compelling, does not exist anywhere in the reality outside of the brain. During dreaming, the dreamer is immersed in a seemingly real perceptual world; she has the fully convincing experience of being physically present in it. Nevertheless, her physical body is actually present in a quite different physical environment. The dream world is thus "virtual" for precisely the same reason as a computer-generated synthetic environment is: in both cases I feel physically present (i.e., I *am* phenomenologically present!) in an unreal place where my physical body is not really present at all.

During immersion in a virtual world, the phenomenal content of the brain is modulated by sensory input not originating in the distal physical environment, but, instead, by input coming from computer-controlled displays (in technologically produced VR) or from internal activation of the brain itself (such as PGO waves in REM sleep dreaming). The phenomenal level consequently brings about a model of the world not corresponding to the model it would have brought about were its sensory states modulated by information generated in the real physical surroundings.

All of the above should be quite uncontroversial. Dreams are virtual realities in the same sense as fully immersed computer-generated environments (although I guess that none as convincing as dreams exist yet). But this is not the main point of the world-simulation metaphor, for it is supposed to capture the phenomenal level in toto. Why, then, should *all* conscious experiences be regarded as world simulations? What is the *further* sense in which also all everyday waking experiences are virtual? To understand this, we need to first grasp that the phenomenal level is designed to produce experiences with a special externalized structure. I characterize the externalization of consciousness as an *out-of-brain experience.* The idea is easiest to grasp when first applied to dream consciousness. Still, the externalization of consciousness works basically in the same manner also when we perceive something during wakefulness. This I call a *telepresence experience.* In the following, these two central ideas implied by the world-simulation metaphor are developed in detail.

Dreaming as an Out-of-Brain Experience

Let us think about the dream world once again. The dreamer experiences being present in a reality where she, as a matter of fact, is not—it may well be a purely imaginary place where no one *could* be truly present. But then, what *is* the reality where the dreamer is located? It cannot be the physical surroundings of the physical body, for the dreaming brain has effectively isolated itself from the sensory information originating in the environment. We know for a fact that the dream is really going on somewhere deep inside the skull (though we do not understand exactly how the brain works to produce the virtual world of dreams).

Nonetheless, despite this indubitable knowledge of the origin of our dreams, we never think about our own dream experiences in the following way: "Well, so *this* is *how my brain looks from the inside*!"

Why are we not inclined to conceive of our dream experiences like that? The answer is the thoroughly deceiving *externalization* of the dream world. Its implications are nearly impossible to swallow from our folk-psychological, naive realist stance (that most of us entertain in everyday life). It certainly does *not* seem to me as if I was trapped inside a living brain when I am dreaming, but still, I know for a fact that that *must* be where all the stuff that dreams are made of is actually coming from. In the same vein, when inside a fully immersed VR system, it does not seem to you that you are in fact trapped inside a small room or inside a head-mounted display and a full-body data suit. When you are *immersed in* the world, your experience of the surrounding world is externalized to be *out there* beyond the boundaries of your mind and body.

Now we approach one rather astonishing implication of the world-simulation metaphor. Although we intellectually know it for a fact that our dreams in some sense happen inside our brains, we never have the experience of being somehow present inside a brain when we dream. Instead, we always feel directly present in the center of an externalized multimodal perceptual reality, the dream world. But the dream world must happen entirely within the confines of the brain and therefore the very sense of presence is but virtual. Everything we experience during dreaming is really happening inside the brain, but the phenomenal level is organized in such a manner as to produce an "out-of-brain" experience for us!

Through this brain wizardry, we, as subjects, experience an immediate but nevertheless only virtual presence in a world outside the brain. The feature of virtual presence is as though it is built into the externalized structure of the phenomenal level: as soon as the phenomenal level is realized in the brain, it involves the inescapable illusion that the events we are directly conscious of are not taking place inside a brain at all, but in a complete, centered, perceptual world definitely external to the body and the brain.

Now we have arrived at the very core of the world-simulation metaphor of consciousness. Whenever the phenomenal level of organization is generated inside the brain, the outcome is a natural form of VR: the sense of presence in and immersion in a world that seems to be outside the brain.

Perception as the Brain's Natural Telepresence System

At this point we need to introduce another concept from VR technology. A *telepresence* system is a specific type of world simulation. When a VR system creates an interactive feedback loop between my perceptions and the real environment somewhere out there beyond the reach of my sensory organs, I enjoy an experience called "telepresence." The feedback could in principle originate from a few meters away, or from very exotic and distant places like the bottom of the ocean or the cockpit of a fighter plane soaring high in the air. In telepresence there is a robot with multimodal sense organs connected to yours. Consequently, your brain constructs the experienced world from the point of view of the robot, not from the perspective of your physical body. Moreover, all the movements of your body are reproduced by the robot: when you move your hand, you see the metal arms or tentacles moving in front of your viewpoint. Telepresence is not pure science fiction: Howard Rheingold (1991) relates his experiences in a tele-existence laboratory in Japan:

> When the apparatus was switched on, I began to look through the eyes of a robot. The world looked like the world would look like if I was located twelve feet left of my body, where the robot was located. . . . The strangest moment was when Dr. Tachi told me to look to my right. There was a guy in a dark blue suit and light blue painted shoes reclining in a dentist's chair. . . . He looked like me, and abstractedly I understood that he *was* me, but I know who me is, and me is *here*. He, on the other hand, was *there*. . . . It was an out-of-the-body experience, no doubt about it. (pp. 263–264)

Telepresence VR is capable of constraining sensory inputs so that my "self" (or rather my viewpoint on the world) is no longer located in the same coordinates with my body image. The perspective to the virtual world, constructed inside the phenomenal level, could be from any angle whatsoever. It is not necessary to have one's own body image in the center of the world to create a virtual world experienced from a certain perspective.

The core message is: All the phenomenal worlds we enjoy—whether those of dreams, computer-generated models, or waking "reality"—are basically the same; the realities we experience are always "simulated" or "virtual," as is our experienced sense of presence within them. Our subjective existence consists in the sense of presence in externalized surrogate worlds, constructed at the phenomenal level of organization somewhere in the brain. The neural mechanisms capable of bringing about any sort of sentience at all are forever buried inside our skulls and cannot reach out from there, whereas the nonvirtual world outside the skull in physical space is, in itself, black and imperceptible. Neither the neural mechanisms of consciousness nor phenomenal consciousness itself is able to travel backward on the causal chains—through the afferent neural pathways—to the real external world out there in physical space, and directly "sense" it, touch it, hear it, or see the objects out there. If there is a phenomenal level of organization realized in the neurobiology of the brain, there is no way it could leak out of the brain. If there is a consciously experienced model of the world constructed in the brain, causal chains from the world outside must travel inward to constrain this model; virtual actions performed on the phenomenal model must immediately travel outward to have effects on the world outside.

Let me illuminate this VR metaphor of consciousness through a thought experiment (Revonsuo, 1995b).

The Black Planet

Imagine that you are an explorer about to land on an alien planet. When you get out of your space capsule and onto the surface of the planet, you are immediately engulfed by an impenetrable darkness and silence. You cannot see anything, hear anything, feel anything. There must be an environment somewhere out there, but you are utterly unable to sense it in any way and, consequently, there is no "organism-environment interaction" to speak of. You feel like floating in a sensory-deprivation tank, unable even to perceive the position of your body, let alone the environment you are surrounded by. Somehow you manage to return to the mother ship. You examine carefully all the data that were collected from the planet's surface. You find out that actually there is a lot of physical activity going on but of a kind you have never encountered before. Consequently, you were not able to perceive anything. Well, you do not give up—you design a suit that has sensors for the alien radiations and vibrations on the planet, translating them into the sort of physical stimuli that your body is able to handle. Thus, a certain sort of alien radiation is translated, by your goggles, into electromagnetic radiation of the visible wavelengths; the vibrations of the planet's strange atmosphere are translated into vibrations of air near your ears, and so on. When you return to the planet, you step into a quite different, spatial and extended world of objects, colors, and sounds. Now your brain can construct an experienced model of the world, which enables you to successfully interact with the world. Of course, the world in itself is still silent and dark, just physical matter and energy hurrying about, but nevertheless, your brain is now clothing it (its model, that is) with properties that do not really exist out there. The phenomenal level of organization is, thus, an illusion created by the brain, but still, a most useful one for an organism that must find its way around. (pp. 50–51)

It should not come as a surprise if I now tell you that actually the strange planet described above is the planet Earth, the space suit is our physical body, especially its sensory organs; the "translation" of alien physical signals into familiar ones is the transmutation from external physical stimuli first into internal neural firings and then into internal phenomenal features at the phenomenal level; and the useful out-of-brain illusion somehow created inside the brain is the thing that we ordinarily call "reality": the simulation of the world with the self as the central actor. "Reality" is only the fully immersive "world simulation" that creates the telepresence experience constrained by current sensory input. For the neurobiological systems realizing the phenomenal level of organization, electromagnetic radiation of any kind or any wavelength is just darkness; the vibrations of any gas or liquid are just silence, and the physical contact of skin with objects is nothing but anesthesia. For the human brain the sensory and motor systems are nothing but a "brain-mounted three-dimensional display" connected with a whole-body "data suit" and a telepresence system which allows virtual movement to be translated into real effects in the world through voluntary muscles.

If the technological variety of VR has made it possible for us to undergo "out-of-body" experiences with telepresence robotics, Mother Nature certainly clothed us, that is, our phenomenal level of organization, with a built-in "out-of-brain" experience. Yet we are not really out of our brains in our experiences—how could we be when all the required neural machinery sits tightly there—no more than Rheingold was really out of his body in the Japanese laboratory. No, we are only virtually out of the brain and in the external world. In fact, we didn't invent the art of world simulation at all—evolution invented it for us millions of years ago. At least since the first mammals evolved, the phenomenal level came into existence in the mammalian brain and ever since has faithfully produced nature's own telepresence experiences—conscious perception—during wakefulness, and virtual presence in internally simulated environments—dreaming—during REM sleep. We have merely invented one fresh way to use and manipulate the natural VR machinery in our brain with the help of computer technology.

During wakefulness, the phenomenal level constitutes a biological telepresence system, enabling the sphere of phenomenal experience—which is what we as subjects consist of—to be virtually present in the external physical reality. The brain permits the internal organization of the phenomenal level to be modulated by the information received from remote sensors located far beyond the phenomenal level itself, on the surface of the physical body. We are virtually present in the external world because the phenomenal level that constitutes us as subjective beings is in online resonance with external objects out there in external physical space. Our direct experienced presence in the external physical world is but a massive, biologically programmed user illusion that the brain has entangled itself with.

Why is it so hard for us to become disillusioned? Obviously, for the very same reason as it was hard for humankind to grasp the fact that the Earth is not flat but round, and that the Earth is not the immobile center of the universe but instead moves around the Sun, not vice versa. Those facts just fly in the face of our naive and seemingly "direct" observations: look around you and the earth on which you stand looks flat, not round; follow the sun and you will see it changing its position gradually while the earth you stand on stays still.

VR technology has now taught us that in order to achieve effective human-computer interaction, it is necessary to hide the actual machinery from the user's view altogether. When that succeeds, the result is full immersion and the feeling of direct presence in the virtual world. Hence, we should expect that the same principle applies to the biological telepresence system in the brain: the less noticeable the interface between consciousness and the external world, and the more invisible the biological machinery required, the more seamless the resulting organism-environment interaction will be, since it is largely guided by the online model of the world in consciousness. In the interest of functionality it was necessary to hide from us the fact that the world we experience around us is actually a phenomenal telepresence model inside the brain. We take our phenomenal simulations for reality, and virtual presence for direct presence in the world. One of the main tasks of consciousness science is to break this compelling illusion for good and thereby reveal consciousness for what it is.

Summary

We examined the world-simulation metaphor of consciousness by connecting it to VR technology. Computer-produced world simulations in the brain aim at fully convincing experiences of being-in-a-simulated-world. "Presence" and "full immersion" are key concepts by which to analyze experiences of being-in-the-simulated-world. When we put together the lessons from dream research and VR technology, we end up with the idea that the brain externalizes its world simulations in such a manner that we seldom realize that we are in actual fact inside our own brains when we experience being-in-the-world. In dream experience we feel present in a world rather than seeing what our brain looks like from the inside. In perception, we feel being present in the external physical world surrounding our bodies. But even perception is just a "telepresence" experience created inside the brain, as the internal world simulation engages in real-time resonance with sensory information. This internalist conception of experience—that the world we experience is a world simulation in the brain—may be hard to accept, as it flies in the face of our naive ideas about perception and awareness. But—as Sherlock Holmes would have concluded—once we have eliminated the impossible—that consciousness could somehow break out from the confines of the brain—whatever is left, no matter how improbable or incredible, must be the truth.

7 The Philosophy of Virtual Presence

In perception and in dream experience, I find virtual objects that are directly present for me. They create the *sense of presence*—the sense that I share a common spatial and temporal framework with the objects in my presence. The idea of a spatiotemporal framework of virtual objects directly present for me—an inner world simulation in the brain—may sound like an intuitively inviting characterization of subjective consciousness.

Unfortunately, once analyzed more carefully, intuitively inviting views are usually packed with philosophical problems. The world-simulation metaphor of consciousness is no exception. On the contrary, many philosophers seem to consider such internalist approaches to consciousness much too problematic to even warrant serious discussion.

In this chapter I defend the world-simulation metaphor of consciousness and show that it is not as problematic as the bad reputation of internalism may lead us to believe. Opponents have ridiculed internalist theories of consciousness as including the problem of an infinite regress, or the problem of an internal homunculus in the brain, or the problem of a Cartesian Theater or a mental screen in the brain, and so on. The world-simulation metaphor, as we shall see, carefully avoids these traditional counterarguments.

Representative Realism

The philosophical theory of perception that underlies the world-simulation metaphor is called *representative realism.* This view holds that the external world is real and exists independently of our experiences and representations of it; that accurately perceiving an external object is to be in causal interaction with it; and that the perception is realized not by any immediate or direct contact with the external world, but indirectly via a surrogate of the external object in consciousness, directly experienced.[1]

Representative realism raises several questions that must be faced in order to find out whether this doctrine offers a plausible footing for biological realism and the world-simulation metaphor. Some of these are epistemological worries that concern the possibility and reliability of perceptual knowledge if, as representative realism holds, our access to the external world is indirect. Some are metaphysical worries that concern the fundamental nature of the virtual objects that form the phenomenal contents of experience, and the nature of the relation between the virtual objects and the perceiver (or the subject of perception).

Common objections against representative realism go along the following lines:

1. Any theory that says we directly know only the world in our consciousness easily leads to solipsism and to skepticism concerning the existence of the external world. If we have direct contact only with virtual objects and a virtual world, then perhaps there *is* no "real" world beyond my own consciousness, or at least I can never be *sure* that there is any such world.

2. Representative realism commits one to the existence of unaccountable phenomenal objects: What are such objects? What are they made of?

3. Assuming phenomenal objects somewhere inside the mind or the brain leads to infinite regression because the phenomenal objects have to be perceived by some perceiving subject or agent inside the head. Thus the theory must invoke the dreaded homunculus somewhere inside the mind or the brain, and explain how the homunculus can perceive the phenomenal objects. Perhaps it has an even smaller homunculus inside its head . . . and so on ad infinitum.

These traditional objections can be refuted without further ado with arguments that strike me as convincing. So, let us see how a defender of representative realism can reply to such objections.[2]

Epistemological Worries

Objection: Representative realism leads to solipsism and external world skepticism, because it is logically possible that no physical objects exist outside the circle of my own conscious experience, beyond the ideas or mental representatives in my consciousness.

Reply: Regardless of one's theory of perception, no one can provide an absolute logical *proof* of the existence of an external world, or of the falsity of solipsism. It is logically possible that solipsism is true, or that we all are just brains-in-vats, or that we are constantly deceived by a Cartesian evil demon. We just have to learn to live with those *logical* possibilities. This is certainly *not* to say that we should have the slightest reason to think that any of those bizarre views have any truth to them. The most reasonable scientific hypothesis for explaining the complex organization we find in our experience is that in fact there *is* an external world out there, causally modulating the structure of experience through sensory systems. For the purposes of any empirical science it is beyond reasonable doubt that the egocentric simulation of the world in consciousness, which provides me with virtual presence in the world, is, in fact, embedded in my brain which is, in fact, embedded in my flesh-and-bones body. However, it is *logically* possible that my consciousness and brain could be embedded God knows where: perhaps in the evil demon's crystal ball, or the mad scientist's laboratory. Philosophers will undoubtedly go on discussing these logical possibilities, but those more interested in contributing to the science of consciousness can focus on other issues.

Objection: OK, if the *existence* of an external world is beyond reasonable doubt, how do we know that the internal surrogate of the external world *corresponds to* the external world *as it is in itself?* The external world is only *indirectly* perceived by inference from the immediate perception of our own mental states. Perhaps the external world is something completely different which bears no relation to our sensation of it; perhaps it is in principle unknowable to us.

Reply: Our internal representation, the transparent surrogate world in consciousness, shows an immensely complex organization and internal consistency. If that coherency does *not* arise by virtue of systematic causal relations to something like the external physical world that science postulates to lie out there, then we do not have the foggiest idea how it could arise at all. Can anyone come up with a rival scientific hypothesis that is different from the far-fetched solipsistic evil demon type of logical possibility, but still would have a ghost of a chance of being true? I fear not. So, again, the most reasonable scientific hypothesis for explaining the complex regularities and coherent organization at the phenomenal level during perceptual states is to suppose that there *is* an organized external physical world out there. It is causally related to the phenomenal level and it modulates the phenomenal contents of consciousness which thereby inform us about the external world. And through these transparent surrogates, we come to *know about* the external physical world. Our sensation does bear a consistent, systematic causal relationship to the external world, and thus renders the world knowable (though it does not of course guarantee the *incorrigibility* of that knowledge).

Furthermore, perception via a representative mechanism is not as indirect as the skeptic tries to lead us to believe, for we do not in everyday perception distinguish between the (virtual) objects in our awareness and the (physical) objects in the external world. The phenomenal world and its virtual objects are wholly transparent, and in our everyday perception the nature of the external world is certainly not somehow indirectly and effortfully *inferred* from them. J.R. Smythies has often compared the way our brain comes to know the world through representative mechanisms to the way we use *external* representative mechanisms, such as television, to gain knowledge of distant external states of affairs in the world. When we watch a live broadcast of a football game on color TV, we actually *see the game,* not a complex arrangement of patterns of luminous phosphor on the TV screen on the basis of which we would have to effortfully infer what is going on in the game. The screen is, as a vehicle of analog pictorial representation, perfectly transparent for our perception. What we perceive are the events going on on the football field, not the physical events going on on our TV screen. The states of the screen *reveal* the remote events for us; they are a perceptual window to the world, not a veil cast between us and the real-world events. In a similar vein, phenomenal representations in consciousness or the transparent surrogates that constitute the world simulation in the brain *reveal* the world for us rather than hide it, and by virtue of them we may say that we have knowledge of the external world (though of course illusions and misperceptions are possible, just as various disturbances in the live broadcasting of a TV signal or malfunctions in our TV set are possible). As to our epistemic access to the external world, the skeptic tends to complain that the glass is not full but half-empty, whereas the representative realist is happy to point out that the glass is not empty but at least half-full.

J. R. Smythies (1965; see also Wright [1993]) presented a thought experiment which shows that we can make our perception even *more* indirect than it naturally is; we can imagine adding layers of representative mechanisms on the natural ones, and our perception of and epistemic access to the world in such a case remains exactly the same. The world is not lost, no matter how many veils (or, rather, transparent windows) of perception are thrown on it. The thought experiment is known by the name of "The Smythies TV-hood analogy of perception":

> Imagine that we surround the head of a young child with a television apparatus cunningly contrived that the child would never find out that it was looking always at a television screen and not 'directly' at the world. [I think that here Smythies has in mind a kind of head-mounted virtual-reality (VR) system that has a camera and a display, and it transmits a picture in real time from right in front of the viewer. VR technology was of course unheard of in 1965.] The child would learn as much about the world as any other child. And if we removed the apparatus, say after 10 years, would we then say that all the knowledge that the child obtained was false, or had to be checked, or was unjustified or suspect in any way? If this is true for one child it could be true for all. Thus we can see how sentient beings could acquire a body of knowledge about the physical world over a period of centuries under the mistaken impression that they were looking, as it were, directly 'into' the physical world. (Smythies, 1965, pp. 255–256).

The crucial point of this argument is that we can add an arbitrary number of levels of transparent representative mechanisms between external objects and consciousness, as long as the mechanisms are faithfully mediating the informational states to our sensory apparatus in real time. No "loss of the world" or loss of knowledge about the world accompanies such maneuvers. Thus, the thought experiment turns out to be a realistic possibility: perhaps in the human perceptual system there already *are* layers of natural representative mechanisms, built in by Mother Nature, without any overall loss of the external world, but instead, creating the wholly transparent sense of presence in the world (this is what I attempted to show with the story of the black planet in chapter 6). The world-simulation metaphor of consciousness is the hypothesis according to which that *is* the case, as a matter of fact. The natural representative mechanisms of our sensory systems and the brain provide us with telepresence in the world.

Objection: All right, perhaps our access to the external world can be accounted for in a satisfactory manner. But doesn't the VR metaphor imply *incorrigibility* or *infallibility* about one's own conscious states? How could we ever be wrong about phenomenal content itself?

Reply: No, incorrigibility is not implied; instead, we should be well aware of the pitfalls of introspection and retrospection. They manifest themselves in, say, empirical dream research. When I report the contents of my consciousness, the report should not be taken uncritically at face value. It is all too well-known that when we use descriptive introspection, we tend to forget, reconstruct, censor, substitute inference for observation, be vulnerable to experimental demands, and so on (for details, see chapter 2). In an introspective report, one must translate a multimodal, temporally progressing, animated phenomenal scene into a verbal, serial, description which necessarily is incomplete and inaccurate and may well be partly false.

Moreover, in order to produce a public ('heterophenomenological') version of one's current state of consciousness (a verbal introspective report), one must take a reflective stance toward the contents of one's own primary consciousness, which may in itself disturb the phenomenal contents that were supposed to be reported. In introspection, two levels of consciousness, primary and reflective, are necessarily involved (see chapter 2 for more details). The phenomenal contents of consciousness at the level of primary consciousness are what they are, and as such they cannot be either "right" or "wrong." Phenomenal consciousness as such is simply *a complex pattern of phenomenal features at the phenomenal level of organization,* and the concept of "incorrigibility" just doesn't apply to it. To ask whether the pattern of phenomenal features in my primary consciousness is incorrigible makes no more sense than asking whether the pattern of calcium in my bones is incorrigible. But the beliefs, reports, and other higher-order conscious states that express claims or judgments about the contents of primary consciousness can be more or less accurate; they certainly aren't incorrigible.[3]

Our reflective states about the contents of primary consciousness can be wholly false if we are allowed to imagine extreme conditions, such as the implantation of instantaneous false memories. Such far-fetched possibilities show why Dennett's (1976) cassette or false-memory theory of dreaming is not *logically* impossible. In a nutshell, Dennett's cassette theory of dreams suggests that dreams could be false memories, unconsciously composed during REM sleep and unconsciously implanted in short-term memory just before awakening (for more on this theory, see chapter 3).

Metaphysical Worries

As we noted above, biological realism and the world-simulation metaphor can ease the epistemological worries that might be raised against them. The world is not lost and we do not become infallible even if our perceptual access to the world is based on an indirect but transparent representative mechanism. However, perhaps the real challenge for the biological research program is metaphysical rather than epistemological. It would seem that the world-simulation metaphor is committed to several metaphysically questionable entities. It postulates the existence of a world simulation or the "phenomenal world" that is widely dreaded in philosophical circles. That world is inhabited by ontologically burdensome virtual objects or phenomenal objects. The critic will immediately raise the following questions that have been raised against every internalist theory postulating an inner phenomenal world.

What are phenomenal objects supposed to be? What are they made of—some strange nonphysical stuff or what? Are they what has been traditionally called *sense-data*? Have they been dyed with some kind of "mental paint?" How are the objects of the phenomenal world perceived? If there are internal objects, then must there not also be an internal perceptual mechanism? And *who* perceives the phenomenal world—an internal observer, the little man in the head, the infamous homunculus? Doesn't all this talk about internal objects, internal perception, and internal perceiver just lead to an infinite regress, a hopeless metaphysical slippery slope from which no internalist theory postulating the phenomenal world can be saved?

These questions surely look devastating for any theory of consciousness adopting the world simulation metaphor. Yet, I shall argue that the philosophy of presence may find a path of its own that does not lead us down these metaphysical blind alleys.

The Philosophy of Presence

To be conscious is to have the *sense of presence* in a world. The most central concept of the world-simulation metaphor of consciousness is undoubtedly that of presence or virtual presence. To have contents of consciousness is to have patterns of phenomenal experience *present*.

Consciousness as simple phenomenal "presence" can be sharply contrasted to consciousness as "awareness of." According to those who take intentionality instead of phenomenality as the basic mark of the mental, every experience is an *awareness of* some object (whether real or purely intentional); consciousness is necessarily *directed at* or is *about* that object. But the notion of presence treats *phenomenality as the mark of the mental,* and the pure existence of patterns of phenomenal features constitutes their presence. Phenomenality as bare presence is nonrelational and self-contained rather than relational and object-directed.

The concept of "presence" has deep-going, respectable philosophical roots. Unfortunately, discussions of the philosophy of presence are few and far apart these days, and most of them appear to be isolated attempts rather than business as usual in the mainstream philosophy of mind. One reason for this is the dominating status of representationalism, functionalism, and other intentional theories in the philosophy of consciousness. Since they take intentionality as the fundamental feature of the mental they are inconsistent with the philosophy of presence, which takes phenomenality as fundamental. I believe, however, that the philosophy of presence provides the biological research program with a metaphysical footing that respects the true nature of subjective consciousness.

Review of Philosophical Ideas Related to the Notion of "Presence"

In the following I explore some ideas in the philosophical literature that are closely related to my concept of "presence." Rather than argue for or against these ideas in this section, my purpose is to first explore and then gather together a set of ideas that could help to define the notion of presence.

What does it mean to be *directly present* right *here,* or for an object to be directly present *for me*? Philosophers have used the concept of "acquaintance" to denote direct awareness or direct presence (for a review, see Sajama and Vihjanen [1993]). Perception is traditionally regarded as the paradigm case of acquaintance; in perception the subject is acquainted with the object of awareness. The concept was first introduced to philosophy by the grandfather of modern consciousness research, William James:

> I know the color blue when I see it, and the flavor of pear when I taste it! . . . but about the inner nature of these facts or what makes them what they are, I can say nothing at all. I cannot impart acquaintance with them to anyone who has not already made it himself. I cannot describe them, make a blind man guess what blue is like. . . . At most, I can say to my friends, Go to certain places and act in certain ways, and those objects will probably come. (James [1890] 1950, Vol. 1, p. 221)

Two important points are implied: acquaintance with a thing provides us with *nonpropositional knowledge,* or *nonconceptual content;* content that cannot be expressed in sentences. Second, as James notes, such content cannot be communicated linguistically; its source can at best be ostensively pointed at or demonstrated to somebody who does not yet possess it. According to him, the object of acquaintance can initially be singled out by the demostratives "this" and "that." James tells us that acquaintance involves the immediate presence of an object to us, and nothing more, whereas "knowledge about" the object comes later on through an active cognitive process.

There is one point concerning acquaintance that James seems not to have been entirely correct about. He regarded the reidentification of the object of acquaintance as an essential feature of acquaintance. We now know that the discriminative capacities of our perceptual system are far greater than the corresponding abilities to conceptualize or recognize past instances of sensory experience. Hence we are fundamentally incapable of reidentifying whether the blueness of the sky today is exactly the same as it was yesterday (although if both shades of blue were present simultaneously side by side, we could tell). Is *this experience* the same as *that experience* 5 minutes ago? Beyond the limits of our rather coarse recognition abilities, we just do not know. We label a wide variety of discriminably different experiences the same if the phenomenal contents are not present simultaneously. We do not *know* what *that experience* was like! We do not even *know* what *this experience* is like, unless we can compare it online with a spectrum of other possible contents of similar experiences. Independently, Diana Raffman (1995) has taken up the same point, though not applying the concept of acquaintance. She talks about "presentation" and "presentational representations" that are more like "showing" than "telling," and whose content can only be communicated by presenting instances.

Thomas Metzinger (1998) develops the notion of presentational content. It is a nonconceptual, maximally simple form of phenomenal experience. It is realized in a dynamic process called "mental presentation." Presentational content involves temporal information: *this* is what is happening *right now.* Therefore, the activation of presentational content is associated with the mechanisms that generate the *subjective window of presence* for the system.

Thisness is a central concept for Ivan Fox (1994) who has put forward an acquaintance theory of phenomenal consciousness. According to his view, phenomenal consciousness is cognition of an object *immediately present* to the thought about it. In consciousness the particular *itself,* as opposed to phenomenal *properties* such as qualia, enters thought. By "immediate presence" he means acquaintance. The objects that enter thought are not physical objects themselves, but their mental, phenomenal surrogates, acting as virtual objects, which in all but philosophical moments are not regarded as states of mind at all, but as part of external reality. An object of acquaintance can only be referred to demonstratively as *this* or *that.* The immediacy of acquaintance comes about because the object of acquaintance is a constituent of the state of affairs in which it occurs. Thus there is something like a *part-whole relationship* between the object of acquaintance and the state realizing it.

Interestingly, Dan Lloyd (1997) also uses the concept of "presentational content" to denote the totality of one's experience of the world. Unlike representational content, which always depends on the dynamic context and external relations to it, presentational content depends only on our internal structure. To clearly distinguish the two distinct domains of presentational and representational, the study of presentational content should be construed as "methodological phenomenology" or the examination of the purely internal component of experience. Methodological phenomenology pretends that we are all brains-in-a-vat and thereby concentrates only on phenomenology and its immediately underlying neurophysiological basis. This strategy resembles the isolation and identification of the locus of control for consciousness, and the exploration of its lower-level mechanisms. The research strategy in biological realism thus conforms to the spirit of Lloyd's methodological phenomenology.

This brief exploration of the philosophical literature shows that the world-simulation metaphor and the notion of "presence" do not inhabit a philosophical vacuum. Concepts such as "acquaintance," "thisness," "mental presentation," and "presentational content" seem to be what are needed for building the philosophy of presence as the metaphysics of the biological research program on consciousness.

In the philosophy of presence, consciousness is an organized whole of transparent surrogates or virtual objects that are immediately present for us in the here-and-now of subjective experience. The organized system of transparent surrogates is what constitutes inner presence. Individual virtual objects are *parts of our being;* we are *not externally related* to virtual objects, but, rather, *our subjectivity is constituted by them.* I develop this fundamental idea further below.

The Metaphysics of Experience

If we want to have a clear and coherent metaphysical basis for the biological research program, the philosophy of presence must face the following questions: What are phenomenal objects? How are they perceived? Who carries out the act of perceiving—perhaps the infamous homunculus?

These questions already presuppose that the phenomenal level has a particular structure and embodies particular relations. But such presuppositions are based on a mistaken construal of the notions of "perception" and "object." To perceive is to have a systematic long chain of causal covariance between an external physical object or event out there in external physical space (as cause) and the state of the phenomenal level in the brain (as effect). *Accurate perception* is a causal chain establishing systematic covariance between distal external states and the experiential states at the phenomenal level. And, as I have argued above, the number of intervening causal links in the chain does not make it any less direct than it already is. The last link in the causal chain establishing accurate perception is the phenomenal level, bringing about or, rather, *being* or *constituting* perceptual *experience.* To have perceptual experience (accurate or not) is for coherent, organized patterns to come about at the phenomenal level of organization, modulated by a causal chain arising outside of it. The phenomenal level is at the *end* of the perceptual line of business: it *simulates* external reality by going into organized experiential states, providing the brain with virtual presence in the world through the simulated environment in which this presence seems to take place.

The important point is this: neither the phenomenal level as a whole nor any of its parts are somehow "perceived" themselves. That is, they do not serve as *objects* of perception in anything like the manner that external physical objects do. The true objects of perception (that is, the mind-independent, external objects of perception) reside at the opposite end of the perceptual causal chain, as its very first link. The phenomenal level incarnates the ultimate *realizer* and *presence* of perceptual experience, not the object of some *further* perceptual process or the modulator of some further state which could still be regarded as perceptual.

We should get rid of the misguided idea that the "object-perceiver" relation between an external physical object and the organism that receives perceptual information from it is somehow *duplicated* inside the phenomenal level. The virtual objects at the phenomenal level are *not* objects in the same sense as external physical objects are. The whole notion of "physical object" refers to something we (as scientific realists) assume exists *independently* of our consciousness or perception of it, and continues its existence regardless of whether anyone's conscious states represent it or not. A so-called phenomenal object naturally cannot be anything like that. Consider the analogy with the TV screen as the representative mechanism informing us about the soccer game. You can see the ball—the small, round, white circular object on the green football field. Does this mean that on your TV screen, there is a small, round, white circular *object* resembling the real ball? Is the ball you see on your TV screen also made of leather and inflated with air? Of course not. There are merely states of electrical activation of luminescent phosphor rapidly succeeding each other, none of which are remotely like the actual ball. In a similar vein, the phenomenal level realizes complex, organized patterns of activation that constitute phenomenal content instead of constructing permanent or substantial objects somehow persisting independently of those activations.

Since the phenomenal level is directly and immediately *present,* we need not (and must not) postulate any kind of mediating perceptual process whereby the subject (or the infamous homunculus) should "perceive" the phenomenal objects. We do not *perceive* phenomenal *objects* at all, we simply *experience patterns of activation* at the phenomenal level of organization. Such patterns are not solid entities ontologically similar to the external objects of perception. Perception itself is a long chain of processes of which the phenomenal level already is a part. The whole perceptual chain with an object and a perceiver cannot and need not be reproduced inside the phenomenal level. There is no bioluminescent light inside the brain emanating from phenomenal objects, and no perceptual apparatus in the phenomenal body image to receive or process the phenomenal glow supposedly emitted by such objects.

What I am driving at here is that phenomenal objects are intrinsically conscious or *self-presenting* (or composed of self-presenting features or particulars). Self-presenting features do not exist without being experienced; they are *constitutive* of experience.

This conception of experience is similar to the idea of "the given" held by C. I. Lewis ([1929]/1956). He said that the given is a *presentation* of the real (external) object; it is the immediate datum given to the mind. Stubenberg (1998) defended a similar conception of qualia as self-presenting properties—he calls them "silver-screen qualia." Qualia are like images on a silver screen: they exist only while being projected to the screen. An opposite notion, to be rejected, is "celluloid qualia," according to which qualia can exist without being experienced.

Barry Dainton's (2000) simple conception of experience follows independently along the same lines: contents of consciousness are intrinsically conscious, and therefore self-revealing or self-intimating. Phenomenal contents become conscious simply by coming into existence. He contrasts this simple conception with the traditional way of analyzing consciousness in terms of an act/object relation where an act of awareness is supposed to reach out to the contents of experience. But he concludes that awareness and content are not separate. He expresses the core idea eloquently by saying that consciousness does not consist in an *awareness of* a passing stream; instead, *consciousness is the stream itself!*

The notion of self-presenting virtual objects rejects the relational view of experience according to which the subject becomes aware of an object through some sort of mediating mental act. In *The Analysis of Matter,* Bertrand Russell (1927a) used the concept of "percept" to denote a self-presenting qualia-bearing state. A self-presenting state need not be presented to any subject or homunculus; therefore, we should get rid of the existence of the mysterious "subject" of experience altogether. Experience is *subjective,* but it is not presented *to* some intangible entity, the mythical *subject,* that would be external to the experience itself but somehow internal to the mind or brain of the individual.

Relation to Sense-Datum Theory and Adverbialism

Philosophers might try to dismiss the philosophy of presence as just some new variety of the old sense-datum theories or adverbialism, both of which are infamous for their difficulties. Therefore, let me make it clear once and for all that I reject both of them. The philosophy of presence is not a sense-datum theory or an adverbialist theory.

Sense-datum theories construe experience as involving three components (see, e.g., Foster, 2000[4]):

1. The sense-datum or the mental, *phenomenal object*
2. *Presentation* or the mental act of immediate awareness (or the acquaintance relation) directed at the mental object
3. *The subject* to whom the sense-datum is presented.

The philosophy of presence rejects this division of experience into three components. Experience is bare presence. There is no separate subject performing mental acts to reach out for phenomenal objects made of sense-data.

Adverbialism is a variety of nonrelational theory that tries to get rid of the phenomenal objects by turning the object into a modification of the subject's mental act; only the subject and its variable mental acts remain. An adverbialist theory would thus still have to assume two separate components for an experience:

1. The subject who performs the mental acts
2. The mental acts performed

This two-component theory leads to the highly contrived descriptions of our experiences: instead of saying that "I sense a red object before me," I should say that "I am *sensing redly.*" Adverbialists cannot allow talk about objects, but only about various ways and modes of sensing.

The world-simulation metaphor follows a different path, such as the one characterized by Stubenberg (1998) as *monism* and the *neutral theory of experience,* which are very close to Russelian neutral monism. According to this line of thought, the act/object distinction must be discarded. Patterns of phenomenal experience simply come about as inherently self-presenting; they are neither acts nor objects (or, if you prefer to put it in this way, they are both the act and the object at the same time). Furthermore, the patterns or bundles of phenomenal experience are not presented to a self or a subject. Instead, the subject *is* the global bundle of coinstantiated phenomenal patterns. *The subject is simply the total collection of simultaneously present phenomenal features;* it is *the totality of spatiotemporally connected phenomenality.* No entity external to the patterns of phenomenal experience and labeled "the subject" needs to be invoked.

The notion of the subject as the sum of temporally simultaneous and spatially connected phenomenality must be clearly distinguished from the notion of the self or what is more appropriately called the "virtual self." The virtual self is *the transparent surrogate of the biological organism itself* (usually located in the center of the world simulation at the phenomenal level). The virtual self is nothing more than another complex bundle of phenomenal features, in particular, ones that form the body image in the center of phenomenal space. This bundle is not special in any fundamental way: it does not carry out acts of awareness toward mental (or physical) objects, its relation to the other virtual objects that are present is not constitutive of those objects being phenomenally experienced. *The virtual self is simply one organized bundle of phenomenality among others,* and were it to disappear (as sometimes happens in dreams and out-of-body experiences) the rest of the virtual world would continue to be present for the subject (i.e., it would continue to constitute the subjective virtual world) as if nothing special would have happened.

According to the world-simulation metaphor, the subject and the (virtual) self are two different sets of patterns at the phenomenal level, connected by a part-whole relation. The subject is the phenomenal level in its entirety (the whole) whereas the self constitutes a part of that whole: the phenomenal body image and the patterns of phenomenal features located within the confines of the body image. Thus, whenever *any* patterns of phenomenality are instantiated, we may say that they are "present for the subject." "The subject" is just the total, spatiotemporally interrelated collection of self-presenting phenomenal patterns that are currently instantiated in an organism's brain. The subject is necessarily present when any patterns of phenomenaility are present, when any conscious experiences happen, but the self is present only when the special phenomenal features defining the body image and its internal patterns are present.

In the light of the above it should be quite clear now why the world-simulation metaphor is entirely distinct from relational theories of consciousness. The simulation metaphor denies that any external relations between subject, presentation, self, and phenomenal objects should be taken as constitutive of phenomenal experience. Both the so-called subject and the so-called mental objects are simply built out of self-presenting features.[5]

The Metaphysical Basis of Biological Realism

We can now follow this metaphysical path to establish the philosophical basis of biological realism. Virtual objects (or "percepts") are nothing over and above complex organized patterns and bundles of self-presenting phenomenal features. The phenomenal world, the world simulation of consciousness, as a momentary subjective reality, is the total organization of simultaneously present or coinstantiated phenomenal features; it is the complex global bundle that they make up. The global unity of consciousness is the unity constituted by all the simultaneously realized phenomenal features. Together, they form a momentary complex bundle and therefore belong to one and the same globally unified bundle, that is, to the same subject of experience.

The above characterization is an idealization (or simplification) which ignores the fact that in any experience of some duration there will also be experienced continuity. Thus, it would be more accurate to say that the world simulation of consciousness is not only the total organization of momentarily coinstantiated phenomenal features but a *dynamic phenomenotemporal pattern* that consists of an experienced *flow* or *succession* of phenomenal content (Dainton, 2000, p. 180).

One of the principal components of this global bundle is the virtual self. It forms the "center" of experiential space, thanks to the constant activation of the bundle of phenomenal features that constitute bodily awareness, or the virtual body. Although there is more to the self than bodily awareness alone—we have an abstract self-conception that includes semantic and episodic knowledge about our personal history, our future goals, our personality, and so on—the virtual self of immediate bodily awareness is the basic phenomenal entity that we primarily identify ourselves with. It creates the sense of "*I*-am-here-now"; "this is *my* presence in a world"; "this is what it is like to be *me* right now." To create this fundamental self-experience, there need be no access to semantic and episodic knowledge or to a persisting self-conception.

Even in the dream world, I feel that *I* am present there, because there is the virtual self of bodily awareness in the center of the dream world, from whose perspective the dream world is experienced. The dream self has only limited access to long-term memory: it does not remember how it got there in the middle of the dream scene; it may even totally forget who it is, or believe that it is an entirely different person than the dreamer actually is in the waking world. Regardless, the dreamer, after waking up, will describe such a dream by saying, "Isn't it peculiar—*I* was a different person in the dream." The experience of being "me," of myself being present in a world, is not constituted by access to particular pieces of episodic or semantic knowledge about a particular person. The dream world is built from the perspective of the virtual self, and whatever kind of bundle of phenomenal features there is in the center, that is where *I* am and who *I* am in the dream.

Following Thomas Metzinger (2000, 2003) we could say that we constantly confuse ourselves with the phenomenal *model* of the self (or, in my terminology, the *virtual* self). It seems that Metzinger has grasped correctly the consequences of this view when he says that "the conscious self is an illusion which is *no one's* illusion" (2000, p. 301). Indeed, there is no hidden *real* "subject" or *real* "self" concealed somewhere in the mind or the brain; nor is there the mythical homunculus somewhere observing the events in the phenomenal world. No, there are only the self-presenting bundles of phenomenal properties that make up the phenomenal body image. Access from the phenomenal level to episodic and semantic information may be missing, limited, or distorted, but whatever it is, the basic experience of me being there is not dependent on that.

According to this analysis, to *have* a percept or a quale is for that quale to be a part of the complex bundle of phenomenal features realized at that moment (Stubenberg, 1998). A phenomenal feature is "had" by "the subject" when the feature forms a part of the momentary phenomenal world; a part of the totality of simultaneously present or coinstantiated phenomenal features that together constitute the self-presenting subjective reality. The "having" of the relational theory of experience boils down to "being a part of" in the nonrelational, monistic account of experience.

What is the *substance* that phenomenal features are features of? If all the phenomenal features are stripped away, there seems to be nothing left at all, at least phenomenally. Therefore, we should deny the existence of *mental* objects or entities (including mental space) that are supposed to *bear* the phenomenal features. No such mental objects exist, contrary to what the traditional sense-datum theories postulated. The bundles of qualities are all that are needed; no superfluous mental objects should be posited.

The phenomenal features themselves, however, must be somehow grounded in the nonphenomenal domain. A hypothesis that is consistent with biological realism and the multilevel explanatory strategy could be like this: At the lower level of organization, there are nonexperiential entities that function as the realization base of phenomenal features. The phenomenal features and the organized bundles they form, the virtual objects, do not themselves reside at that level but at a higher one. The phenomenal level of organization is a system of self-presenting phenomenal features. This higher level of organization is realized in the brain by some lower-level neurobiological and electrophysiological phenomena whose precise nature remains to be discovered by experimental research on the direct neural correlates (or rather constituents) of consciousness. Thus, it is the task of empirical research to discover the phenomenal level in the brain, and to figure out what the immediately underlying lower-level phenomena are. Like discovering the double helix structure of DNA, it is simply outside of the domain of armchair philosophy.

The postulation of organized patterns of self-presenting phenomenal features is not in conflict with the mechanistic explanatory program, even though such entities are not a part of current neuroscience. The history of scientific explanation shows that the entities and activities that are acceptable change with time:

> At different historical moments, in different fields, different mechanisms, entities, and activities have been discovered and accepted. The set of types of entities and activities so far discovered likely is not complete. Further development in science will lead to the discovery of additional ones (Machamer et al., 2000, p. 15).

If in neuroscience consciousness is to be taken seriously as the phenomenal level of organization in the brain, then self-presenting phenomenal features will have to be taken seriously as well.

Summary

I have now thrown into the cauldron the philosophical ideas that seem appropriate for and in harmony with biological realism on consciousness (this is not to say that all of these ideas would be directly *entailed* by the basic commitments of biological realism). Let me summarize briefly what the metaphysical blend is composed of. I ended up with a nonrelational monistic theory of experience with the help of which it is possible to get rid of a number of metaphysical nuisances: the elusive subject, the mysterious phenomenal objects, and the mental act of the subject (or the infamous homunculus) somehow "grasping" the phenomenal objects through internal awareness or perception. Instead of these widely dreaded metaphysical traps, I endorse a much simpler account regarding the basis of phenomenal consciousness. There are self-presenting phenomenal features that constitute the phenomenal level of organization in the brain. They make up every phenomenal entity that surfaces at that level; everything that my conscious life as a subject consists of—the entire sphere of subjective experience. In short, they constitute me as a conscious subject. My body image or the phenomenal self-model is built out of these features, too; so are all the surrounding virtual objects, as well as the entire world simulation that I find outspreading all around my body image whenever I am conscious at all.

I believe that this metaphysical blend is not quite as bad as the rather vile concoctions offered by the opponents of internalism or biological realism. Although none of the available philosophical alternatives are going to be easy to swallow, I find the philosophy of presence the least intolerable option.

8 Paths Not Taken: Contemporary Alternatives to Biological Realism

Biological realism and the world-simulation metaphor represent only one possible approach to the explanation of consciousness among a number of other lines of thought in contemporary approaches to the study of consciousness. So far I have mentioned some of the alternative approaches only in passing, but in this chapter they will be at the focus of enquiry.

The views discussed in this chapter can be regarded as contemporary alternatives to biological realism for the following reasons:

1. All of them have been put forward specifically as theories or explanations of consciousness.
2. All of them are explicit about their philosophical commitments, so it is possible to point out in a straightforward manner how they differ from biological realism.
3. All of them have been put forward and defended recently during the brief history of multidisciplinary consciousness studies (roughly, after 1990).

The review is not exhaustive—there are many more alternatives than those covered in this chapter. I believe, however, that the ones mentioned here are the major alternatives that have been recently defended and vigorously discussed in the literature. General philosophical theories concerning the classical mind-body problem (such as functionalism, interactionist dualism, reductive and emergent materialism) will not be reviewed here. They have already been covered thoroughly in a number of introductory textbooks, and I have nothing new to say about them. I am more interested in exposing the *specific* claims made by *specific* recent theories of consciousness, and evaluating the plausibility or acceptability of those claims from the viewpoint of biological realism. I will try to be as explicit as I can to lay open what the crucial differences are between biological realism and these views.

My impression is that scientists without philosophical training often have a hard time trying to understand why philosophers say what they say about consciousness. To understand that, one should understand what the underlying philosophical worldview is that is being defended. Thus, I hope to clarify, especially for the reader who is not a professional philosopher, what kinds of philosophical views about consciousness are on offer these days, and why they make the philosophical commitments they do. Without such a basic understanding it would be difficult to determine where one wants to stand, philosophically, in the study of consciousness. As our philosophical commitments tend to guide the empirical science we make, the commitments concerning consciousness will ultimately guide the empirical science of consciousness.

This chapter necessarily delves rather deeply into philosophical issues and concepts. Some of them may be alien to the empirical scientist, but I will explain them as clearly and simply as possible without compromising accuracy. I start off by describing some of the deepest philosophical commitments of biological realism, and then proceed to review and analyze a number of competing theories.

Biological Realism and the Reality and Place of Phenomenal Consciousness

Perhaps the most fundamental question for any approach to explaining consciousness concerns the existence and reality of subjective phenomenal consciousness. Biological realism takes phenomenal consciousness as the basic explanandum for the science of consciousness and thus accepts the following realist thesis:

Subjective phenomenal consciousness exists.

This expresses the ontological commitment to *realism* about the phenomenal realm in its most general form, a form that even dualists and idealists would be happy to embrace. But I want to distance myself from them and therefore I also accept a stricter thesis which basically says that consciousness is part of the physical universe rather than some otherworldly domain:

Subjective phenomenal consciousness exists in physical space and time.

A pattern of phenomenal features, say the dream image from which I suddenly wake up, existed somewhere in the physical universe, came into existence at some point in the history of the physical universe, and disappeared at some later point. There is a *where* and a *when* for each and every bundle of phenomenal features.

If phenomenal consciousness exists in space and time, a research program must specify in more detail the spatiotemporal regions in which consciousness is to be found. Biological realism locates consciousness within the confines of the brain. According to biological realism, if the neural realizing basis of consciousness comes about, then the phenomenal level of organization, consciousness, is necessarily realized as well. Consciousness supervenes on the internal biological entities and events in the brain: nothing but those are required to bring consciousness into existence. The causal or logical relations of the crucial events in the brain to other phenomena external to the brain are inconsequential as to whether consciousness itself exists. Consciousness is ontologically dependent only on its lower-level mechanisms, not on anything external to that microlevel basis.

Therefore, according to biological realism, consciousness would be realized also in the following imaginary cases (drawn from Strawson [1994]):

1. *Brains-in-a-vat* A fully functional brain, even in complete isolation from normal sensory and motor connections, could in principle have the phenomenal level of organization realized inside it, given that some form of artificial or internal stimulation is provided (say, similar to the internal activation during REM sleep and dreaming).

This thought experiment strips away all the causal connections between the brain and the reality outside the brain. The thought experiment of brains-in-a-vat becomes much more feasible if we remind ourselves that, during REM sleep, we in fact turn out to be brains in a natural biological vat! REM sleep effectively realizes this sort of an isolated but internally activated brain, and we know for a fact that the phenomenal level is realized during REM sleep.

Imagine that NASA should find out that there is an alien starship on the dark side of the moon, full of incomprehensibly advanced technology and, among other things, a huge storage of brains-in-vats (abducted mostly from America during the latter part of the twentieth century). The abducted brains are kept in a state reminiscent of constant REM sleep. The close relatives of the victims would bombard NASA with the questions: *But does that mean that they are dead or alive? Are they conscious or are they gone? Do they still feel something? Can they still think? Do the persons we once knew and loved still exist?* If the NASA scientists were to rely on biological realism, they would have to conclude that all those people are still alive, and all of them still enjoy more or less normal conscious experiences, although the world where each one of them lives is just a massive hallucination inside the brain. But in actual fact they are no less and no more detached from our shared world than each and every one of us is during REM sleep and dreaming every night.

2. *Instant people* They are physiologically fully normal people who suddenly came into existence 5 minutes ago by cosmic coincidence or by the feats of a powerful demon. They are not products of a long history of evolution or individual development.

Imagine that aboard the alien mother ship on the dark side of the moon we find a device that can build physiologically complete and fully functional adult humans, given only sufficient amounts of the basic elements that a human body consists of. Note that the brains of the instant people would resemble the mature adult brain, and even the long-term memory systems would be equipped with manufactured memory traces or false memories. If we ourselves should have come into existence only 5 minutes ago, the experiential content we have right now would be just the same, regardless of whether any such past believed by us ever existed.

Biological realism holds that instant people are capable of having subjective experiences in just the same sense as you or I, although we do have both an evolutionary and an individual social history behind us, while our instant friends do not. This thought experiment strips away all causal connections to evolutionary history, or to a history of social or physical interaction with an external reality, as logically necessary conditions for the presence of purely experiential content. It distinguishes the phenomenon itself from the long backward-looking etiological pathways (ontogeny, phylogeny) and shows that the phenomenon itself can in principle be dissociated from any particular etiological pathway leading to it.

3. *Instant brains-in-a-vat* This case is merely a combination of (1) and (2): we can at the same time strip away both causal relations to external stimuli and causal relations to evolutionary or individual history, and imagine a perfect duplicate of a fully functional brain, created 5 minutes ago. If you believe that consciousness has a physical basis in the brain, that consciousness supervenes on brain states, and that any physical thing is potentially perfectly duplicable, then you must admit that an instant brain-in-a-vat must have a phenomenal level of organization if all the microlevels of organization have been perfectly duplicated in the process.

There are several philosophical positions that deny biological realism; some of them deny phenomenal consciousness altogether, or at least locate it elsewhere in the world, wholly or partly outside the brain. Many of these theories also deny that consciousness supervenes on the brain, and consequently the in-principle possibility of brains-in-a-vat is rejected as well.

If these ideas are dismissed, what is offered in their stead? That is what we will try to figure out in the rest of this chapter.

Antirealism about Phenomenal Consciousness

The clearest example of an approach that flatly denies the reality of phenomenal consciousness is Daniel Dennett's philosophy. In his ontology, there are only "judgings" or "takings" in the brain, expressed in introspective verbal reports, but no actual qualitative phenomenology (in Dennett's language, there are no "real seemings").

> There is no such thing as really seeming—over and above the phenomenon of judging in one way or another that something is the case. . . . But what about the actual phenomenology? There is no such thing. . . . *There seems to be phenomenology.* . . . But it does not follow from this undeniable, universally attested fact that there *really is* phenomenology. (Dennett 1991, pp. 364–366)

Dennett's philosophy shows many other features that are in line with antirealism about phenomenal consciousness: he denies that there is any important difference between humans and (behavioral) zombies, and he further denies the existence of the qualitative properties of experience (or qualia). Dennett (1991) also goes to considerable lengths in arguing that there cannot be any such thing as a definable space and time ("the where and the when of consciousness") in which the content of consciousness is determinate and subjectively present. In some of his earlier writings, he has even tried to cast doubt on the idea that dreams are subjective experiences occurring during sleep. (But as discussed in chapter 3, his position is rather difficult to defend in the light of the results of modern dream research.)[1]

The reason for this skepticism about the existence of the internal world derives from the fact that Dennett tries to avoid committing himself to the first-person point of view in the science of consciousness. He firmly sticks to the third-person point of view of the physical sciences and consequently resists the temptation to postulate inner phenomenal entities in the brain, because such things cannot be objectivey observed from the third-person point of view. The study of consciousness, for him, is the study of objective behavioral patterns and measurable patterns of brain activity. Furthermore, an important part of the study of consciousness is the interpretation of the recordable verbal behaviors and texts produced by subjects (what Dennett calls "heterophenomenology"). The existence of these data can be objectively observed and verified from the third person point of view, whereas the existence of a phenomenal world inside the brain is, for Dennett, merely an unacceptable, speculative metaphysical hypothesis.

This strategy leads him to deny (or misconstrue) the principal explanandum of consciousness research: phenomenal consciousness, the internal world-for-me. As that world does not exist as a pattern of behavior or brain activity whose existence could be objectively verified from the third-person point of view of the physical sciences, therefore it does not exist anywhere inside or outside the brain as far as science is concerned. For Dennett, the world-for-me is merely a fictional world, the Middle Earth of the brain that is nowhere to be found in actual reality.

Biological realism holds that phenomenal consciousness exists and is located within the confines of the brain; thus, it rejects all forms of antirealism about phenomenal consciousness, including Dennett's. To grant the reality of the internal world-for-me may be metaphysically somewhat adventurous, but to deny its existence seems just absurd.

The Sensorimotor Theory of Consciousness

Kevin O'Regan and Alva Noë (2001) have recently put forward a detailed and much-discussed theory that mostly concentrates on visual consciousness. They call it the sensorimotor theory of visual consciousness.

The position of O'Regan and Noë (2001) is closely related to Dennett's views, but they take care not to deny the reality of phenomenology directly. They do deny, however, that experiences are states or events or occurences that have qualitative properties—thus, like Dennett, they deny the classical philosophical idea of qualia. In their view, experiences are "ways of acting" or "something we do" (p. 960), and the qualitative features of experience are aspects of this activity. Vision, they say, is the mastery of sensorimotor contingencies, and the subset of the contingencies or rules being currently exercised constitutes what you are seeing.

My understanding of their theory of visual consciousness is that they deny phenomenal consciousness, and they preserve a different concept of consciousness that is devoid of phenomenality. Their concept of consciousness is based on action or behavioral interaction, and it is this peculiar action-based notion of consciousness that they regard as the principal explanandum for consciousness research. In any case they are rather explicit about rejecting phenomenal consciousness and qualia:

> Rather, we argue, as should by now be clear, that the concept of phenomenal consciousness must be (and can be) rejected, and so there is no longer any puzzle about how to explain that. . . . [O]ther aspects of consciousness can indeed be explained according to our view. (p. 963)

> Although we reject accounts of phenomenal consciousness as a property of subpersonal states, we do not deny that there are experiences and that there are facts about what experiences are like. But these . . . are not facts about a person's qualia . . . They pertain, rather, to the person's . . . active engagement with the world he . . . inhabits. They are facts at the personal (as opposed to subpersonal) level. (p. 965)

They seem to locate consciousness outside the brain, and deny that experience would be produced by brain activity (see also Noë & Thompson, 2004a[2]):

> An important advantage of this view is that it allows us to escape from the problem of having to explain how brain activity could give rise to experience. We escape from the problem because we propose that experience does *not* derive from brain activity. (p. 968)

In brief, their fundamental commitments differ from mine in the following respects: I take phenomenal consciousness as the most important and the most essential form of consciousness; they deny its existence. I take subjective experience to be located at some subpersonal, biological level inside the brain; they deny that and propose that consciousness only exists at the higher, personal, and behavioral levels. I take the search for the neural correlates of consciousness (NCC) in the brain as a crucially important empirical project to be undertaken in consciousness research; they argue that the search for the NCC is a philosophically misguided project, doomed to failure for philosophical reasons.

This list exposes the rather profound disagreements between biological realism and the sensorimotor theory of consciousness. Due to the wildly dissimilar background assumptions, biological realism excludes the sensorimotor theory of consciousness, and vice versa.

Radical Embodiment of Consciousness

Another avenue to the view that consciousness is not in the brain goes through the currently popular ideas in cognitive science that cognition is "embodied" and that cognitive science should be "enactive." The claim in this approach is that "the processes crucial for consciousness cut across the brain-body-world divisions, rather than being limited to neural events in the head" . . . "consciousness depends crucially on the manner in which brain dynamics are embedded in the somatic and environmental context of the animal's life, and therefore there may be no such thing as a minimal internal neural correlate whose intrinsic properties are sufficient to produce conscious experience" (Thompson & Varela, 2001, pp. 422, 425).

This "radical embodiment" approach leaves it uncomfortably unclear where exactly the explanandum of consciousness science is supposed to be located. All we get from the supporters of this view is a vague idea of the complex, mutually embedded systems of brain, body, and environment which (they say) cannot be said to be internally or externally located with respect to one another (Thompson & Varela, 2001). This makes one wonder how obscurity about the spatial location of not only consciousness but the whole brain, the body, and the environment in relation to each other is supposed to be an advance in clarifying the explanation of consciousness. On the contrary, it seems to lead us into an even deeper mess.

I fear that the radical embodiment theory of consciousness confuses the internal spatial relations and locations *within* the phenomenal level with those of the external physical counterparts of the phenomenal entities. This suspicion is strengthened by the arguments that have recently been put forward to deny that experience could even in principle be an internal property of neural systems. Noë and Thompson (2004b) argue that a visual experience presents how things are *in relation to oneself* and in relation to one's potential movements in the surrounding world. They believe that no neural system could be the "bearer of this sort of content"; only a whole perceiver as an intentional agent could.

But as the data from dream experiences show, we now know for a fact that *some* system strictly confined to the brain *can* present experiences where perceptual objects are related to oneself in exactly the same manner as in conscious visual perception. What Noë and Thompson probably have failed to appreciate is the fact that the "oneself" in relation to which the other contents of consciousness are presented in subjective experience is *not the physical organism* but the phenomenal body image (or the "virtual self").

The phenomenal level contains the phenomenal body and the surrounding phenomenal world, and in that sense consciousness surely is inherently embodied and embedded in an environment. But all of that has nothing to do with the location of any physical events external to the brain. Unless that point is made crystal clear, the very location of consciousness itself is easily confused with the locations of those external bodily and environmental entities with which consciousness happens to be in intimate, real-time interaction during wakefulness.

Biological realism by no means denies that the phenomenal level has tight interactive loops with the brain, body, and environment. But no matter how tight the interaction may be, it cannot magically transport the phenomenal level out of the brain. In specific conditions (such as REM sleep), the interactive loops can be carved off entirely while the full sphere of subjective experience still remains inside the brain. Any plausible theory of consciousness must clearly differentiate the location of those things with which consciousness is in tight causal interaction from the location of consciousness itself. The radical embodiment view fails to do so.

Intentional Accounts of Consciousness: Representationalism and Content Externalism

In philosophy one of the principal reasons for resistance to biological realism and internalism about consciousness is the belief that *intentionality,* not phenomenality (or consciousness), is the most fundamental feature of the mind. The phenomenological school in philosophy has traditionally claimed that there is a conceptual or necessary relationship between consciousness and intentionality (Gillet & McMillan, 2001). "Intentionality" was understood by Edmund Husserl to be the unique peculiarity of experiences to be the consciousness *of* something. The influence of Husserl's ideas are still widespread in the philosophy of mind, also outside the phenomenological tradition. A number of current philosophical theories of consciousness seem to take intentionality as their starting point. In one way or another, they are based on the idea that there is a necessary relationship between consciousness and intentionality; therefore consciousness always is consciousness *of* something. In other words, whenever we are conscious of anything, there must be a mental act of consciousness directed at its object.

The widespread acceptance of intentionality as the basis of mind has led to intentional theories of consciousness, many of which also nowadays appear under the label of representationalism.[3]

All intentional theories differ from biological realism in at least the following respects: First, they take intentionality or intentional mental states as fundamental to the mental realm, and phenomenality as only derivative from them. Second, because of their commitment to the doctrine of intentionality, they construe phenomenal states as inherently bipolar or essentially *relational.* Awareness is always awareness *of* some object. Every psychological experience contains an intentional object toward which the awareness is directed. Fundamental to mentality is a subject-object relation; object-directedness or aboutness. The object involved in the relation need not really exist; it can be a mere intentional object.

By contrast, biological realism holds that *phenomenality is the fundamental form of mentality.* Genuine intentional mental states (perception, belief, etc.) are only possible if there is first a phenomenal mind that can realize organized patterns and bundles of phenomenal features, say in visual awareness, in mental images, in inner speech, and so on. Only conscious creatures have genuine beliefs, percepts, or thoughts, because such mental states are tied to the first-person subjective viewpoint. Take away the conscious mind and you take away the subject in whose phenomenal and reflective consciousness the beliefs, percepts, or thoughts occur. Zombies or systems devoid of phenomenal states are also devoid of intentional mental states, because there is no subject there in whose consciousness a belief could be entertained or a percept realized. External observers may erroneously attribute intentional mental states to nonconscious zombies, applying the Dennettian "intentional stance" to the interpretation of the behavior of the system, just as we attribute mental states to our computers or toy robots. Zombies may "process information," "represent the environment," or engage in "organism-environment interaction," but none of this nonconscious physical activity has anything to do with genuine intentional mental states.[4]

According to biological realism phenomenal experience need not necessarily involve any *intentional objects* toward which something mental is *directed.* Phenomenal experience consists in patterns of phenomenal features at the phenomenal level of organization; those patterns themselves are the phenomenal content of experience. The phenomenal patterns simply *are;* they are not necessarily *directed toward* something external to themselves; they are not objects (either intentional or physical); they are temporary bundles or patterns of phenomenal features. If experience in addition to its phenomenal content, also has intentional content, the latter is dependent on the former.

Modern intentional theories of consciousness usually replace talk about mental acts and intentional objects with talk about representations and their vehicle-content relations. A representation has a *vehicle* (that which represents) and a *content* (that which is represented), and the relation between the two is intentional (again, in the philosophical, not in the everyday sense of the word): the vehicle *refers to,* or *is about,* or *reliably indicates the presence of,* or *covaries with,* the content. According to representationalist theories of consciousness, phenomenality is secondary to and derives from intentionality and representation; phenomenal consciousness is constituted by the existence of the intentional or representational relation.

Intentional theories can be divided into two broad categories: externalist and internalist theories. Most of the current intentional theories of consciousness are externalist. The externalist-representationalist answer to the localization problem (where is consciousness located in the natural world?) is ambiguous. It might be something like the following:

> Well, the neural *vehicles* of conscious mental phenomena are, of course, in the brain, but the *contents* of consciousness are out there in the external world. Therefore, consciousness does not reside in the brain. You cannot find the contents of consciousness within the brain, because they are not there. The neural vehicles that are in the brain in no way resemble the contents of consciousness. In fact, any neural state of the brain may be the vehicle of any content of consciousness as long as the state of the neural vehicle (e.g., its spiking frequency) reliably indicates, or covaries with, the presence of the content in the sensory environment. Thus, we should not search for consciousness in the brain, because we would be looking in the wrong place.

When intentional theories talk about the "content" of consciousness, they are using a philosophical notion of "content" which is "intentional content," "semantic content," or "representational content." In this context, "content" means something *external* to the physical entity (the vehicle) that has or carries the content (it could mean such things as "reference," "reliable indication of," or "causal covariation with"). This usage is the first step in the external localization of consciousness. According to externalist theories of content, the contents of consciousness do not reside within the mind or the brain (where the vehicles of representation are), but in the causal or logical relations that obtain between external physical objects and the mind/brain.[5]

Representationalists sometimes manage to be explicit about their peculiar solution to the localization problem. Fred Dretske (1995) asserts that

> A better understanding of the mind is not to be obtained by knowledge—no matter how detailed and precise—of the biological machinery by which the mind does its job. (p. xiv)

Michael Tye (1995) is even clearer about this when he says the following:

> The lesson is . . . that phenomenology ain't in the head. Just as you cannot read semantics out of syntax, so you cannot read phenomenology out of physiology. This is why you cannot find any technicolor qualia, any raw feels, by peering around inside the brain . . . . They simply are not in there. To discover what it's like, you need to look outside the head to what the brain states represent. Phenomenology is, in this way, externally based. . . . systems that are internally physically identical do not have to be phenomenally identical. (p. 151).

The above views are only intelligible if we keep in mind that for the externalist, phenomenology is identified with representational content. But for biological realism, phenomenology is phenomenal content, and phenomenal content is included in what for the representationalist is only the vehicle of representation. For the representationalist, then, biological realism would be a *vehicle theory* of consciousness.

Representationalist theories of consciousness are not compatible with the basic assumptions of biological realism about consciousness. When talking about the contents of consciousness, the externalist philosopher is not talking about that which is literally contained within the phenomenal level of organization in the brain; about patterns of phenomenal experience. Just as Dennett and O'Regan and Noë use the concept of "consciousness" to refer to something other than phenomenal consciousness (and then go on to "explain" their notion of consciousness as organism-environment interaction, sensorimotor contingencies, and the like), representationalists use the concept of "contents of consciousness" to refer to something other than internal patterns or bundles of phenomenal experience contained within the sphere of consciousness. And then they go on to "explain" their notion of the contents of consciousness by referring to brain-world relations.

Theories that exorcise consciousness from the head with such conceptual sleight of hand usually cheerfully conclude that no explanatory gap exists: the problem of explaining consciousness has been solved. I doubt that explaining consciousness is going to be quite that easy. What the theories in actual fact have done is first eliminated inner phenomenality and then explained something else. The disagreement between biological realism and externalism is thus not only about the internal vs. external *location* of the explanandum (consciousness), but also about the basic *nature* of the explanandum.

One conspicuous difference between representationalist theories and biological realism concerns the question of what we should expect to find in the brain when we try to explain consciousness. According to biological realism, since consciousness is a biological level of organization in the brain, it follows that the structure of neurobiological phenomena, at some higher level of physiological organization and description, corresponds to the structure of the phenomenal level or consciousness itself. Thus, for example, a visual experience consisting of complex organized patterns of form and color necessarily implies a phenomenon of corresponding complexity and organization in the brain. By contrast, in representationalism the structure or complexity of a representational vehicle in the brain need not in any way reflect the structure or complexity of the represenational content in consciousness (Lloyd, 1997). A very simple vehicle (e.g., the firing rate of a single neuron) could, in principle (and perhaps also in practice), reliably indicate the presence of a complex visual scene and therefore constitute its representational vehicle. Hence, for externalist representationalism there is nothing in the brain that could explain the content of consciousness. In the brain, there are only neural representational vehicles that correlate with the presence of external stimulus objects that constitute the true contents of consciousness.

Neurophenomenology

In consciousness studies the research program called "neurophenomenology" is associated with the work of the late Francisco Varela and his intellectual legacy. This research program attempts to combine, as the name suggests, aspects of phenomenology (the school of thought in philosophy following Brentano and Husserl), especially first-person descriptions of lived experience, with modern neuroscience and "embodied cognition."

The tradition of phenomenological thought is much too complex to be discussed in any detail here. Let me just try to summarize some basic ideas and commitments that separate neurophenomenology from biological realism. The ideas about the structure of mind and consciousness in neurophenomenology are firmly based on Husserlian phenomenology. Hence, intentionality or object-directedness is also here regarded as the mark of the mental. This further involves a commitment to the act-object structure of consciousness. In Husserlian terms, experience involves not simply awareness of its objects (or "noema") but tacit awareness of itself as mental act or process (or "noesis") (Lutz & Thompson, 2003). In any instance of conscious experience, an act (of awareness) must reach out to some (intentional) objects.

The philosophy of presence adopted by biological realism posits that consciousness consists of patterns of phenomenal features as such; no acts of awareness or objects to be reached out by such acts are needed. This seems like a fundamental disagreement between these two approaches.

Neurophenomenology further involves a theory of how phenomenality in its basic form comes about. The most elemental form of phenomenality is believed to be *reflexive consciousness* or a *primitive, nonintrospective form of self-consciousness.* Reflexive consciousness is a primitive form of self-awareness believed to belong inherently to *any* conscious experience: any experience, in addition to intending (referring to) its intentional object is reflexively manifest to itself (Lutz & Thompson, 2003).

According to biological realism, simple phenomenal presence is the most basic form of consciousness. Higher-order, reflective, or self-aware forms of consciousness, are dependent on the basic forms of phenomenality. Underlying phenomenality are nonconscious neurophysiological mechanisms, not complex forms of mental phenomena, such as any kinds of reflexive or self-aware states. These states postulated by neurophenomenology as the basis of consciousness are empirically problematic, for they are not accessible introspectively (so there can be no *psychological* evidence about their existence), and I cannot see how their existence could be empirically tested by neuroscience either.

Biological realism thus differs from neurophenomenology in some fundamental commitments about the basic structure of consciousness—simple presence vs. act-object structure—and about the basic form of consciousness—immediate presence of phenomenal features vs. primitive reflexive or self-conscious states.[6] Yet, biological realism and neurophenomenology share the interest in phenomenal data and systematic phenomenological description of subjective experience, and the project of combining the phenomenal data with the neuroscientific data, but the differences in their fundamental commitments may render their theoretical integration difficult.

HOT Theories of Consciousness

The term *HOT* refers to *h*igher-*o*rder *t*hought theories of consciousness. Like representationalism and neurophenomenology, HOT theories take intentional mental states as primary and try to derive phenomenal states from them.

HOT theorists view consciousness along the following lines. Mental states are either conscious states or unconscious states. For our mental state to be a conscious state we must be conscious *of* the mental state or we must be aware *of* the state. Thus, conscious mental states are mental states of which one is conscious.[7]

What renders an otherwise unconscious mental state a conscious mental state is that it falls under the scope of an inner awareness. This higher-level inner sense or higher-order inner thought takes the unconscious mental state as an object and thereby transforms it into a conscious mental state. For me to have the conscious mental state of seeing X, for example, means that I am aware that I am seeing X or I am conscious that I am seeing X. According to this logic, then, "seeing X" as such is not yet a conscious mental state if I am not at the same time *aware of* seeing X.

The general idea behind HOT theories thus appears to be that there are first nonconscious, sensory (mental) states ("seeing X" as such). Only when a nonconscious higher-order intentional mental state or thought takes the first-order sensory states as an *object* and generates the awareness *that* "I am seeing X," does phenomenal consciousness result.

It is not entirely clear how the unconscious first-order mental states differ from the conscious mental states.[8] Either the unconscious state (the "seeing X" as such) already possesses all its phenomenal features, or they are brought about only when the spotlight of awareness falls on the unconscious state. If the phenomenal features exist all along, then it is difficult to see what the difference between the conscious and unconscious states consists in. If the unconscious states already possess all the experiential features, what do we need the "awareness of" for? The first-order mental state appears to be equipped with all it needs to be a phenomenal state, which makes the postulation of an extra process of awareness superfluous.

In the context of biological realism and the philosophy of presence, the notion of a state that is at the same time phenomenal and unconscious is incoherent. It would amount to the state possessing nonphenomenal phenomenality, which is, of course, nonsense. Thus, genuinely unconscious mental states cannot possess any phenomenal features. If this conclusion is granted, the only coherent alternative that is left for a HOT theorist is to claim that somehow the spotlight of higher awareness brings about phenomenal features in the first-order states it falls upon.

The question that then arises is, How exactly does the touch of higher awareness turn nonphenomenal states into phenomenal states? What evidence do we have that a higher awareness is really at play here? As the higher-order thoughts and the "awareness of" are themselves totally nonconscious mental entities, we cannot have any direct phenomenological evidence, any subjective data, concerning their existence or operation. To show that such things exist at all must thus be done by using objective empirical data.

One possibility would be to assign nonconscious mental states to someone on the basis of external behavior and its functional role (this is what Gennaro [1996] suggests). In that case, we simply decide that functionally adaptive behavior is "mental" by definition. We do not thereby *discover* that the internal causes of such behavior have some special mental features, we simply use as the basis of HOT theory our folk-psychological ability to externally attribute mentality to any adaptive behavior. This strategy boils down to using Dennett's (1987) "intentional stance" and treating mentality as an observer-relative, behaviorally based feature. This move might be acceptable for someone who has a prior commitment to metaphysical functionalism as a theory of mind, but not for someone who treats mentality as an intrinsic biological rather than an observer-relative behavioral feature. Biological realism therefore rejects purely externally based attribution as an adequate basis for the existence of nonconscious mental states.

If behavioral data cannot be used as an objective basis for establishing the mentality of nonconscious internal states, perhaps neurophysiological data can. But it seems that their mentality could not be objectively tested or demonstrated by any kind of neurophysiological measurement either. How could it be empirically shown that some neurophysiological activity detected by, say, EEG is in fact a nonconscious higher-order thought or an unfelt awareness directed at a nonconscious first-order state, as opposed to being just a nonconscious, purely neurophysiological state? On what basis can we rule out that some other electrophysiological activities do not also constitute unconscious mental states? How could we tell apart those neurophysiological responses that are nothing over and above purely neurophysiological activity from those that are in fact higher-order unconscious mental states or processes? Of course, we can *interpret* some neurophysiological activity as being an "unconscious mental state" by simply labeling it as such. But any interpretation like that would have to be based on the prior acceptance of HOT theory rather than forced upon us by the neurophysiological data alone.

Therefore, if the nonconscious mental states postulated by HOT theories have neither any subjective phenomenal nor any objective neurophysiological reality to them, it is not clear what the empirical grounds for postulating such states at all are supposed to be.

HOT theories create many further problems: Are animals devoid of higher-order thoughts, and therefore nonconscious creatures, zombies? If they are zombies, do they perhaps enjoy unconscious experiences nonetheless? Furthermore, it is possible to construct convincing counterexamples where phenomenality results in the absence of higher-order thoughts, or fails to result in its presence (Siewert, 1998).

There is a lively debate going on about the merits and the problems of HOT theories. However, I shall not go into those discussions in more detail. HOT theories include fundamental assumptions concerning the nature of consciousness that are very different from biological realism. They build phenomenality on the complex interplay of unconscious or nonconscious mental states, whereas biological realism builds phenomenality on the complex interplay of nonconscious neurophysiological processes that are totally devoid of mentality.[9]

In biological realism the notion of "reflective consciousness" (see chapter 2 for a definition) and the interplay between primary and reflective consciousness, also involving selective attention, might easily incorporate most of the ideas on the basis of which HOT theories may seem intuitively plausible. Reflective consciousness, by engaging selective attentional mechanisms, takes the contents of primary consciousness as objects. But the contents of primary consciousness involve phenomenality *before* reflective thought touches them; their phenomenality is in no way dependent on them being the objects of thought. Unlike in HOT theories, in biological realism reflective consciousness is *secondary* to phenomenality, not *constitutive* of it.

Incidentally, the dream researcher David Foulkes in his book *Children's Dreaming and the Development of Consciousness* (1999), adopts a notion of consciousness as a "self-reflective act," and cites HOT theories as lending philosophical support for the notion. Consequently, this philosophical background assumption leads him to deny that children under the age of 5 years and all nonhuman animals dream, or that they are conscious even in the waking state. He does not accept the notion of nonreflective, purely phenomenal consciousness; thus, there cannot be phenomenal dreams of which one is not conscious of:

> One counterproposal . . . is that maybe dream imagery is present all along, even in infancy, but children aren't yet consciously aware of it. Well, if there is imagery, there has to be conscious awareness, because you have to be consciously aware of something for it to be "imagery." And, if there are supposed to be narrative simulations of which the person is not consciously aware, then they can't be "dreaming," since dreaming necessarily implies consciousness (awareness of a mental state). (p. 120)

As this passage makes clear, bare phenomenality (such as "imagery") in the absence of an "*awareness of* a mental state" is just not conceivable for a HOT theorist. Foulkes's theory of dreaming vividly exposes the decisive role of one's philosophical background assumptions in guiding a research program. In his worldview, children and animals are nonconscious zombies deviod of dream life or waking consciousness. This in turn leads him to the view that the functions of dreaming "cannot have anything to do with elementary tasks of biological and social adaptation" (p. 138). By contrast, biological realism sees children and (many) animals as phenomenally conscious both during wakefulness and REM sleep, and tries to identify the biologically adaptive functions of dreaming and consciousness (see chapter 24).

Direct Realism: Are Colors in the World or in the Brain?

Direct realism is primarily a philosophical theory about perception, but it has some straightforward implications also for the explanation of consciousness.[10] Direct realism holds, as its name suggests, that we have experience of objects out in the world directly. Thus, when we see colors, for example, that seem to be out there on the surfaces of objects, the direct realist says that then we are in direct touch with some physical property residing in the physical object. He denies the contrary view, that the colors we experience would be psychological properties generated inside the brain.

Direct realism has had influential supporters in modern philosophy of mind (e.g., Armstrong, 1961) and in the psychology of vision (Gibson, 1979). However, it seems that the modern science of color vision rejects direct realism. In a leading textbook called *Vision Science,* Palmer (1999) explicitly states that colors are not in the world but in the head:

> Neither objects nor lights are actually "colored" in anything like the way we experience them. Rather, color is a *psychological* property of our visual experiences when we look at objects or lights, not a *physical* property of those objects or lights. (p. 95)

Yet Ross (2001) has recently defended a direct realist theory of colors, which he calls "color realism." He claims that the colors we experience are really the external physical properties of the surfaces of objects out there in the world: colors are located on the surfaces of external physical objects. This theory illustrates the problems associated with direct realism (see Revonsuo [2001b]).

One trouble for the direct color realist is that there is no well-defined physical property to be found in the physical objects out in the world that would correspond to different instances of the experience of the *same* color. "In general, merely from perceiving something to be red, you cannot say anything about its physical constitution or its mode of production of the 'red' light. Your perception of it as red is not the detection of some property characteristic of it. . . . Two things can look the same color and be producing completely different spectra of light" (R. J. Hall, 1996, p. S126). Thus, the external physical properties that constitute a certain color have no intrinsic feature in common by virtue of which they should constitute the color. The only thing they do have in common is relative to the states they can causally bring about in the human sensory system: two surfaces that cause experiences of the same color may share no property specifiable independently of the fact those two surfaces happen to affect our sensory systems in the same way (Clark, 1996, p. S148).

The usual solution to this problem is to claim that colors are wildly *disjunctive* physical properties, and the terms of the disjunction are specified in relation to their effects on the human visual system. The color red, for example, thus becomes the disjunction of all those heterogeneous physical properties that happen to *cause* red experiences in the human visual system. Such an infinetely long, artificially constructed disjunction hardly qualifies as a genuine "physical property" which we are supposed to directly grasp when we enjoy the visual experience of the color red.

The lack of unique external physical causes for color experiences can, however, be accommodated by biological realism: The phenomenal quality "red" is a psychological property of experiences, and it resides only at the phenomenal level in the brain. There are, however, a multitude (perhaps an infinite amount) of different possible immediate etiological pathways, originating in different types of external physical conditions, that could lead to the realization of "red" at the phenomenal level. From the biological realist's point of view, direct realism confuses the *causal origin* of color experience (which *is* physically heterogeneous) with the *experience itself* (which has a unique constitutive basis inside the brain).

Another difficult problem for color realism is the prediction derived from it that colors would spread to new physical objects in the external physical world if these physical objects, in interaction with our sensory system, should start to produce color experiences in us. Such a situation could conceivably come about if a genetic mutation affecting human color vision were to spread in the population. A condition called *synesthesia* (see chapter 12) in fact presents a situation where phenomenal color experiences are produced by atypical causes. For a synesthetic, sounds, tastes, or other sensory stimuli may be experienced as inherently colored. If all of us suddenly became synesthetic, many physical phenomena that are not colored now would, according to the direct color realist, suddenly be so. In the physical world outside the brain absolutely nothing has changed, yet external physical objects that were not colored before humankind became synesthetic are now colored. Where did those colors suddenly come from if not the brain, and where are they supposed to be located if not in the brain?

The problems of direct color realism do not end here. The color realist would also have to explain how the perceiver gets *access* to the colors that are out there in physical space, far beyond the brain and the body. The only thing that the perceiving organism can have any access to outside the brain is the pattern of stimulation in the retina (the proximal stimulus field). According to color realism, however, colors are constituted by a process called "perceptual access" which is supposed to run mysteriously backward on the causal chain from the phenomenal and neural states in the brain to the (wildly heterogeneous) physical conditions in the distal stimulus field where the physical colors themselves are deemed to reside. This maneuver is carried out in order to exorcise phenomenal colors from the mind-brain and locate them in the external physical world, and thereby provide direct access to the physical world through perception.

The color realist's idea of perceptual access is inconsistent with the facts of perception, but the inconsistency is hidden under an ambiguous and confused concept of "the visual field" in direct realism. The direct realist identifies the visual field with the physical objects (or their surfaces) and light sources out there in the external world. But once this identification is made, it becomes impossible to give a coherent causal account of perception. When a person visually perceives something, the correct scientific description includes at least the following (J. Smythies, 1996): (1) The external or distal stimulus field (the physical objects and surfaces that reflect light and other external light sources); (2) the retinal image or the proximal stimulus field; and (3) the events in the brain that give rise to subjective visual awareness or the phenomenal visual field. But direct realism does not make these distinctions, which leads to a confused view of how perception is supposed to work. Direct color realism holds that phenomenal qualities are physical properties of the external physical objects perceived. But given the causal theory of perception, how could that be the case? The external stimulus field is ontologically distinct from and causally antecedent to the phenomenal visual field, and yet direct realism incorrectly identifies the two. No coherent account of perception can hold that the *input* to the visual system (distal physical stimuli) *is identical with its output* (subjective visual awareness) (J. Smythies, 1996). Direct color realism confuses the explanandum (phenomenal color experiences) with (certain parts of) the etiological, backward-looking pathway that describes the chain of events that led to the phenomenon to be explained.

Furthermore, color realism is in difficulties in coming to terms with the fact that there are colors in dreams. The dreaming brain shows us that colors can be totally dissociated from all external physical objects and from all of their physical properties, as well as from neural processing of visual input at the retina and in the visual pathway. As is shown by the vivid colors in our dreams—and even in the dreams of adventitiously blind people, who do not have any perceptual access to anything visual anymore—colors can exist and they do exist even in the complete absence of external physical objects and in the complete absence of any neural processing of visual input. Those things cannot be necessary for (and even less can they be identical with) color.

The failing of direct realism to make the fundamental distinction between the *external causes* and the *internal constituents* of consciousness is reminiscent of the confusion in the history of biology when theorists failed to make a clear distinction between the *genotype* and the *phenotype,* but somehow treated these as one and the same phenomenon (Mayr, 1982). Theoretical progress in genetics became possible only after this confusion was resolved. My prediction is that no significant theoretical progress can be made in the scientific understanding of consciousness unless the internal/external confusions included in direct realism are left behind for good.

Panpsychism

Panpsychism (or panexperientialism) is the view that phenomenality is a fundamental feature of the physical universe and therefore consciousness is widely distributed everywhere.[11] Consciousness or some primitive form of it is a fundamental building block of the world; thus, there is no need to explain how consciousness *arises* from nonconscious components or lower-level phenomena; consciousness is already involved at the microphysical levels. One specific theory (Chalmers, 1996) proposes that all physical *information* has a conscious aspect; whenever an information state is realized physically, the corresponding phenomenal state is realized as well. (For a recent defense of panpsychism, see also Lehar [2003a].)

Panpsychism disagrees with biological realism about the location of consciousness in the physical world. According to panpsychism, consciousness is just about everywhere: in rocks, trees, electrons, toasters, tennis rackets, protein molecules, toilet paper; you name it! The brain is not a special phenomenal engine. Of course there has to be *something* different about the brain (it may, say, combine or amplify the already existing bits of phenomenality in a novel way), but it is far from being the only seat of phenomenality in the world.

Since panpsychism points to fundamental physical levels and forces as on a par with phenomenality, its supporters are often interested in fundamental physical theories such as quantum physics rather than neuroscience. If consciousness exists in its basic form already at the level of elementary particles or fundamental physical forces, then perhaps that is where we should look for the features of consciousness. Some features of the quantum world may be seen as resembling significant features of consciousness and mind. If consciousness is a fundamentally unified phenomenon, perhaps this is because it is based on quantum coherence or entanglement or instantaneous action-at-a-distance: perhaps these could be the quantum mechanisms of consciousness. If we have a truly free conscious will, perhaps it is based on the fundamental indeterminacy found at the quantum level.

Panpsychism and biological realism have in common the view that phenomenal consciousness exists and that it is the basic form of mentality. They seem to agree about the nature of the explanandum. But, obviously, they disagree about the location of phenomenality in the world: Does it exist only in the brain or just about everywhere? They also point toward different empirical investigations as the most central: panpsychists try to find a place for phenomenality in fundamental physical theories and in all sorts of even very simple physical systems, whereas biological realists confine their search for phenomenality within biological organisms and the brain.

According to panpsychism there is no *radical* discontinuity between any physical systems as to the possession of consciousness; it is just a matter of degree (Revonsuo, 2003a). Everything is more or less conscious; simple physical systems to a lesser degree, the human brain perhaps to the highest possible degree. This smooth continuum of consciousness across all physical entities is supposed to have the following explanatory strengths: (1) Consciousness is a *fundamental* property of physical matter and therefore need not be explained in terms of (nonconscious) physical matter (or anything else physical); (2) there is no radical conscious/nonconscious dichotomy to be found anywhere in the natural order (in phylogeny or ontogeny, for example).

Panpsychism raises some severe problems. There are clear, well-demonstrated dichotomies between the presence and the absence of the state of consciousness (caused by anesthesia, epileptic seizures, fainting, and coma) and between the presence and absence of particular contents of consciousness even though the stimuli are implicitly processed (as in blindsight or neglect). Any theory of consciousness should be able to explain these radical subjective differences between the presence and absence of consciousness. The panpsychist is, however, forced to say that these are not really cases where the presence and total absence of consciousness in the brain could be strictly contrasted. The contrast is only between *primitive* and *more sophisticated forms* of consciousness. The idea that simple physical systems only display very elementary forms of consciousness is called *protopanpsychism.* According to the protopanpsychist the primitive form may be something so simple that we would hardly recognize it as consciousness at all. Thus, what we thought was the total absence of experience is actually the presence of a primitive form of experience; we just cannot recognize it as experience.

Unfortunately this move will not help us to understand the radical contrast between the presence and absence of conscious experience in the above cases. Regarding everything as conscious (to some degree) does not remove the radical conscious/nonconscious contrasts. In fact it leads to a position as difficult (but the exact opposite) as the eliminativist position defended by Dennett. If we take either the panexperientialist position that phenomenal consciousness is *everywhere* in the world, or the eliminative position that it is *nowhere,* we are no closer to explaining the radical empirical differences that we want to understand.

Furthermore, protopanpsychism smacks of a misuse of the concept of experience. It is difficult to see why the postulated "primitive form" of consciousness—which we might not even *recognize* as experience—should be placed in the same category as our vivid phenomenal experiences. There seems to be no clear idea what such "protoconsciousness" could be, whether it exists at all, or how the claims for its existence could be empirically tested or theoretically modeled, and how exactly the primitive form of consciousness relates to our ordinary vivid phenomenal consciousness.

Hence I do not regard panexperientialism as a wise metaphysical commitment for a research program on consciousness. I would rather postulate that the sphere of subjective experience only exists at particular levels of biological organization, and in those creatures whose brains can realize such levels. Otherwise the physical universe is devoid of phenomenal consciousness. When we totally lose consciousness, as we do during general anesthesia, for example, our brain is temporarily incapable of supporting the phenomenal level. No lesser forms of phenomenality remain: our brain is in a totally nonconscious state.

Physical matter at lower levels of organization perhaps may be said to contain the *potentiality* of being conscious, but only in the weak sense in which all physical matter contains the *potentiality* to be alive. The mere potentiality does not make simple physical systems (say carbon atoms or diamonds) alive, and it would be a waste of time to study the microphysical structure of diamonds in order to understand the biology of living systems. In a similar vein, I fear that the assumption that all physical systems (diamonds, toothbrushes, bacteria, and so on) are conscious (or "protoconscious") is going to be a useless, untestable hypothesis for the science of consciousness.

Protoconsciousness seems to be comparable with "ether," the invisible form of matter that was once believed to fill all physical space (Revonsuo, 2003a). The idea of a vacuum devoid of physical matter was unimaginable. Perhaps the idea of a "phenomenal vacuum" or the total absence of conscious experience is equally difficult to accept, at least for panpsychists. But while there were genuine empirical phenomena that the ether models tried to account for, there seem to be no phenomena (either nonconscious physical or conscious phenomena) that the phenomenal ether of panexperientialism accounts for. Furthermore, as far as we know there *are* total phenomenal vacuums, total absences of phenomenal experience, and we should not try to fill them by postulating a phenomenal ether that pervades all physical matter. Instead, our theories of consciousness should explain the definitive differences, both phenomenal and biological, between the total presence and the total absence of consciousness in the brain.

Projection Theory and the Reflexive Model

Projection theory is an attempt to make sense of the transparency of consciousness. The intuitive logic behind projection theories is approximately the following: the mind (or the brain) produces the qualitative features of our experiences. However, we experience the qualities not as spatially located in the mind or the brain, but out there in the world: pains and tickles located in parts of our bodies, colors located in distal external objects. How do they get out there? There must be some sort of *projection* going on, which transmits the qualities from their original source (mind/brain) to where they are experienced (in the external objects of the world). The projection theory seems to lead to the curious view that the results of sensory processing somehow get projected back out of the brain to be superimposed on the external world.

Max Velmans (1996) has recently advocated this sort of theory. He recognizes the need to identify the locus of control for consciousness when he says that "in order to learn *what* something is, it is useful in the initial instance to know *where* it is, so that one can point to it. . . . But where does one point, when one is pointing at consciousness?" (p. 183). Velmans argues that, in order to decide where consciousness is, one has to attend to its actual phenomenology. Thus, if you stick a pin in your finger, you experience the pain in your finger: "The pain one experiences is in the finger. If one had to point at it one should point at where the pin went in" (p. 184). In his view, which he calls "the reflexive model," experiences are where we experience them to be, and there is no other or second experience of pain in the brain or anywhere else. Velmans agrees that there is information about the pain in the finger encoded in a mental model realized by a brain state, but the mental model is not identical with the experience.

A puzzle for this view, as Velmans admits, is the question, If the neural causes and correlates of pain are in the brain, *how does the resulting experience get to be in the finger?* Velmans says that a psychological (as opposed to a physical) process of "perceptual projection" takes place and results in conscious experience. The experience is "projected" in the sense that from the perspective of the subject, it is located in the phenomenal space beyond the brain, rather than in the region of its neural causes or correlates. However, this projection should not be understood as a mechanism that actually broadcasts something somewhere; it is rather a description of the subjective effect itself. The central notion of his theory, "perceptual projection," remains somewhat obscure: it refers not to a physical, but a *psychological* process, he explains, and yet he says that "psychological processes may, in part, *be* physical processes" (p. 194).

Velmans treats the first- and the third-person views as complementary, and he distinguishes two meanings of "physical": the phenomenal physical (roughly, the experiential and externalized world that is located outside of your perceived body; the simulated world that naive realism treats as the physical world, directly perceived) and the physical world as described by physics. He also believes that the phenomenal world is a biologically evolved representation of the world as described by physics. He does not disagree with the view that the entire sphere of phenomenal experience—our own bodies and all externalized objects included—is a construct of the brain.

Perhaps the only point about which I disagree with him is this: Velmans denies that there is *any* sense in which the sphere of phenomenal experience is actually located *in* the brain. According to him only the proximal causes and direct correlates of conscious phenomenology are in the brain, but the subjective effects—consciousness *itself*—are not. He says that "one can safely conclude . . . that although a neural encoding of the world is within the brain, the phenomenal world is outside the brain" (Velmans, 2003, p. 429).

As far as I can tell, Velmans does not tell us *where* in the world as described by physics the sphere of phenomenal experience is located, if it is *not* located in the brain. Perhaps the question does not make sense for him; or perhaps it presupposes the (for him unacceptable) idea that the third-person point of view is ontologically primary and the first-person point of view has to be located *somewhere* within it. Be that as it may, in the case of the location of consciousness we just agree to disagree. In many other respects our views are very close to each other.

One reason why a projection mechanism might be invoked may be the naive realist view of the transparency of conscious states. Since it seems so obvious that the pain is in my finger and not in my brain or that the red traffic light is out there and not in here, then the experiences just *have to be* somehow projected outward from the brain, even if we have no idea how this is done. The spatiality of experience is mistaken for the spatiality of the world as described by physics, directly perceived (however, I do not think that Velmans commits this mistake). But if we turn again to our model system, the dreaming brain, it becomes obvious that the transparency of conscious states should not be interpreted as showing that experiences somehow mysteriously reach out from the brain to a space beyond. Consider the following dream experiences of pain in dreams (reported by A. L. Zadra, Nielsen, & Donderi, 1998a):

> I'm listening to a colleague and I begin to scratch my left forearm. Its itchy and it burns. I look at my left arm and I see that I have many "pimples." I try not to scratch my arm but it's really burning [41-year-old woman]. (p. 158)

There is a painful sensation in this dream, clearly located in the left forearm. The subject could look at and point to the location of the pain within the dream: Where is she looking and pointing? Certainly not to her left forearm of flesh and bones, which was probably lying entirely paralyzed on the bed. The location of the pain is defined purely at the phenomenal level of organization which remains in its entirety within the brain. The flesh-and-bones body need not necessarily have anything to do with the experience and location of the pain, as in the following example, where an excruciating pain only exists at the phenomenal level and evaporates completely as the phenomenal level becomes connected with its waking perceptual input:

> I dreamt that I had been in a train crash. Most people had died and I was stuck in an unknown wooded area. The woods are really thick and I couldn't find a path. A group of "primitive" people (loincloths, painted faces) start yelling at me. They grab me and tie me down to the ground with my hands above my head. One of the men takes this long spear with a metal arrow on its end and holds it over my chest. I'm really scared that they're going to kill me. I start to plead with them but then he plunges into my rib cage and begins to twist. I scream in pain and beg them to stop. The pain is just excruciating and I try to wiggle around but it doesn't help. The man just keeps on twisting and pushing in further. I can't stand it anymore and beg them just to kill me but they won't. My wife then woke me up saying that I was making moaning and grunting noises. *When I woke up I was surprised and relieved to note that the pain, which had been absolutely horrible, had completely disappeared* [28-year-old man]. (A. L. Zadra et al. 1998b)

Where, according to the projectivist theory, is the pain located in this case? We know for a fact that dreams take place within the brain (where else could they be?). Therefore, all the phenomenal contents of the dream—including the body image of the dream self and the pain located in that body—have to be inside the brain. The transparency or externalization of experience is a trick pulled on us by the phenomenal level of organization: the irresistible out-of-brain illusion. We should not fall for it and wonder in bewilderment how all those experiences get out from the brain, because they do not and there is no way they could or reason why they should get out of the brain. If we take seriously the evidence from dreaming, then we can become disillusioned and begin to see the transparency of consciousness for what it is: nature's conjuring trick, not, as it is naively supposed to be, our direct access to the external physical world or the brain's projection miraculously cast out and superimposed on the world outside the brain.

As far as I know, no version of the projection theory exists that would give a clear and plausible account of the nature of the projection mechanism, or of the location of consciousness in the physical world, once the content of consciousness has been projected somewhere out of the brain.

How to Solve the Location Paradox without Miraculous Projection?

The phenomenal level is a reality of its own, and talk about the "location" of various experiences only refers to the *internal* organization of this level. Thus, pains and other bodily sensations are experienced at various locations of the phenomenal body image. Objects are experienced as located outside the phenomenal body image. Thoughts are experienced as located inside the head of the phenomenal body image, and so on. This whole phenomenal system itself, however, is realized by and located within the confines of the brain, as empirical evidence from dreaming shows.

Objects, pains, and thoughts retain their relative location within this phenomenal system even in dreams, although online causal connections with the world external to the brain are temporarily severed. The experience of pain is located *in the finger of the phenomenal body image,* not in the physical finger of flesh and bones, where the *distal cause* of the pain may be located. There is no paradox involved; it is just that the notion "in the finger" is ambiguous as to whether it refers to the phenomenal body image or to the flesh-and-bones biological body part. There are two entirely different coordinate systems in which we could locate the referent of the everyday concept "my finger." As long as one does not realize this, there is no hope of construing a coherent story of the location of conscious experiences in the physical world.

The fact that the phenomenal level is the brain's model or simulation of the world is effectively hidden from subjective experience. It does not look like a model; it looks like a world. That is why we do not *experience* the world to be in our head; it would simply make a disastrously poor model of the world for the brain. At the phenomenal level, *we have no experience whatsoever of our brain* (as an internal organ within the biological head). Consequently, we do not have (and could not have) any idea of what it *would* feel like to experience something to be inside the brain. One's own phenomenal body image simply does not include any phenomenal content that could be thought of as a brain. Hence it could not include any experience that is located "inside" the brain, for at the phenomenal level *there is no phenomenal image of the brain for an experience to be located in.* This is just another reminder of the fact that the phenomenal body image is not identical with the biological body.

If on the basis of purely phenomenal content we have no idea what kind of experiences should be counted as occurring inside the brain, then neither do we have any idea what kind of experiences should be counted as *not* being inside the brain. *The structure of purely experiential content does not reveal its own location* (or the location of its realizing ground) *in the wider context of physical space.* The structure of purely experiential content cannot really be used as an argument against the empirical scientific hypothesis that, as a matter of fact, the phenomenal level resides in and is brought about by processes going on entirely in the brain.

Phenomenalism

I will consider one further example of philosophically motivated resistance to locating consciousness in the brain that also has gained some support recently. Phenomenalism takes patterns of subjective experience (sensations) as basic and given, and casts doubts on whether physical objects are anything else but sequences of actual and possible patterns of phenomenal experience. Perhaps physical objects are not concrete entities inhabiting an independent, unperceived world when conscious beings are not present. Perhaps the only concrete entities and activities that exist are just organized sequences and patterns of subjective experience, but behind them there is no imperceptible physical world of the kind that science suggests. Whitehead ([1925] 1997), in this spirit, criticized the conception that physical matter is something with a simple location in space and time. He calls this the "fallacy of misplaced concreteness," meaning that we mistake the abstract for the concrete. The conception of the universe as composed of configurations of soundless and colorless bits of matter forever hurrying about is merely a figment of our imagination in our effort to make the abstract mathematical and physical theories concrete. The paradoxes of trying to fit mind into a system of matter only arises because we have mistaken an abstraction for a concrete reality.

In this view the core of the explanatory gap can be traced back to the external physical world: consciousness should not be located inside the brain because *there may be no such concrete material object as the brain.* In a phenomenalist spirit, Hut and Shepard (1996) suggest that we start with subjective experience instead of an "objective reality," for the latter is only an inference whereas the former is indubitably given. According to this view, the biggest mystery is no longer consciousness, but the objective physical world, which is never directly experienced but only inferred on the basis of order and correlations within subjective experience. Therefore, consciousness should not be thought of as located in the brain because the brain is merely an inferred, abstract physical system that might not even exist.

> As for regularities and correlations, that are often interpreted as pointing to the brain as the seat of consciousness, we can think of many other explanatory avenues. After all, effectively jamming the printer does not "prove" that computer processing takes place in the printer heads; nor does switching channels on a TV "prove" that the information in the channels is produced inside the TV set. This is not to suggest that the "source" of experience is outside the brain, in some other physical location; rather, the whole notion of a source that is reducible to spatio-temporal-physical terms is something we question. . . . we should no longer speak of conscious experience as taking place "in the head" or "in the brain." (pp. 317–318)

Hut and Shepard are prepared to give up scientific realism about physical reality, and opt for some sort of phenomenalism (or perhaps even idealism). They do not deny the possible existence of a world behind the phenomena we directly experience, but they treat any notions about such a world as hypotheses that are useful to the extent that they predict and explain the regularities in our experience. That sounds like an instrumentalist or phenomenalist interpretation of science.[12]

Giving up the realist interpretation of science to explain consciousness is a high price to pay. After all, the whole point of a scientific research program on consciousness is that we wish to be able to understand how subjective consciousness as a real mental phenomenon is possible in the equally real "objective" physical reality, as revealed by natural science. We would like to understand the connection between the two realities: our undeniable, subjective psychological reality, and the reality described by the natural sciences. Elimination, crude reduction, or instrumentalist interpretation of one or the other of these realities equals changing the original rules, for then there are no more two realities to be related to each other: one of the realities has simply been dismissed as an illusion or a mere abstract hypothesis.

I am not prepared to give up either of the two realities: there really is an external physical world, and there really is phenomenal experience. If you deny the reality of one or the other, you have not solved the problem of consciousness; you have given up on it. Biological realism is realism not only about subjective phenomenal experience but also about the entities postulated by the best available scientific theories; therefore, it is a variety of scientific realism (see Niiniluoto [2002]).

Summary

The current wave of interest in consciousness has produced a wide variety of philosophical approaches to the study of consciousness. In philosophy, internalism and biological realism are minority positions. Therefore, it is important to know what the mainstream philosophical views are currently, and how exactly do they differ from the views advocated by biological realism. First, there are a group of views that simply deny the existence of phenomenal consciousness (Dennett, O'Regan, Noë). It goes without saying that such views differ radically from biological realism. Second, there are a variety of views that do not deny phenomenal consciousness, but that locate it (or its contents) outside the brain. Many of these views construe consciousness as derivative from intentionality, and regard object-directedness, or an "act-object" or "vehicle-content" structure as the fundamental feature of consciousness, and of all mental states in general (representationalism, neurophenomenology). By contrast, biological realism takes simple phenomenality as fundamental and denies that phenomenal consciousness in any way depends on, or should be analyzed in terms of, intentionality. Some other views that locate consciousness outside the brain seem to confuse the spatial organization of phenomenal experience with the spatial organization of the external physical world (radical embodiment, direct realism, projection theory). They point out that we experience phenomenal features and objects as out there in the world and therefore they come to the conclusion that experiences cannot be located inside the brain. All in all, a review of the current philosophical approaches to consciousness reveals that biological realism and the philosophy of presence offer a novel philosophical footing for the science of consciousness that might transcend the current confusion about the basic nature and place of consciousness.

III The Phenomenal Level

In parts I and II the cornerstones of the biological research program were laid: biological realism and the world-simulation metaphor. In part III, we explore the *internal* structure and organization of phenomenal consciousness in more detail to get an accurate picture of the phenomenal level on its own terms.

9 The Virtual Space around Us

This chapter deals primarily with the *experience of space:* the phenomenal space that we see and feel all around us. The chapter opens with a general description of "empirical phenomenology," the attempt to establish systematic, empirically based descriptions of the phenomenal level. Then it proceeds to describe one of the most fundamental features of phenomenal experience: spatiality. The idea that all experience has at least *some* spatial features is first put forward, then its implications are explored, and finally it is defended against counterarguments. In the world-simulation metaphor of consciousness, the virtual space in which all experiences take place forms a bridge between nonconscious biological mechanisms and phenomenal consciousness.

Phenomenology as an Empirical Inquiry

The term *phenomenology* is usually associated with the philosophical study of experience, and particularly with the Brentano-Husserl tradition in continental philosophy. But as the science of consciousness is an *empirical* science rather than a philosophical exercise, it requires guidelines as to the empirical study of subjective experience; it requires an empirically based phenomenology. I suggest that the principal goals of *empirical phenomenology* be outlined as follows:

1. Empirical phenomenology involves systematic description of the *normal* contents, structure, organization, dynamics, and unity of the phenomenal level. The "normal" contents are those that predominate in the *baseline state* of consciousness (as it was defined in chapter 2).

2. Empirical phenomenology also involves the systematic description of *pathological* or otherwise *anomalous* distortion or breakdown of the contents, structure, organization, dynamics, and unity of the phenomenal level. The "abnormal" contents of consciousness are those that appear in *altered states* of consciousness (for a definition of altered states, see chapter 2).

A theoretical model of the phenomenal level should be able to accommodate the actually observed cases of distorted or altered phenomenology reported in neuropsychology, dream research, and other relevant sources of phenomenological description. Furthermore, on the basis of the model we should be able to *predict* the scope and the limits of *possible* cases of anomalous phenomenological organization that in principle may be found.

First, a provisional model of the *normal* structure of the phenomenal level is required. Subsequently this description can be applied to describe and explain the anomalous cases where phenomenal organization is disrupted or somehow distorted. The anomalous phenomenal organization can then be used to constrain the original model and to propose mechanisms and principles possibly underlying the integration of the phenomenal level.

A similar modeling strategy is widely used in cognitive neuropsychology (Ellis & Young, 1988), where functional models of the cognitive architecture of mind are applied in the description and explanation of normal and pathological cases. This strategy has proved to be very fruitful in that domain. I see no reason why the same approach would not work in consciousness research, if all the empirical findings are related to one unifying theoretical framework.

Anomalous phenomenal organization is often a result of some nonpathological altered state of consciousness (such as dreaming, meditation, or hypnosis) or the result of some pathological process in the brain: organic injury to brain tissue (such as those underlying visual agnosias), the transient disturbance of electrophysiological phenomena in the brain (such as those that bring about experiential epileptic auras, or those caused by the direct electrical stimulation of cortex), or changes at the neurochemical level (drugs, hallucinogens).

There may be significant differences between *reversible* and *irreversible* forms of altered consciousness. The *transient,* completely reversible distortions take place in the absence of any structural damage to brain tissue. *Permanent* phenomenal distortion takes place only when nonreversible tissue damage has occurred. One of the goals of empirical phenomenology is to figure out what these differences are. The temporary distortions possible in transient nonpathological states of consciousness reveal the *flexibility* of the phenomenal level and its underlying mechanisms. In altered states of consciousness a range of variations and recombinations are possible in the patterns of experience. The alterations in the phenomenal contents of consciousness take place in the absence of any permanent structural changes in the neurons or synapses at the lower levels of organization. Reversible altered states of consciousness show that *even when the configuration of the neural hardware remains relatively constant, radical changes can occur at the phenomenal level.* The permanent distortions that are only possible once the structure of the system at the neural level has irreversibly changed give insights into the contribution of the underlying mechanisms which have been damaged. Their contribution should have something to do with those aspects of phenomenal content and organization that have been lost due to the damage.

The multilevel approach includes the assumption that phenomenal organization is (at least to some extent) *decomposable:* it consists of features or parts or subsystems which are largely independent of each other and can therefore be dissociated from each other. A dissociable part or feature of phenomenal organization can be temporarily missing or even permanently abolished without hindering the rest of the phenomenal level from being realized, even if without that feature or part. Moreover, the remains of the phenomenal world are assumed to retain their original organization.

Hence a kind of subtraction logic can be used to analyze the composition of the phenomenal level: whatever feature or part that can be selectively abolished from the phenomenal level, the rest being left much as it was, must have a realizing basis largely independent of the other features. By distinguishing dissociable features and parts of the phenomenal level in this way, we make it more tractable for empirical modeling. Subsequently, the independent features of the phenomenal level may each be investigated separately. The task is to understand how each of the features is normally generated and seamlessly integrated into the whole.

I call this idea the *decomposability hypothesis* of the phenomenal level. It will be applied to several aspects of dream experience in the following chapters.

Phenomenal Spatiality

The rest of this chapter deals not with the decomposable parts of the phenomenal level, but rather with what *unifies* the phenomenal level as a whole: phenomenal space. Phenomenal experience has several features: quality, intensity, location, and duration (as discussed in chapter 2). But if we think about the phenomenal level as an entire simulated world, then perhaps the most pervading global feature of the world of consciousness is its all-embracing *spatiality.*

Spatiality in Visual Experience

Qualitative differences are not the only ones we can make at the phenomenal level: we can also discriminate phenomenal features from each other on the basis of their *spatial location* within the phenomenal field (Clark, 2000). Colored surfaces always lie in a particular direction and at a particular distance in relation to the center of perceptual space. We can discriminate two visual objects from each other purely on the basis of their distance, even if they have identical color and fill the same visual angle. Also sounds are localized at particular directions and distances. Our discriminative powers show that there is a phenomenal feature corresponding to depth (Clark, 1993). Sensory experiences are located at particular regions in the simulated world and they have a *voluminous character.* Every sensory modality presents phenomenal features that have at least *some* spatial characteristics (such as location, shape, or depth)— the qualities appear as if spread out in space, filling a volume (Clark, 2000). Furthermore, all phenomenal events take place within what is experienced as being a *single* spatial volume. This *singularity* of virtual space is the reason why we find ourselves in the center of exactly *one* world, although this world can contain a multitude of different virtual objects and phenomenal qualities.

Spatiality in Other Sensory Modalities

Also the phenomenal body image is a spatial entity; I experience my body as filling a volume, and the space it fills is a part of the same space where the visual objects I see around me are embedded. Some of the visual objects around me are associated with sounds. The auditory qualia are experienced as if coming from the same place where the objects are located in visual space. Both auditory and visual qualities thus seem to inhabit the very same space. The chirping of the bird in the tree, the sound of the alarm clock on the desk, the hum of the bumblebee in the flower: the experience of these sounds is not only an experience of auditory phenomenal features but an experience of those features at specific locations within the single spatial volume that constitutes the whole world of experience. Furthermore, what applies to visual and auditory qualities seems to apply to all kinds of qualities across the board. The experience of touch is not just the experience of tactile phenomenal qualities, but those qualities as having a specific location with respect to the organization of the body image, which itself is embedded in the center of the world.

What about other types of experiences, such as feelings, emotions, and moods, whose spatial location is not as obvious? We return to these cases at the end of the chapter.

The Centeredness of Phenomenal Space

The phenomenal fact that the virtual world is *centered* or that it is constituted by an egocentric reference frame has also been called its *perspectivalness* (Metzinger, 1995b), or the first-person perspective (1PP; see chapter 2). The centeredness of phenomenal space means that the spatial volume surrounding us is experienced as spreading outward in every direction from a region which itself is immersed in the space. That central region is like the origin of a coordinate system: wherever it moves, it is always in the same centered position with regard to the other coordinates of the system. The center of phenomenal space anchors the rest of the coordinate system.

We typically identify our own self, an observing ego, as residing in the center of phenomenal space (that is why it is called an *egocentric* reference frame). What there is in the center, in fact, is just our phenomenal body image. To be more precise, there is a particular part of the phenomenal body image: the phenomenal head. My nose and eyes and teeth, as I feel them within my body image, are very close to the center of the phenomenal world, whereas my knees and toes, although parts of my body image—parts of *me*—are somewhat more distant from the center, and can change their position in relation to the center.

The organization of the phenomenal level is thus primarily a spatial organization around a center of gravity of sorts. Even though the center can at different times relate differently to the surrounding virtual objects (they can be first far, then near; first on the left, then on the right, and so on), the center cannot relate differently to itself and the coordinate system of phenomenal space. Whenever the centerpoint moves, it changes its relation to every phenomenal object in the surrounding phenomenal space, but wherever it moves (in relation to the objects), it never changes its relation to the center of phenomenal space: it remains in the core, the self-presenting phenomenal qualities spreading out in every direction in the spatial volume around it.

The Phenomenal Horizon

The basic organizational principle of the phenomenal level is, therefore, that of a three-dimensional expanse that has a center and an outer boundary (or four-dimensional, if the temporal dimension is also taken into account). There is an ultimate limit to the experience of spatial distance from the center. Virtual objects at the outer boundary are experienced to be as far from the center as the space itself extends. In the perception of natural scenes, the horizon, the zenith, the sun, the moon, and the stars on the dome of the sky are all located at the *ultimate spatial distance* from the center of virtual space. They are at the *phenomenal horizon.*

It makes no phenomenal difference that the external objects (the actual celestial bodies in theoretical physical space, for example) that constitute the distal external *causes* of the perceptual experience of the sky are at wildly differing distances from the position of the organism in the external world, ranging over several orders of magnitude. The horizon, a few kilometers away; the moon, hundreds of thousands of kilometers; the sun, millions of kilometers; and the stars, light-years away. Yet, in the spatial organization at the phenomenal level, the surrogates of celestial objects are at the same distance from the center: they are at the phenomenal horizon. It is impossible to have the experience of something being spatially farther away than that.

No wonder it was difficult for humanity to get rid of the intuitive idea that the heavens must be an outer sphere on which celestial bodies are fixed, and the Earth must be an inner sphere that stands motionless in the center of the universe. This worldview seems to reflect faithfully the egocentric structure of phenomenal space rather than the structure of the external physical universe.

The Relationship between Phenomenal and Physical Space

What is the relation of the phenomenal spatiality of consciousness to volumes of "real" or theoretical physical space? The spatiality at the phenomenal level is categorically distinct from the "real" or "physical" space that *surrounds* the biological organism.

Phenomenal spatiality is directly present in experience (it constitutes experience), whereas the idea of theoretical physical space is an abstraction in physical theory, not anything directly experienced. The phenomenal level literally resides within the confines of the brain, and therefore, whatever the spatiotemporal basis of the phenomenal level turns out to be, the physical space-time in which those properties are realized is the physical space-time inside the brain.

One exciting possibility (also mentioned by Dainton, 2003) is that the neural activity in the brain is somehow using the physical space-time it occupies from moment to moment to realize phenomenal qualities with inherent spatiality.The problem of how the spatial (or spatiotemporal) organization of the phenomenal level is actually realized, however, remains to be solved by the empirical research program that discovers the phenomenal level of organization in the brain. All that can be said with certainty at this point is that the experience of space is a *transparent surrogate of external physical space.*[1]

Phenomenal Space: Fundamental to the Phenomenal Level

I propose that the existence of phenomenal space is a fundamental requirement for the existence of the phenomenal level. At bottom the phenomenal level consists of the direct presence of spatially organized and interrelated qualities. For several qualities to be present at the same time they must share the phenomenal space that interrelates them. Thus phenomenal space is necessary for the global unity of consciousness. And for any single quality to present itself, it must be spatially located *somewhere* in experiential space. Thus phenomenal space is a prerequisite of any qualities at all to spring into existence.

Dainton (2000) calls this kind of commitment to the primacy of phenomenal spatiality the S-thesis: simultaneous experiences are coconscious solely by virtue of occurring at the same time within a single unified 3D phenomenal space. Still, nonspatial forms of consciousness might not be entirely inconceivable. However, such forms are certainly extremely difficult to imagine; therefore I will proceed on the basis of the assumption that spatiality is fundamental to consciousness. Apparent counterexamples to this principle (such as emotions, moods, and thoughts; see discussion below) can be construed as somewhat unusual forms of phenomenal spatiality rather than as entirely nonspatial forms of experience.

The qualia-bearing level of organization is arranged in what can be described as a 3D, centered, bounded volume. Each point or region in this volume has a specific location. Each region also has the capability to realize a characteristic variety of self-presenting, qualitative features and thereby to construct transparent surrogates or virtual objects. The phenomenal fields of different sensory modalities are spatially coordinated, so that a colored object, defined by visual qualia, may occupy the same spatial location as a sound, defined by auditory qualia. Thus, the buzz of the gadfly flying around you is coming from the same location where the visual percept of the rapidly moving insect is experienced. The song of the nightingale is emanating from the location where the bird is visually perceived. There are not two different locations, one for visual and the other for auditory space; there is just one location where both the auditory and the visual features are realized; therefore, they are seen as features of the same object.

The Nature of Phenomenal Space

Phenomenal space is a 3D coordinate system that allows qualities to present themselves for us. The issue concerning the intrinsic nature of phenomenal space could be expressed in terms introduced by Dainton (2000). He distinguishes between P-space and V-space. P-space is a spatially extended phenomenal space: even empty P-space has its own intrinsic phenomenal character. If phenomenal spatiality is based on a P-space, then the spatial coordinate system itself may be present for a subject without realizing any qualitative features. In that case it would generate the subjective sense of pure spatial extension: an experience of pure, empty space. But it is doubtful that such experiences of pure empty space ever happen. Therefore, perhaps phenomenal space is not a P-space, but another type of space altogether.

V-space, by contrast, has no intrinsic phenomenality. If a V-space is empty, there is a phenomenal void or vacuum or absence of the experience of spatial extension. If the spatial coordinate system of consciousness resides at a nonphenomenal (or subphenomenal) level, then our phenomenal space is a V-space. This means that the coordinate system merely *allows* us to experience the spatial relations between the contents of consciousness, but there is no *intrinsic* phenomenal spatiality; the subphenomenal space itself remains hidden. By contrast, if the spatial coordinate system is the first genuine phenomenal level, then it is a phenomenal spatial medium (a P-space), and even empty regions of this space have an intrinsic phenomenal spatiality.

The position I find most inviting regards the spatial coordinate system of consciousness as not per se at the phenomenal level of organization, but at the immediately underlying level. Thus, empty phenomenal space as such resides at a level that is ontologically nonphenomenal (or, more accurately, *sub*phenomenal). The coordinate system merely *allows* phenomenal features to be realized in a spatially unified and organized form. We never experience the contentless coordinate system as such, as it is entirely subphenomenal in itself. We merely observe its phenomenal consequences in the spatial organization manifested by patterns of qualitative phenomenal experience. Thus, our phenomenal space is a relational V-space rather than a substantive P-space.

In this view, phenomenal space is regarded as the mechanism that *mediates* between the conscious and the nonconscious domains. Whenever it is present, it allows qualitative experiences to come about and it compels them to be spatially organized. Yet the space as such can never be experienced directly, its existence can only be inferred on the basis of the spatial organization of experiential qualities. Phenomenal space as such is not self-presenting, but it is the crucial underlying mechanism that allows self-presenting qualities to spring into being.

Therefore phenomenal space is not purely conscious, nor is it purely nonconscious. It lies at the very interface between the phenomenal and nonphenomenal realms. It might be properly called "subphenomenal" space. Yet, it manifests itself at the phenomenal level in the ways in which the qualities of experience are necessarily spatially located and organized. For the sake of simplicity, I will continue to call it "phenomenal space" (rather than "subphenomenal space"). Irrespective of its somewhat misleading name, phenomenal space does not as such lie at the phenomenal level, but at the subphenomenal level. It is the link between the objective neurophysiological levels of organization and the subjective phenomenal level of organization.[2]

Phenomenal Space and the State of Being Conscious

This conception of phenomenal space connects it to the concept of the conscious state (see chapter 2). The state of being conscious is not something that we could experience as such. We only experience particular contents, particular qualities, but whenever we experience anything at all, we necessarily are in the conscious state. Thus, the concept of "conscious state" also refers to something not experienced as such, yet it refers to something that in general enables all experience. I suggest that in fact "phenomenal space" and "the conscious state" are connected. To be in a *conscious state,* to be conscious at all, is for a creature to have the phenomenal coordinate system realized in its brain at a higher level of neurophysiological organization (the subphenomenal level). To have specific *contents of consciousness* is for this coordinate system (or regions defined within it) to materialize (or to allow the materialization of) phenomenal qualities at the phenomenal level.

The state of being conscious is defined in terms of the realization of the spatial coordinate system itself, independently of the phenomenal values that the various regions in this system incarnate. Phenomenal contents of consciousness are ontologically dependent on the existence of the state of consciousness, that is, on the spatial coordinate system that constitutes phenomenal space. If this hypothesis is on the right track, then there cannot be any subjective qualitative experiences in the absence of the spatial coordinate system that expresses the qualitative properties. Qualities require the subphenomenal space that allows patterns of phenomenal experience to be realized in an inherently spatial form.

Phenomenal Space and Time

Although I have emphasized the spatiality of consciousness, I should point out that the temporal dimension appears to be extremely important for the phenomenal level as well. Phenomenal experience has temporal features: there is some moment at which the experience commences and before which it did not yet exist. It endures across time and then disappears. Patterns of phenomenal experience are extended in the temporal dimension. Phenomenal consciousness totally frozen in time is a theoretical fiction or an idealization; actual consciousness never stops changing and moving forward. The flux of phenomenal patterns coming and going cannot be stopped. Immobilizing the stream of consciousness may be something that some forms of meditation aim at, but it is doubtful whether such a state can truly be achieved without losing the state of being conscious altogether.

Are there any constraints as to how the total subjective experience at time *t* can change over the next few seconds? In principle it might be possible to have a system whose content of consciousness varies randomly from one second to the next, so that *any* two momentary experiences from the class of all possible human experiences may follow each other. In fact sometimes our contents of consciousness do radically change from one moment to the next: when we all of a sudden wake up from an exceptionally vivid dream, for example. Unlike external physical objects, the patterns of phenomenal features that define virtual objects are not necessarily spatiotemporally continuous and therefore they do not follow the same physical constraints—just as the picture on the TV screen at time T_1 may change to *any* other picture at time T_2.

Representationalism and Phenomenal Spatiality

Austen Clark (2000) has developed the view that modeling the contents of sensory experience can only be captured by a framework that acknowledges two independent dimensions: the qualitative and the spatial. According to him, the schema by which it is possible to characterize the facts of subjective experience must be of the form: "Appearance of quality Q at region R."

In other words, two kinds of terms are needed. One identifies a *location* and the other attributes *qualities* to that location. Reference to the regions or volumes at which the qualities are located is necessary to capture the nature of experience. Clark calls this "feature-placing": "Sensing proceeds by picking out place-times and characterizing qualities that appear at those place-times" (p.74).

This sounds like a reasonable characterization of the fundamental spatiality of the phenomenal. However, Clark interprets this model of sensory experience in an externalist—representationalist framework. He says that the places where the qualities reside are physical places, physically in front of the sense organs; they are place-times in or around the body of the sentient organism. According to his theory, to transport the qualities out of the brain and into the external physical world, there must be an information channel that reaches from the organism's brain to the physical region; there must be something going on in that region that can be reliably detected by the sensory systems of the organism. Thus, sensory processes *pick out, identify, refer to, represent,* or are *about* those space-time regions where their qualities appear to be: "The intentional character of the experience is nothing more or less than its spatial character" (Clark, 2000, p. 117).

As usual, this commitment to externalist representationalism serves to drive the contents of consciousness out of the brain and into the external world (or into the relations between the brain and the external world). Therefore, the metaphysical commitments that Clark advocates are not consistent with biological realism, nor can he say anything informative about the phenomenal level of organization in the brain. When the relations of subjective experience to the external world are carved off (as happens in dreaming, hallucinations, brains-in-a-vat, etc.), the very experience itself, our explanandum proper, stays exactly the same, but for the representationalist it ceases to be anything that should be taken very seriously because it no longer bears the proper intentional relations to the external world. Thus, the representationalist labels it a "misrepresentation" that has *mere* "intentional objects" or *mere* appearances, and these nonveridical appearances identify nothing, and therefore one should not "quantify over" the intentional objects of visual misrepresentations.

This is just philosophers' technical jargon for expressing the belief that consciousness reduces to intentionality and representation, and when the representational relations are carved off, nothing of importance remains (or whatever remains should be eliminated or denied rather than "quantified over").

But biological realism aims at understanding precisely the subjective experience that still *remains* even when all its external relations have been carved off. To label our vivid dream experiences as a "mere intentional object" or a "misrepresentation" hardly offers a proper scientific explanation of those experiences. In a causal-mechanical model of consciousness, labels such as "misrepresentation" or "intentional object" have little, if any, explanatory power. They cannot illuminate the actual mechanisms that bring about patterns of phenomenal experience in the absence of external stimulus objects.

Thus, although Clark's phenomenological analysis of the dimensions of sensory qualities and the spatial nature of experience is valuable in itself, his metaphysics is unacceptable for biological realism. Phenomenal qualities and phenomenal spatiality should not be externalized to physical space in the way Clark attempts to do. The Gestalt psychologist Wolfgang Köhler ([1929] 1971) realized this long ago:

> Under no circumstances has the phenomenal object anything to do with the place in physical space where the "corresponding" physical object is located. If it has to be localized at all at some point in physical space, then obviously it belongs most properly to that place in the brain where the directly corresponding physiological process takes place. (p. 128)

The representationalist externalization of consciousness allows one to characterize consciousness in any way one wishes, for the features of experience have been found to be features of something external to consciousness itself, and what remains as consciousness itself must have some completely different characteristics (or perhaps none at all).

In this way, Colin McGinn (1999) discards the idea that consciousness has anything to do with spatiality:

> . . . our world is thoroughly spatial, but . . . our consciousness is not spatial. . . . [W]e need to make a distinction between the object of awareness and the awareness itself. Consider the visual experience of seeing a red sphere. . . . The object of this experience is of course a spatial object with spatial properties, but the experience itself does not have these properties . . . [T]he spatiality that is inherent in our experience of the world, can be seen to belong to the object of experience, not to experience itself. . . . When we reflect on the experience itself, we can see that it lacks spatial properties altogether. Your visual experience of red . . . has no particular shape or size. Nor does it stand in spatial relations to other experiences . . . [C]onsciousness *could* not have spatial properties. (pp. 109–110)

McGinn applies intentionality (or the act/object dichotomy) to drive consciousness out from the brain and, eventually, to mystify its properties beyond all conceivable empirical investigation:

> The nonspatiality of consciousness is connected with another feature of it, namely its imperceptibility. . . . [C]onsciousness is necessarily not perceptible. We cannot even conceive of a type of sense organ that would enable us to perceive consciousness. (pp. 113–114)

If the representationalist (or the intentional act/object) analysis is taken as the philosophical basis of a research program on consciousness, the prospects for a biological science of consciousness look dim. As the features of our experiences are not features of consciousness, then consciousness itself will be stripped of all features and, eventually, nothing is left; at least nothing that would count as a *positive* characterization of consciousness. Instead, only a set of negations remain: consciousness is *non*spatial, it is *im*perceptible. This reminds me of the Cartesian way of characterizing consciousness as *im*material substance, as the negation of physical matter. Nothing remains that empirical science could try to seriously search for.

Other Views on Phenomenal Space

Although the externalist-representationalist interpretation of the spatiality of consciousness is probably the mainstream view in current philosophy of mind, also views that are not dissimilar from the world-simulation metaphor have been defended recently.

Steven Lehar (2003a,b) advocates a version of indirect realism that comes close to the world-simulation metaphor. On this basis he has developed a modernized version of Gestalt theory, which respects the original philosophical commitments of the Gestaltists. Lehar calls it a perceptual modeling approach to consciousness. He suggests that the phenomenal level uses a bounded spherical coordinate system that allows a finite representational space map the infinity of external space. The resolution of depth reduces as a function of distance and beyond a certain limiting depth, all objects are flattened into two dimensions, with zero extent in depth. Viewed from the inside, this geometry produces exactly the kind of perspectival effects we have in vision. Lehar proposes that visual consciousness should be modeled as a spherical volumetric matrix of dynamic computational elements that can encode transparent or opaque states. The opaque states can vary in all the subjective dimensions of color. Conscious visual perception is defined as the turning on of the appropriate pattern of elements in the volumetric analogue representation, or the "Gestalt bubble model," as he calls it. He argues that it must be an analogue representation, a miniature, virtual-reality replica of the external world inside our head. However, it need not be literally a spherical entity, but only computationally spherical or functionally isomorphic to a spherical coordinate system.

Lehar's proposal appears to be largely consistent with biological realism and the world-simulation metaphor of consciousness. Still, Lehar (2003b) does not accept biological realism, but defends panpsychism as the ultimate metaphysical position on the nature of phenomenality. As I have explained in chapter 8, there are several weighty reasons why the biological research program should reject panpsychism. Thus, on this question I am afraid I must part company with Lehar. I also think that it may be misleading to say, as Lehar does, that the phenomenal level is or contains a "replica" of the external world. The phenomenal level contains a transparent surrogate of the world, but it is unclear to what extent the internal model truly resembles the external world that it models. If we accept that physics tells us the correct story about external physical objects out there in physical space, the resemblance is limited to structural similarity. External physical events are known "so far as their space-time structure is concerned, for this must be similar to the space-time structure of their effects upon percipients" (Russell, 1948, p. 229). When we see a luminous dot through a powerful telescope and interpret it as a vast nebula existing millions of years ago in some far-off regions of physical space, it is quite clear that what we visually experience is entirely different from what we have inferred to be the cause of that experience (Russell, 1948).

Barry Dainton (2000) has developed a sophisticated treatment of descriptive phenomenology, concentrating mostly on the unity of consciousness. His methodological approach is exactly the kind of "objective phenomenology" that will be needed to develop a systematic phenomenal level of description. In addition to this valuable methodological approach, Dainton arrives at a conception of phenomenal consciousness not unlike the world-simulation metaphor. He defends the view that our experiences at any given moment are simply bundles of self-revealing phenomenal items, and that there is no experiential substance to bind those items together. Furthermore, he admits that spatiality is a very important ingredient of all conscious experience, but he does not regard it as necessary or essential for all forms of experience (hence we have a slight disagreement in this respect). Dainton arrives independently at a view not dissimilar from the one I defend, that although consciousness is unified, it is also decomposable into parts:

> The unity we find in our streams of consciousness, both at and over time, consists in the simple fact that our experience divides into parts and these parts are co-conscious. Since a given stretch of experience can be divided into parts in any number of different ways, and whatever parts can be discerned can themselves be regarded as wholes consisting of further parts, the unifying relationship of co-consciousness is all pervasive. (Dainton, 2000, p. 236)

Is the Spatial Disunity of Consciousness Conceivable?

How fundamental is the spatiality of consciousness? Couldn't we imagine cases of spatially disunified phenomenal contents that nevertheless are parts of a single subject's consciousness? Dainton (2000) believes we can (for a continuation of this discussion, see Revonsuo [2003b], and the response in Dainton 2003). Although he admits that spatiality is a very important factor in phenomenal unity, he suggests that there is reason to believe that experiences, although altogether dissociated phenomenospatially, could somehow be coconscious (i.e., being experienced together as synchronous component parts of a single stream of consciousness). He describes a science-fiction scene in which a subject's audiovisual experience comes from sensory organs located on a mountaintop while at the same time bodily experience (including voluntary movement) is fed into the subject's consciousness from a body diving and swimming at the bottom of the ocean. This bizarre arrangement would lead, according to Dainton, to a situation in which the two channels of experience would be coconscious but still entirely unconnected in any spatial manner. The subject of course would pay more attention to either one or the other channel of information at any one time but both streams would be conscious at the same time.

This argument is weakened by the well-known fact that our perceptual system (and our consciousness) abhors incoherent sources of input. For example, if two different objects or images are presented to the two eyes, either they are merged into one, if coherent enough (binocular fusion), or only one of them will be seen at any one time (binocular rivalry). Thus, a more plausible prediction as to Dainton's thought experiment would be that (1) either the two coherent streams of information compete for access to consciousness and therefore only one of them is experienced at any one time or (2) they will be merged together into a very unusual phenomenal world: You seem to be on a mountaintop as regards your audiovisual experience, but somehow you also seem to have an invisible body located there; furthermore the whole space around you seems to be filled with a cold, invisible liquid surrounding your body. The entire invisible liquid world seems to be moving in relation to the visible world, rather than you moving inside the liquid world. Thus, in this case of streams of information merging into one there would be experience of only one phenomenal space, albeit a very peculiar one: an audiovisual phenomenal space filled with transparent liquid moving in relation to your invisible body and the surrounding invisible objects.

There seem to be cases of altered states of consciousness in which people experience themselves in two places at once (e.g. out-of- body experiences). Are they good evidence for fundamental spatial disunity in consciousness? As far as I can see, such experiences seem rather more like a dissociation between visual perspective and bodily awareness. The experience is usually described as one where "I could see myself from the outside," which indicates that the visual field is constructed from a disembodied perspective, but a human character identified as "me" or as "my body" appears as one distinct object among others in the visual field. Sometimes the two spatial frames of reference (the normal embodied and the abnormal disembodied perspectives) can alternate or one can rapidly turn into the other. Still, at any one time the world is seen either from the embodied or the disembodied perspective, not from two perspectives at once. Thus, these cases do not seriously challenge the fundamental spatial unity of consciousness.

Of course one can always argue that spatially dissociated experiences might still be possible in some alien nonhuman consciousness. Perhaps, and perhaps not. I would be inclined to say that in such cases the alien creature possesses more than one single center of consciousness or that it houses more than one subject. Each distinct phenomenal coordinate system defines a different subject: the global bundles of phenomenal features synchronously present within each single coordinate system are the momentary phenomenal contents of one subject. Thus, I am inclined to treat phenomenospatiality as the basic unifying feature of human consciousness, and also as an explanation of why the relation of coconsciousness holds. Furthermore, I believe that the postulated phenomenal spatiality must in turn be explained by referring to even lower, nonphenomenal levels of organization. By contrast, Dainton takes coconsciousness to be the ultimate explanation of binding and the unity of consciousness, and says that there is no need to postulate any unifying principle over and above experience and interexperiential relations.

There are some further counterexamples that might be raised against the spatiality (or spatiotemporality) of consciousness. Emotions, feelings, moods, and conscious thoughts, for example, do not seem to be spatially localized in the same manner as visual percepts.

Emotions—attacks of fear, pangs of jealousy, bursts of joy, and so on—are experienced in and with our bodies. Their experiential part consists of various qualitative features presenting themselves within the internal phenomenal space of bodily awareness. Although emotions also require some cognitive interpretation, there is no doubt that the primary experiences are qualitative, bodily, and located (though not necessarily precisely localizable) within the phenomenal body.

In my view, moods (feeling good, depressed, anxious, etc.) are bodily feelings in the phenomenal background or peripheral consciousness. Being in a good mood is equivalent to experiencing a moderate or high level of pleasure whatever activity one engages in. Moods are not momentary experiences but extrapolated with reflection from longer sequences of experiences and from the pleasure, indifference, or fearfulness that forms the phenomenal background of momentary experiences and activities. Moods are thus experiences that have a low level of intensity, remain in the periphery, but form the context for other experiences; they change slowly, have fuzzy temporal borders, and are located in the body (or at least extrapolated from bodily feelings). It would not make any sense to say that my good mood is located in visual objects around me, or that my depressed mood has nothing to do with the fact that my body reacts with indifference and an absence of pleasure no matter what I do.

The case of conscious thoughts is easier: they are more clearly located in time and they are often in the focus of attention. Now, where is that inner voice located? It certainly is not located in my toes, or in the television set, or in my teeth (people who believe so are usually psychotic—they suffer from a pathological altered state of consciousness). Thus, I would say that the inner voice which is the phenomenal surface of my conscious thoughts is located inside my head. Anyone who disagrees should have to propose a more appropriate location. I cannot come up with any plausible rival hypothesis.

Summary

Empirically based phenomenology should be built on a model that takes the spatiality and centeredness of consciousness as its fundamental structural and organizational property. The phenomenal level is based on an egocentric, bounded coordinate system whose regions can instantiate qualitative features. When that coordinate system is present in the brain, the brain is in the conscious state (i.e., capable of realizing phenomenal contents); when it is absent, the brain is in an unconscious state (i.e., incapable of realizing phenomenal contents). Phenomenal space lies at the interface between the nonconscious and the conscious realms: the space as such remains nonconscious, but it can be indirectly experienced through the spatial features of qualities and the spatial unity of the phenomenal level. This view of phenomenal space narrows the explanatory gap, because it establishes a direct link between phenomenal and physical space.

10 The Phenomenal Contents of Consciousness

The phenomenal level consists of phenomenal space and the contents of that space. The phenomenal contents of consciousness make up a world of subjective experience: a world simulation. This phenomenal world consists of meaningful objects embedded in an overall egocentric space. Throughout our waking and dreaming lives, we find ourselves in the center of such a phenomenal world simulation.

Empirical phenomenology describes the basic components of this world and the basic principles of organization that the phenomenal contents of consciousness follow. The analysis of the contents of experience reveals that consciousness involves a hierarchical structure. First comes phenomenal *space,* then *qualities* in this space, then *organized bundles* of qualities, then *meaningful* bundles of qualities. The organized, meaningful patterns of qualities are what we normally take as the objects surrounding us. The *world-for-me* is primarily a world consisting of meaningful virtual objects.

The Structure of the Phenomenal World

So far, we have been calling consciousness *the* phenomenal level, or *a* level of organization in the brain. Now that we venture deeper into the phenomenal realm, we will discover that as a matter of fact there is a complex *system* of levels involved. We know that the nonconscious biological levels in the brain form hierarchies where macrolevel phenomena are based on microlevel phenomena. The very same principle applies to the biological levels where phenomenality is involved. Higher-level phenomenal entities are based on the complex organization of lower-level phenomenal entities.[1]

At the bottom of the experiential hierarchy is phenomenal space: the spatial coordinate system that mediates between the objective and the subjective domain. It lies at the subphenomenal interface. Without it, no contents of consciousness, no qualitative experiences, would be possible at all, because it is the subphenomenal medium whose regions bear qualitative features. Once this coordinate system for realizing phenomenal qualities is in place, then it is possible to build higher levels of organization on it.

The experience of visual shape is an example of a phenomenon that resides at a higher level of phenomenal organization. Visual shape is more than just the presence of simple, isolated qualities. It is the presence of an *organized pattern* of qualitative features in the phenomenal coordinate system. The phenomenal world is largely constituted by a multitude of organized patterns of qualities. The objects we experience around us are nothing but complex ordered patterns of phenomenal qualities (mostly visual, auditory, and tactile). The emotions experienced within our bodies are patterns of bodily qualities (associated with cognitive interpretations). The thoughts within our minds are patterns of phonological imagery (and sometimes imagery in other sensory modalities) associated with semantic interpretations or *understanding experiences.*

The higher-level organization of qualities is at least as important an aspect of the world-for-me as the qualities themselves. Of course, qualities as such are terribly important, too: without them, there would be *nothing-for-me.* Given qualities, there will be at least *something-for-me.* But unless the qualities manifest higher-level organization, there will not be a world-for-me, only a random mass of qualities, chaotically jumping around in a whirlwind, a phenomenal maelstrom in the stream of consciousness.

It is the beautifully precise *organization* of qualities that makes phenomenal experience worth having at all. Qualities in the absence of the slightest order are not particularly enjoyable. Chaotic, totally disorganized, and discontinuous phenomenal contents—a world of random sounds, colors, touches, emotions, tastes, smells—would be worthless, even irritating: a mere pandemonium of qualitative noise. I am doubtful that it would be even by a hairsbreadth preferable to the complete absence of consciousness: death, coma, or total, irreversible zombiehood.

But I am positive that mere qualitative noise cannot compare with the beauty of organized phenomenal states: the patterns of green you experience as the canopy of trees in the forest, the patterns of sounds you experience as a Bach composition, the kinesthetic pattern experienced within your body image when you perform a perfect move in sports. Our lives as subjects are based on the complex patterns of phenomenal organization realized in the brain. The world-for-me as a *world* is ontologically dependent on the emergence of such organized patterns at the phenomenal level.

Much of empirical phenomenology, therefore, will be the study of the organized patterns of phenomenal experience, rather than atomic, unanalyzable, maximally simple qualia. It is doubtful whether qualities *ever* exist in an atomic, isolated form at the phenomenal level. We always seem to have a whole phenomenal volume present, with patterns of qualitative features realized in it.

Basic Contents of the Phenomenal World

What are the phenomenal contents that structure the phenomenal level throughout our dreaming and waking lives? To figure that out, let us exercise some "commonsense phenomenology."

Commonsense phenomenology of our dreaming and waking experience suggests that the world-for-me may be coarsely divided into three main categories of organized experience: the virtual world, the virtual body, and mental phenomena. These categories can be clearly distinguished by way of their mutual spatial relationships within the world-for-me.

The virtual world consists of the qualitative features realized in the volume experienced as being spatially located *out there, beyond* the boundaries of the virtual body (the phenomenal body image). The virtual world is perceptually experienced through multiple sensory modalities. We see objects and surfaces and hear sounds "out there," far beyond the reach of our bodies. Many objects near the boundaries of the body image can be brought to bodily contact and thus their spatial location and three-dimensional form can be experienced by touch.

The virtual body or the phenomenal body image consists of proprioceptive awareness of the body, or the experience of the body as from the inside (Eilan, Marcel, & Bermudez, 1995), coupled with visual awareness of the body as an object perceived from the outside. The virtual body differs from virtual objects at least in the following respects: First, it is the only object in the virtual world that can be experienced not only from the outside but also from the inside. The posture of the body and its volumetric extent, as well as its boundaries with the external world, are experienced from within this special object. Second, bodily sensations and emotions only occur within the boundaries of the virtual body, and sensations are usually clearly localized in a specific region. Third, we feel very close to our own virtual body; we have a sense of *ownership* toward it, and a sense of *control* over the paths it takes in relation to other phenomenal objects. Fourth, the virtual world is construed from the perspective of the virtual body, which stands in the very center of the virtual world. Consequently, the sense of self is firmly attached to the virtual body—the self is experienced as located within the boundaries of the virtual body, and exerting its control directly on the body and indirectly on the external world through voluntary action.

The mind houses all phenomena we normally call "mental." Mental phenomena are felt to be located *within* the phenomenal body, right behind the perspectival point of view from which the visual virtual world is construed, within the volume of space that in proprioceptive and visual awareness is construed as the head of the virtual body. Inner speech and mental imagery are felt to take place inside the head, not within the stomach or limbs or out there inside the external objects. The quality of mental images, such as our inner silent speech, is otherwise quite similar to externalized percepts—inner speech does sound almost as if somebody were speaking—apart from the fact that the phonological imagery involved is experienced as located entirely within our head, not outside of it.

Dissociations of Phenomenal Contents

Given the considerations above, it is thus established that the phenomenal level involves qualitatively and experientially distinguishable parts which bear certain spatial relations to each other within the simulated world. Can these parts be dissociated from each other in such a way that the rest of phenomenal organization does not collapse? It seems that they can. Such curious dissociations do occur every now and then in connection with various sleep-related phenomena.

A Virtual World without a Self

The virtual world can be represented without any virtual body or self. This sometimes happens in dreams. About 10% of dreams are experienced from an observer or "camera's-eye" perspective—as if seeing the dream world from a detached, disembodied third-person perspective—but there may be large individual differences in the frequency of such dreams (Foulkes & Kerr, 1994). In some of these disembodied dreams, there is a specific character identified as the dreamer herself, but of course in such cases the dreamer perceives herself exactly the same way as all the other characters are perceived: from an external point of view. No proprioceptive awareness is involved; the point of view is not incorporated into any phenomenal body image that would be experienced from the inside.

Usually, in camera's-eye dreams there is no self-character involved at all; the dream unfolds for the dreamer as a 3D movie would. The dreamer is uninvolved and, in fact, not explicitly present within the virtual world at all. The perspective or point of view only implicitly involves the dreamer, as an empty point from whose perspective the visuo-spatial virtual world is constructed. The point of view, however, still constitutes the *center* of the virtual space, from around which the phenomenal features spread outward. The center of the phenomenal coordinate system is still there, even though not clothed in the disguise of a body image. The rest of the virtual world remains otherwise entirely normal: there may be objects, events, characters, and verbal communication that are subjectively experienced. The phenomenal world is still spatially structured around a centered coordinate system, but it is not an *ego*centric system. The ego (the virtual self) need not be in the center of the reference frame, nor need it be present at all.

In these dreams the virtual world lives a life of its own, completely oblivious to the absence of the dreamer. The possibility of such a dissociation confirms that the experience of phenomenal objects is not a *relation* between the self (or some other type of homunculus) and objects (or at least it is not a relation obtaining between the phenomenal self and phenomenal objects as we experience them). On the contrary, patterns of phenomenal features are experienced as such; they are self-presenting in no way dependent on any relations to a self or a perceiver external to those patterns.

The phenomenal body image can thus be missing at least during dream experiences, but is it possible to have comparable waking experiences? There is a rare pathological condition (extensive sensory polyneuritis) in consequence of which proprioceptive awareness, the virtual body, can be permanently lost. One such case is described by Oliver Sacks (1985) in *The Man Who Mistook His Wife For A Hat* as "the disembodied lady."

She feels that her body is blind to itself, or dead and unreal; there is only sensory darkness or silence, a bottomless void where once there was virtual body. Of course she still can *see* her body—there still are visual qualities forming the appropriate bodily boundary at the appropriate location in the virtual world, but the external visual knowledge does not provide her with true embodiment, with the feeling of actually *being inside* her body. To some extent she can feel light touch on her skin, and if exposed to a strong wind, she can faintly sense her arms and legs through this stimulation. Two similar cases are described by Cole and Paillard (1995). Below the neck the persons have no perception of their body from the inside, or of its movement. Without extensive attention paid to visual input from the moving body parts, these persons without the virtual body have no control over where a moving limb ends. One of them describes her body as being a machine to which she imposes commands.

These cases vividly demonstrate that phenomenal embodiment not only provides the sense of being inside the sensory volume of the virtual body, it also provides the necessary template for carrying out intentional action smoothly and effortlessly. Action is normally felt unfolding from the inside toward its goal, with sensorimotor predictions and feedback loops monitoring the success in reaching toward the intended goal.

As the above anomalies show, virtual body or virtual self is entirely dissociable from virtual presence. It is perfectly possible to be conscious, to have the phenomenal level realized, and patterns of phenomenal features experienced, even though none of those patterns depict the biological organism itself, the individual whose phenomenal states they are.

This empirical fact seems to refute Antonio Damasio's (1999) theory of consciousness, insofar as it is erected on the accuracy of the following statement:

> The neural patterns and images necessary for consciousness to occur are those which constitute proxies for the organism, for the object, and for the relationship between the two. (p. 20)

Bodyless contents of consciousness constitute empirical counterexamples against Damasio's theory, or, indeed, against *any* theory of consciousness claiming that the body image and its relation to object images is a *necessary* condition of consciousness.[2]

Dream research and neuropsychology provide us with undeniable evidence of fully realized subjective experience not accompanied by any representation of self. According to the philosophy of presence, no *particular* phenomenal pattern, whether presenting the virtual self or virtual objects or their mutual relationships, is necessary for the realization of consciousness. Instead, the underlying phenomenal coordinate system is. Only this system can support any kinds of patterns of phenomenal qualities at all, and any pattern of self-presenting features realized in it is, by definition, immediately experienced. No *special* patterns, such as the self, with magical powers to somehow *add* subjective experience to other patterns, are required.

Can the Virtual World Disappear?

If the virtual world can be present without the virtual self, then the respective realizing grounds of the virtual body and the virtual objects have to be able to work independently of each other. In fact, this hypothesis is further supported by an opposite dissociation, the loss of virtual world but the presence of virtual body and self and mental phenomena. Such a condition—a rather frightening experience in fact—can sometimes occur in connection with *sleep paralysis*. It is a state of consciousness on the borderline between REM sleep and waking, and therefore involves a curious mixture of those states. In sleep paralysis proprioceptive awareness is preserved or regained when one partially awakens from REM sleep, but all voluntary muscles (apart from the breathing muscles and those controlling eye movements) are still as fully paralyzed as they normally are during REM sleep. Sometimes hallucinatory dream imagery (also called hypnopompic imagery) may emerge in this state:

> Sleep paralysis is an unforgettable experience. The paralysis, which prevents limb movement and eye opening, is frequently accompanied by a sensation of struggling to move or speak or of fighting to wake up. The subject may believe that he or she is dying or unable to breathe. Frightening illusions or hallucinations, such as visions of animals or monsters in the room or a sense that persons are about to enter the room, often accompany the paralysis. The subject often feels awake or half-awake and is usually aware of being in bed. The sensations accompanying the first episode of sleep paralysis are often so vivid and terrifying that the person recalls them clearly for years afterward. (Aldrich, 1993)

Sleep paralysis is not an uncommon experience: up to 5 % of people report having experienced it (especially during adolescence). It is not usually a sign of pathology, but it may be a symptom of the sleep disorder called narcolepsy, because it occurs in 60% of narcoleptic patients.

The following experience was reported by a female student in a home dream diary she wrote when she participated as a voluntary subject in our dream research. It clearly is a case of sleep paralysis (though the subject did not recognize it as such because she had probably never even heard of it). It serves as a fine example of the loss of the phenomenal world:

> I lie still and am unable to move. All around me there is just emptiness, nothing. First I try to lift my arms and then my legs, but they are numb and so heavy that they do not rise. I feel very anxious, desperate and powerless. (subject 23/20-year-old woman/20 September 1997)

Here we have no virtual world of objects in the center of which one could place oneself, only an awareness of being inside the virtual body which cannot be moved by will, floating in an emptiness or void. It is interesting to note that the self is experienced as residing inside this virtual body and that bodily sensations (e.g., numbness, heaviness) and emotions (anxiousness) are experienced too. This is unlike in selfless dreams where the virtual body is absent; no embodiment whatsoever is experienced.

As the above examples show, the organization of the phenomenal level can thus consist of either nothing but the virtual world with only a disembodied point of view, or, conversely, nothing but the embodied self floating in an emptiness without a world surrounding it. There is a *double dissociation* between virtual world and virtual body at the phenomenal level of organization.

Mental Phenomena in Isolation

Can mental phenomena be dissociated from the virtual body? Some dream reports consist of nothing but repeated thoughts in phonological imagery (traditionally called "sleep mentation" rather than dreams). In such cases subjects report the phonological imagery as "thinking" rather than "hearing words being uttered," which suggests that the phonological imagery is experienced as going on within the mind, in the center of the phenomenal coordinate system, rather than coming from somewhere outside. This type of internal verbal imagery was reported by the Israeli sleep researcher Perez Lavie (1996):

> But the greatest surprise awaited us after the sleep recordings of November 28–29, 1984. Mr. R. awoke from his fifth REM sleep and reported that he did not remember a dream. He muttered one word which he said was "stuck in his mind": the word was "carbide." (p. 96)

The word was experienced as located in the mind rather than coming from a perceptual space outside the self. That is enough to demonstrate my point: even when there is no experience of the body image, patterns of phenomenal properties have an experienced location, in this case in the center of the phenomenal coordinate system, experienced by the subject as a word "stuck *in his mind.*"[3]

The Transmutable Virtual Self

In a dream the nature of the dream self is sometimes vague or unstable. It may change abruptly from one dream character to another, or from a disembodied perspective to an embodied perspective or vice versa. Consider the following excerpts from our students' dream reports:

> It's the Second World War and *I am a dark-haired, strongly built, Finnish male soldier.* The enemies are probably German." . . . [Later in the same dream):] "I could see myself in a mirror. *Now I was a blond, strongly-built woman.*" (Subject 05 / 25-year-old woman / 10 March 1993).

This dream shows a sharp discontinuity in the nature of the self: the sex and the color of the hair change during the course of the dream. The next dreams are perhaps even more weird, showing the changeable nature of the virtual self:

> I was on my way to the campus; it was late in the evening. On my way I stopped off at a nearby shop. They had a sale. I remember buying at least some lettuce. Suddenly my mother was working in this shop, and somehow *I was my mother.* The boss gave me permission to go home. When

I was biking home, the road was full of wet snow. Somehow my big brother also came to the shop and then with me. When I got to my place at the campus, *I was myself again.*" (Subject 03/ 21-year-old woman / 27 September 1997)

It is not entirely clear what happens when "suddenly" the dreamer's mother was working in the shop. Perhaps that was only a *belief* the dreamer arrived at suddenly, and subsequently interpreted herself as being the mother who she believed was working there. Or did she actually see her mother in the shop and then became one with her? In any case, at some point after leaving the shop she ceases to be her mother and is back to her own self. Whether this is based on some sort of perception of herself, or only on beliefs and interpretations of the situation, remains unclear.

I was walking (*apparently it was me*) in a suburban area, past a house whose yard was about one and a half meters above the street level. In the yard a girl I know from medical school was leading a big bearlike dog. I was leading a dog that actually was my female classmate from medical school. The girl suddenly attacked the bear-dog and they fought. *The person in the dream that so far had been me was suddenly my classmate J. Somehow I became (physically) detached from myself and I noticed that I was not me but him.* This was accompanied by a funny feeling." (subject 19, 22-year-old man, 23 February 1993)

Here the dreamer's point of view gets suddenly dissociated from the normal frame of embodied reference. In fact it seems to be an out-of-body experience of some sort. The dreamer sees the person that he detached from and notices to his surprise that it looks not like himself but rather like his friend. It is noteworthy that after detachment from the body, *the dreamer construes "himself" as being the detached disembodied point of view* rather than the person from whose body image the perspective did detach.

In neurology and psychiatry, the experience of seeing oneself from the outside, from the third-person perspective, is called *autoscopy.* It is not uncommon as an aura, a warning sign of an approaching migraine attack or epileptic seizure. Here is one typical description of such an experience connected with migraine:

This sensation came just before a violent headache attack and at no other time. Very often it came as I was serving breakfast. There would be my husband and children, just as usual, and in a flash they didn't seem to be quite the same. I felt as if I were standing on an inclined plane, looking down on them from the height of a few feet, watching myself serving breakfast. It was as if I were in another dimension, looking at myself and them. I was not afraid, just amazed. I always knew that I was really with them. Yet, there was "I," and there was "me"—and in a moment I was one again. (Lippman, 1953, p. 346, cited in Blackmore, 1992, p. 160)

The phenomenon of a detached perspective is also common in autobiographical memory imagery, and not uncommon in waking fantasy. In fact, Freud was one of the first to write about this field/observer perspective distinction in memory. In one study, over 40% of autobiographical recollections were experienced from a detached point of view. The older our memories are, the more likely we are to experience them from a camera's-eye perspective, as a detached observer of events in which we see our own self engaged (Schacter, 1996). In another study 15% of spontaneous visual imagery elicited during relaxed wakefulness was experienced from a similar see-oneself perspective. One subject reported remembering an experience by a campfire, but in the imagery her vantage point of herself was as if from up in a tree, watching (Foulkes, 1994). This tendency, to see the events of the past from the camera's-eye view, shows that memory images are *constructed during the recollection process,* not simply played back as if they were some sort of accurate videotape recordings replayable in consciousness.

The commonsense phenomenology we have exercised above establishes that the organization of the phenomenal level that is *typical* during waking perception is far from *universal* or *necessary.* Virtual world, virtual body and self, and mental phenomena do not need to go neatly hand in hand, but may be completely detached from each other.

What Is the Virtual Dream World Made Of?

Dreams occur in the brain's virtual world. What does such a world consist of? How is it put together? In their classic study, Calvin Hall and Robert Van de Castle (1966) distinguished broad classes of dream content such as "physical surroundings," "characters," "social interactions," and "activities." Physical surroundings include settings and objects. "Setting" is the general background of the dream events; "objects" are the various figures that stand out against the background.

In one study (Revonsuo and Salmivalli, 1995) we developed a classification system where we divided the phenomenal content of dreams into three general classes: (1) dream setting (self, place, time); (2) surrounding dream elements (characters, animate objects, inanimate objects); and (3) dream events (passive events, intentional action, speech and language, thought and cognition; emotion; sensation).

Virtual Places

In the Revonsuo and Salmivalli (1995) study we defined the place of dreams as the immediate surroundings of the dream self such as a room, a vehicle, a building, a yard, a street, a garden or a forest. The place is the overall context that spatially surrounds the dream self. The place forms the overall background for the more specific objects in the dream. Most dream reports simply begin by identifying the place as the context in which the self finds itself within the dream. Here is a collection of such opening lines from dream reports of students:

"I was in my grandmother's kitchen."

"I was in some restaurant with my two sisters."

"Together with my grandmother we got on a bus which was quite full."

"I was in the living room of our former apartment."

"We were at our summer cottage."

"I was driving a big car."

"I was walking around a big house."

"I was somewhere with three other persons. We looked down from a hill."

Thus the general nature of the surroundings is each time immediately transparent for the dream self: there is an immediate orientation to the place. Whenever we are present in a virtual world, we are instantly aware of the general nature of the scene surrounding us. The same is not true of the wider geographical context where the immediate surroundings are thought to be located. Sometimes it is difficult or impossible for the dreamer to locate the dream place in any geographical coordinates; the place is just "somewhere." By contrast, sometimes the sensory content of the dream is extremely limited, and yet the dream self knows fully well where she is located:

I am at my aunt's house, upstairs in a long and narrow closet where there is also a freezer. It is dark there. I try to be quiet, but all the time I happen to stumble on something. I try to spy on the woman in the next room." (subject 4 / 22-year-old woman / 11 March 1993)

Here the dream place is a dark and small closet throughout the dream, and yet the dream self has a full interpretation of its location in a larger geographical frame of reference. Thus, a virtual place consists not only of a certain overall sensory content that forms the background to all the objects in the vicinity but also of a certain orientational and geographical *interpretation* of that content. The interpretation involves a kind of background anchoring of the perceived environment in a spatial map in long-term memory. A virtual place thus involves a map location: a tacit, immediate understanding of where in the world the perceived place is supposed to be located.

Sometimes the interpretation of the dream place includes the general nature of the place (house, forest, foreign country, ship, beach) but leaves it open where such a place is supposed to be located in real-life geographical coordinates. Dream places need not necessarily have any map location. Obviously, such geographical localization is not necessary for the dream self to mistake the place for a real one, and for the dream to carry on. In our waking lives we practically all the time know exactly where we are and how we came to be there. People who tend to lose their map location during wakefulness are usually suffering from severe neurological problems such as dementia.

But in the dream world we often have no idea of our map location although we do know what *kind* of place we are in. Also, we do not realize that we did not arrive at the dream place from anywhere in particular; there was no route from our previous whereabouts (or from our bedroom) to the place where we suddenly find ourselves. The dream place just came out of the blue—the dream began when we simply found ourselves suddenly in a place, no matter where the place is located and how we ended up there.

Virtual Objects

The virtual world where we are directly present in dreams (and waking perception) is, above all, a world of *objects*. The dream place forms the overall background and context of our virtual presence in a dream, and the individual objects form all the parts of the environment that somehow stand out as coherent patterns or figures against the background. Virtual objects stand in a part-whole relationship to the virtual place: take all the objects out, and the place loses its identity. A place is labeled as a certain *kind* of place because it contains a configuration of objects that belong together. If a dream place contains walls, floor, ceiling, and furniture, we will immediately categorize it as a room; if trees, grass, sky, and a horizon, we will categorize it as forest. A virtual place is a coherent configuration of virtual objects.

In the Revonsuo and Salmivalli (1995) study, we separated three classes of objectlike elements in dreams: inanimate objects, animate objects (animals, plants, and body parts), and persons (human or humanlike animate objects). Let us first take a look at what inanimate objects in dreams are like. C. S. Hall and Van de Castle (1966) described dream objects in the following way:

> An object is a thing. It has tangibility, palpability, and dimensionality. It also has definite physical boundaries or limits . . . any object we encounter in waking life can be represented in dreams . . . (p. 43)

The last claim certainly seems to be true. C. S. Hall and Van de Castle (1966) present an impressive list of 1170 objects, encountered in 1000 dreams, and their frequencies for male and female dreamers. Their list shows that virtual objects of all sizes, shapes, and categories abound in the dream world: the dreamers had encountered, for example, 9 cats, 19 dogs, 103 doors, 5 islands, 6 magazines, 149 automobiles, 20 buses, twice the moon, once an octopus, 125 rooms, 12 times the sun, 2 tomatoes, and so on.

Recognizing all the objects in a scene requires what cognitive psychologists have called "scene segmentation." Segmentation involves the decomposition of the scene into objects. In visual perception it is a process that attempts to extract from the stimulus image those structures that correspond to significant objects and parts or portions of objects (Ullman, 1996). Many objects in a natural scene cannot be seen completely, but are occluded by other objects, so recognition must be based on the visible parts or portions.

Is it reasonable to talk about "object recognition" when we consider the purely virtual objects of dreams? Although there is no external physical object behind the causal chain that brought about the virtual object in our dream, even in dreams we surely see a scene segmented into separate objects, and we treat the purely virtual object as an external physical one. Thus, surely even the purely virtual objects have been segmented from each other and *recognized as* particular *types* of objects—they have been semantically *categorized.* Surely similar cognitive operations are required to make a dream scene a meaningful array of objects as is required when a stimulus field is analyzed into a similar scene.

Virtual Objects as Gestalt Windows and Semantic Windows

How is the formation and semantic categorization of virtual objects supposed to happen? According to Treisman's (1988) feature integration theory, attention to a location binds all the features in that location and creates a temporary representation of the object in an *object file.* In conscious perception the contents of the object file are matched with stored descriptions in memory, allowing recognition.

The object file defines the boundaries of the object. The boundary separates the figure from the ground and makes the object a perceptual unit, located in the phenomenal coordinate system. The object file also combines all the phenomenal features that fall inside those boundaries into a coherent object representation. The object file thus consists of all the directly present phenomenal features of the object and its overall Gestalt.

If the object happens to be a novel, unfamiliar object that has no match in long-term memory, then the object cannot be recognized as a specific kind of object, as a member of any particular semantic category. If a hunter-gatherer, who is living in the Amazonian jungle and who has had no contact with technology, should find a mobile phone or a laptop computer in the jungle, those objects as visual stimuli would surely cause coherent gestalts in his subjective visual field, but he would possess no category in his semantic memory in which to place the alien objects.

Let us call the visuospatial pattern that such directly visible, spatially extended and bounded features make up, a *Gestalt window.* To be experienced at all, a visually perceptible object must open its own Gestalt window in the phenomenal visual field. Only then does it become a virtual object in the subject's phenomenal world. However, in order to render the virtual object subjectively meaningful in the same sense that the world of objects is immediately meaningful for us (both in dreams and awake), the Gestalt windows need to be semantically categorized. Categorization requires that the proper semantic representations in semantic memory become activated and that the Gestalt window makes and retains a connection with that information as long as the Gestalt window persists as a part of the virtual world.

Now we are ready to define a "virtual object": a full-fledged virtual object is a *semantically categorized Gestalt window,* or *semantic window* for short. The virtual world is a complex hierarchical system of such semantic windows, immediately present for the subject and making up (most of) the surroundings of the virtual body, in dreams and awake.

The Hierarchical Organization of the Virtual World

The virtual world consists of the following hierarchy: phenomenal space, qualities, patterns of qualities, virtual objects (Gestalt windows and semantic windows), virtual place, and map location.

The highest level in the hierarchy of semantic windows consists of *map location* or geographical orientation. It provides an answer to the question, Where is the currently present place located in relation to other places not currently present? This level may be missing or vague in dreams, for it is tightly tied to real-life coordinates and the pathways we necessarily have to take to get from one place to another. In dreams we may all of a sudden become present in a place (or a place suddenly becomes present for us). Under those circumstances we may forget about geographical orientation altogether. But in almost all other cases, the virtual place we find ourselves in also automatically opens up the semantic window for our map location. Sometimes, when waking up in a foreign land far away from home the first morning after arrival, one may have to wait for a moment or two to open up the proper semantic window for one's current location. Patients suffering from severe dementia have to struggle with much more severe and persisting forms of disorientation.

The next level of semantic windows is the level of the *virtual place,* the immediate surroundings, the *kind* of surroundings we are in. This consists of the largest semantic windows filling the perceptual background: if we find ourselves in a room, the walls, floor, and ceiling; if in a forest, the trees, the ground, the sky, and so on. Usually these need not be categorized or named at the level of conscious reflection in order that we immediately grasp what the nature of the place really is. Our semantic system is very efficient in recognizing object configurations, and this fact is an important part of our ability to deal with natural scenes effectively.

After the level of place comes the multitude of individual *virtual objects* that are contained in the place. Many objects are further organized hierarchically into parts (or features) and their parts, all of which can be construed as separate virtual objects or semantic windows in the scene. In waking perception, the part-whole organization is coherent. Once an object has opened a certain semantic window, it retains its semantic value as long as it stays in view. This despite the fact that the actual Gestalt window radically changes in shape and color when, for example, the object moves from central to peripheral vision, or becomes too close to be fixated on, or when the lights go out and all objects become obscure and dark gray.

This can be easily demonstrated. Hold this book about 5 to 10 centimeters from your face, keep your eyes fixated on the middle of the book, and then, without changing your eye fixation, pay attention to the Gestalt windows that occupy the periphery of your vision. What you see there are various more or less shapeless patches and regions of different colors and levels of luminance, yet you have no difficulty in recognizing those distorted patches as a chair, a table, a window, a lamp, a tree, and so on. The Gestalt windows, though grossly disfigured from what they were when you fixated them, nevertheless retain their semantic values and still constitute the very same semantic windows and, consequently, the same virtual objects.

The persistence of semantic windows despite the constant transformation of Gestalt windows is why we do not lose the world and its meaningful objects when we do not pay attention to them. Virtual objects may lose their coherent shape and organization at the phenomenal surface, but they persist as determinate semantic windows at the fringe of our consciousness. Should we suddenly need to pay attention to them, it is as if we knew and perceived all the time what kind of objects they were and where they were located in relation to ourselves.[4]

A semantic window is, above all, the brain's way to access huge amounts of semantic knowledge very quickly. Once a semantic window is open at the phenomenal level, the brain has within immediate reach a huge knowledge base about (1) all the different kinds of attributes of the object (is it edible? dangerous? valuable? alive?); (2) the contexts in which such objects usually are encountered (does it belong in the kitchen? street? forest? bathtub?); (3) readily available motor programs to use or cope with the object (should I sit on it? run away from it? take a bite of it? say hello to it?); (4) readily available names to communicate about it (hey, there's a ______! what do you think about this ______? beware of the ______!). Virtual objects as semantic windows are an interface between the phenomenal level and long-term explicit memory. Through semantic windows all the wealth of semantic and autobiographical knowledge is brought to the phenomenal level of organization where it is immediately accessible if needed, establishing conscious understanding (semantic interpretation) of the content of perception.

This highly efficient way in which consciousness presents semantic information has been recognized by Mangan (1993). He compared it to menu bars on the computer screen:

> . . . the bar functions to indicate the existence of potential information, information not, itself, on the screen. . . . This . . . allows some information to be displayed in radically summarized form, indicating information that can be *potentially* called to the screen in detail—just as the fringe radically summarizes information that can be called into focal attention. (p. 98)

Even when in the focus of attention, virtual objects function as icons for further information retrieval. Merely visually attending to an object does not automatically provide us with information other than what is currently needed. Mere attending does not necessarily bring additional semantic information to consciousness; it simply sharpens the Gestalt window—its shape, boundaries, feature combination, and exact location. But if we need to interact with the attended object or communicate about it, then the more detailed semantic information becomes immediately available.

Furthermore, there are everyday situations in which we may notice that our brain has, without us paying any attention, opened a *misleading* semantic window. This kind of a situation may happen in a department store in the clothing department if you are totally absorbed in finding the right shirt or whatever piece of clothing you are looking for. You notice somebody in one corner blocking your way. You do not want to go too close, that would be impolite, but what's that guy doing all the time in the same place anyway? Then you look at him more closely and—lo and behold—it was only a manikin all the time! What a relief! Nobody was spying on you—your brain had just opened the semantic window "person" or "man" for that vague person-like blur in the periphery of your vision, and after that you automatically behaved as if that virtual object really were a living person.

Our brain probably does this kind of automatic categorization all the time, without us even realizing it. When we enter a crowded elevator or bus we do not have the time or courage to look closely at every single person. It might take quite some time to discover a lifelike puppet or two among the virtual objects that our brain straightaway categorizes as "living persons," mostly on the basis of vague Gestalt windows and expectations based on previous similar situations.

Summary

The inquiry into the contents of phenomenal consciousness revealed some fundamental facts about phenomenal space and phenomenal objects. First, the all-pervading spatiality of experience implies that the phenomenal level in the brain is organized around an underlying egocentric spatial framework: phenomenal space. That system is responsible for the fact that qualitative experiences have definite spatial locations in relation to each other. It also accounts for the overall unity or singularity of the phenomenal level: consciousness forms exactly one experiential world. Second, regions or points of the phenomenal coordinate system can realize the whole range of qualitative, self-presenting features. They constitute subjective experience entirely on their own (i.e., nonrelationally). The organized patterns and bundles of such features constitute object-like wholes, virtual objects, that are present in subjective experience. The three main categories into which the patterns fall are virtual body (self), virtual world (virtual objects), and mental phenomena. Third, virtual objects consist of two types of information: the concrete surface pattern of phenomenal features (the Gestalt window), and conscious access to a large body of semantic and autobiographical information that turns the Gestalt window into a familiar, meaningful object: a semantic window.

IV Binding and the Phenomenal Unity of Consciousness

One of the most conspicuous features of consciousness is its unity. Part IV of this book is concerned with the description and explanation of the phenomenal unity of consciousness. The underlying *mechanisms* that account for the phenomenal unity of consciousness are believed to somehow *bind* together the phenomenal contents of consciousness and they are therefore called mechanisms of binding. The *binding problem* is the difficulty of seeing how *any* brain mechanisms could really account for the phenomenal unity of consciousness.

The binding problem is first clarified and defined specifically for the purposes of a science of consciousness (chapter 11). Then fascinating data concerning the disunity of consciousness and the breakdown of the mechanisms of binding are reviewed from the viewpoint of the science of consciousness. Such data originate especially from neuropsychology (chapters 12 and 13) and dream research (chapter 14). Then the cognitive and neural mechanisms of binding are explored (chapters 15 and 16).

11 The Binding Problem and the Unity of Consciousness

One may come across the terms *binding* and *binding problem* in neuroscience, cognitive science, experimental psychology, and consciousness research. It is not entirely clear whether all usages of the term refer to the *same* process (of binding) or even to the *same* problem. In this chapter we distinguish between several different formulations of the binding problem. While all of them have something to do with *unity* and *integration,* not all of them have something to do with the unity of consciousness. As the science of consciousness is interested in unity of consciousness specifically, rather than unity of phenomena unrelated to consciousness, we need to formulate the binding problem anew. The chapter closes by introducing the new, more precise formulation of the problem that defines the binding problem for the science of consciousness.[1]

What Is the Binding Problem?

The binding problem appears in several different formulations in current cognitive neuroscience. Some of these formulations refer directly to the unity of consciousness, but others are silent about the role of consciousness. Thus, there is no *single* binding problem, or any *single* definition of the problem to be found. Instead, the label "binding" refers to a confusing variety of different problems at different levels of description (Revonsuo, 1999).[2]

The job for consciousness science is to make it crystal clear which of these discussions are about consciousness, whether directly or indirectly, and which are about the unity of cognitive and neural mechanisms that have little, if anything, to do with the phenomenal level. Instead of simply giving my version of the definition of the binding problem right at the outset, I think it will be more enlightening to see how several different people have characterized it recently.

Stimulus-Related Binding

One classic version of the binding problem refers to the *relation* between *brain activity* and external physical objects as *sources of stimulation.* Now, if one single physical object can trigger a number of input processes in our sensory systems, how does the brain know that the multiplicity of neural activity that was triggered by the stimulus originated in a *single* external object? And if the stimulus field contains several different physical objects, then how does the brain sort out which set of stimulations originated in *this* physical object *over here* and which set in *that* one *over there*? How is it that the complex packages of sensory input do not get thoroughly mixed on their way to the brain?

> There is, next, what is commonly referred to as the binding problem, a critical problem for visual physiology. The problem is that of determining that it is the same (or a different) stimulus which is activating different cells in a given visual area or in different visual areas. (Zeki, 1992, p. 321)

> The "binding problem" refers to the means by which the brain "knows" that signals depicting such perceptual features as visual orientation, movement, colour, and sound all come from that one object. (Kahn, Pace-Schott, & Hobson, 1997, p. 20)

This conception of binding I shall refer to as *stimulus-related binding* (figure 11.1). The binding problem is here depicted as follows: How do external physical objects, as physically unified entities, end up being mapped as coherent neural entities in the brain, although input processing first segregates the activities elicited by the single object across a multitude of distinct neural maps? Binding is seen as the problem of finding the mechanisms that map the external physical entities out there in the world to corresponding internal neural entities in the brain. The key issue is to reveal the ways in which neurons "code" or "respond to" the features of external physical objects.

Note that in this formulation of the binding problem, no reference whatsoever is made to consciousness. Binding is seen rather as *any process or mechanism that in some sense recovers the unity of the stimulus object,* a unity objectively existing out there in the external physical stimulus. Stimulus-related binding refers to any neural processing that represents (or reconstructs) stimulus unity, regardless of whether the neural activity in question is conscious or nonconscious.

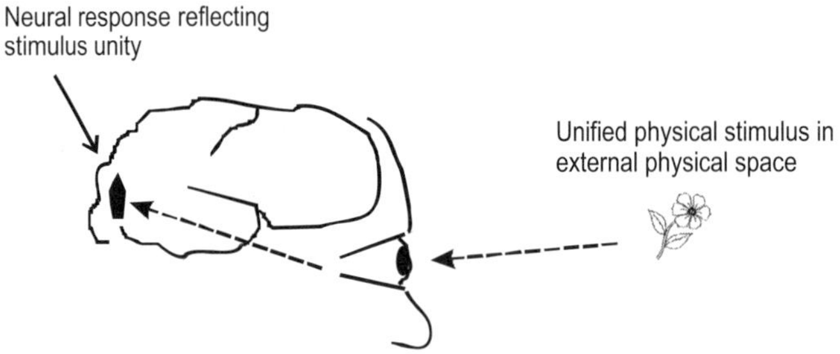

Figure 11.1
Stimulus-related binding. In stimulus-related binding, an internal neural representation correlates with the unity or holistic properties of an external physical stimulus object. Note that consciousness or phenomenal unity need not be involved in any way in stimulus-related binding. It primarily answers the question, Which neural processes in the brain covary with the holistic properties of external physical stimuli?

Consciousness-Related Binding

Phenomenal unity is the unity of experience—the unity of phenomenal consciousness. The science of consciousness should primarily be interested in phenomenal unity—not the unity of external physical objects or the unity of neural assemblies per se. Some formulations of the binding problem are explicit about this:

> Current knowledge from neuroanatomy and neurophysiology of the primate nervous system indicates unequivocally that any entity or event that we normally perceive through multiple sensory modalities must engage geographically separate sensory modality structures of the central nervous system. . . . The experience of reality, however, both in ongoing perception as well as in recall, is not parcellated at all. The normal experience we have of entities and events is coherent and "in-register," both spatially and temporally. Features are bound in entities, and entities are bound in events. How the brain achieves such a remarkable integration starting with the fragments that it has to work with is a critical question. I call it the binding problem. . . . The brain must have devices capable of promoting the integration of fragmentary components of neural activity, in some sort of ensemble pattern that matches the structures of entities, events, and relationships thereof. (Damasio, 1989, p. 29)

Here Damasio quite clearly refers to our *experience* of reality, entities, and events, which normally is unified. How the brain brings about *that* unity—the unity of consciousness—is the binding problem for the science of consciousness. This has been recognized by Searle (1992) at least:

> It is characteristic of nonpathological conscious states that they come to us as part of a unified sequence. . . . Unity exists at least in two dimensions, which . . . I will call "horizontal" and "vertical." Horizontal unity is the organization of conscious experiences through short stretches of time. . . . Vertical unity is a matter of the simultaneous awareness of all the diverse features of any conscious state. . . . We have little understanding of how the brain achieves this unity. In neurophysiology it is called "the binding problem," and Kant called the same phenomenon "the transcendental unity of apperception." (Searle, 1992, p. 130)

This variety of binding I call *consciousness-related* binding (figure 11.2). Consciousness-related binding concerns the relationship between phenomenal unity experienced in consciousness and its directly underlying mechanisms. Our phenomenal experience of a world of objects is in many ways unified or holistic. Phenomenal unity is a feature of the contents of consciousness residing at the phenomenal level of organization in the brain. Lower-level neural mechanisms should in some way account for the fact of phenomenal unity. Phenomenal unity must be *somehow* related to binding mechanisms resting at the lower, neurophysiological levels. A multilevel explanantion of phenomenal unity requires reference to the lower-level binding mechanisms.

If we take into account our current knowledge of neuroanatomy and neurophysiology, it is by no means obvious how an explanation of phenomenal unity could be reached. The neural mechanisms necessary for creating different phenomenal contents (e.g., color, movement, vision, audition, touch) are distributed all around the cortex.

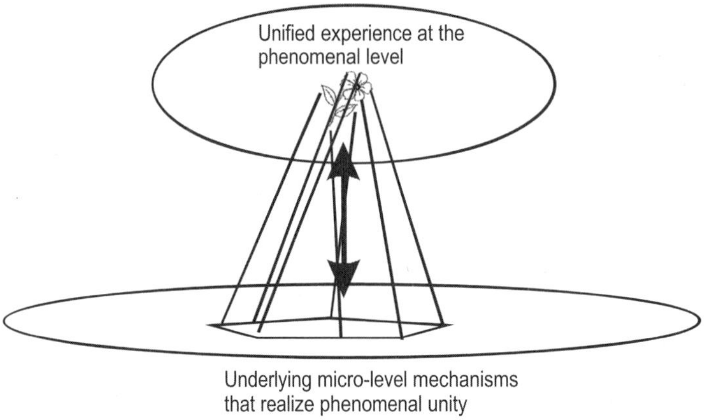

Figure 11.2
Consciousness-related binding. Consciousness-related binding describes the underlying cognitive and neural mechanisms that directly realize phenomenal unity. Note that external physical stimuli or neural responses to such stimuli need not be involved in any way. The unified phenomenal object as such is independent of external stimulus objects, and may be realized in their absence, as in hallucinations or dreams. The explanation of consciousness-related binding tends to be a *constitutive, downward*-looking explanation. It primarily answers the question, Which neural processes directly underlie the holistic properties of phenomenal experience?

There is no anatomical center in which phenomenal binding could occur. At present hardly any neurophysiological mechanisms are known that might account for the phenomenal unity of consciousness (however, more on the potential neurophysiological mechanisms in chapter 16).

It is important to recognize that stimulus-related binding and consciousness-related binding do not *necessarily* have anything to do with each other. Some physical stimulus may be received by the visual system and a unified representation of the object may be formed somewhere in the visual cortex, but entirely outside of consciousness. Conversely, some unified phenomenal experience (say during dreaming or during the perception of illusory unity) may be constructed by the consciousness-related binding mechanisms in the absence of any unified physical stimulus. In the brain there probably are nonconscious but unified representations of stimuli, as well as unified phenomenal contents bound together without any stimulus input. When we consciously perceive external objects during wakefulness, the consciousness-related mechanisms become also stimulus-related. Thus, in perception the operation of consciousness-related binding reflects both the unity of experience and the unity of the stimulus.

Binding at Different Levels of Description

The above distinction between stimulus-related and consciousness-related binding is a good starting point, but we should additionally distinguish between the different levels of description at which binding and unity can be conceptualized.

I shall distinguish the following principal levels of description: phenomenal, neural, and cognitive.

1. *The phenomenal level.* This level of description only applies to concepts referring to the subjective experience of unity, rather than to concepts referring to cognitive or neural mechanisms. Thus, the phenomenal level of description involves an account of the elementary phenomenal contents of consciousness, the local binding of the elementary contents to unified wholes (coherent virtual objects), and the global unity of consciousness (the unity of the simulated world in which all the virtual objects are embedded).

2. *The level of neural mechanisms* involves description of functionally unified neurophysiological phenomena, especially ones that correlate with the perception or representation of unified stimuli. For neuroscience the binding problem is the problem of the integration of single neuron activity to functional neuronal groups and assemblies. The elements are microlevel entities and activities studied by basic neuroscience (single neurons and their spiking frequencies or firing patterns), and the unified wholes are higher-level neural assemblies (single neurons temporarily interacting in some manner that integrates them into larger functional clusters).

Crick and Koch (1990) define the binding problem in a way that refers to purely neural-level unity:

> . . . it is highly reasonable to assume that seeing any one object often involves neurons in many different visual areas. The problem of how these neurons temporarily become active as a unit is often described as "the binding problem." (p. 269)

According to this formulation the binding problem is the problem of finding out the neural mechanisms that can transiently unify an ensemble of neurons. Exploring the neural mechanisms that are involved in creating transient, unified neural assemblies certainly constitutes a major issue for neuroscience. But we should take note of the fact that consciousness need not be mentioned at all when such mechanisms are discussed or investigated.

3. *The level of cognitive mechanisms* involves the description of input-output transformations (information processing) that produce unified representations for perception, memory, and action in a cognitive system. Note that "the cognitive system" need not be a biological system: the cognitive binding problem applies to computer vision as well as to biological vision.

In cognitive science and cognitive neuropsychology the binding problem is typically clothed in purely cognitive concepts. How can a distributed, modular architecture of information processing produce unified representations? According to the modularity hypothesis (Fodor, 1983; Ellis & Young, 1988), the input processing of perceptual information is handled by a multitude of isolated, specialized, mandatory, fast, nonconscious, neurologically specific modules. How does our cognitive system unify the results of the multitude of distributed modular processing to create unified representations of objects for perception, recognition, and memory? This is the binding problem for cognitive science.

The Binding Problem in the Science of Consciousness

Phenomenal consciousness presents itself in the form of one world—a single experiential space or the world-for-me. The unity of the sphere of subjective experience equals the unity of consciousness. It unifies all the different sorts of phenomenal contents into a single phenomenal world. This *global unity* of the sphere of phenomenal consciousness is not the only type of phenomenal unity. The individual phenomenal contents within the sphere of consciousness are also *internally* integrated. Any phenomenal object that presents itself within the sphere of consciousness is a tightly unified package of phenomenal features that appear together in a well-organized form. Thus, individual phenomenal objects show considerable *local unity.* A solution to the binding problem requires the discovery of the underlying mechanisms that support the global unity of consciousness and the local unity of the phenomenal contents of consciousness.

In the science of consciousness, binding refers to the integration of phenomenal contents into unified phenomenal wholes, and the immediately underlying mechanisms that explain phenomenal binding. In the science of consciousness the unity of consciousness is regarded as the truly problematic phenomenon. The cognitive- and neural-level descriptions are treated only as descriptions of the (possible) lower-level mechanisms of phenomenal binding. Cognitive- and neural-level descriptions are of interest to consciousness research only insofar as they can be, directly or indirectly, related to integration at the phenomenal level, insofar as they can be regarded as the possible underlying explanatory mechanisms of phenomenal binding. In such cases we may hope for *explanatory shifts* to take place from the higher, phenomenally unified levels to the lower neurocognitive levels. A multilevel explanation of binding should show how the unity at the higher level arises from the integrative mechanisms at the lower levels.

In our everyday, baseline state of consciousness we take it for granted that our consciousness is unified; we experience one seemingly coherent world around us which is just there for us, without any effort on our part. Furthermore, the single unified world contains internally unified objects. We have no indication that all this unity is the construction of complex neural mechanisms in the brain. Like any smoothly operating complex biological system, the phenomenal level does not reveal its compositional structure easily.

The history of biological science has shown that one of the best ways to figure out how a system is put together is to take it apart. It may sound outright absurd to talk about "taking" consciousness "apart," but, as a matter of fact, there are many ways in which consciousness can become disintegrated in altered states of consciousness or in consequence of brain injury. These exceptional forms of consciousness are crucial sources of evidence for empirical phenomenology in the science of consciousness.

A systematic account of phenomenal disunities is therefore indispensable as a body of data about the unity and binding of consciousness. The scope and limits of phenomenal unity and disunity impose top-down constraints on the underlying mechanisms. Once we know the ways in which phenomenal unity may break down, we can probably rule out some potential mechanisms as unlikely or impossible because they could not account for the data. Conversely, we may be able to identify some potential mechanisms that show promising explanatory power, in that they could support local or global types of phenomenal unity. Furthermore, when they break down in their characteristic ways, the kinds of phenomenal disunity that follow should correspond to the available empirical evidence concerning known disunities of consciousness. Perhaps it will even be possible to predict some novel phenomenal disunities that have not yet been observed, or rule out some other types of disunity as impossible because the binding mechanisms just cannot break down in ways that would produce those types of phenomenal disunity.

Summary

In this chapter we distinguished three different levels at which the process of binding may be described:

1. Binding as a process that integrates the contents of consciousness and results in the (local, global, or both) phenomenal unity of consciousness.
2. Binding as a neurophysiological process that integrates the activity of single neurons to larger functional units such as neural assemblies and results in coherence and unity of large-scale neural activity.
3. Binding as a cognitive process that integrates the outputs of information processing from a multitude of independent processing modules, to form unified cognitive representations to be used in recognition, memory, and action in the cognitive system.

We furthermore distinguished two different ways in which the binding problem may be framed:

1. Stimulus-related binding: the problem of understanding the relationship between the physical unity of external stimuli and the neural representations that internally recover or represent the unity of the stimuli.
2. Consciousness-related binding: the problem of understanding the relationship between the phenomenal unity of consciousness and the immediately underlying mechanisms that could explain phenomenal unity.

We concluded the chapter by stressing that for the science of consciousness, the binding problem is first and foremost the problem of consciousness-related binding.

12 Binding and Phenomenal Disunity I: What Visual Disorders Tell about Consciousness

Empirical phenomenology describes the ways in which the normal unity and organization of phenomenal experience may break down. The decomposition hypothesis states that different phenomenal features may be independently disrupted. In this chapter we put empirical phenomenology and the decomposition hypothesis to work. We meet patients suffering from various types of brain injury that have resulted in curious disruptions of visual phenomenology. Here, we are particularly interested in cases where the perception of form, color, and motion (or their integration) is compromised. (In the following chapter we consider other kinds of deficits.) The subjective worlds of patients who have lost the visual experience of coherent form, qualitative color, or the sense of visual motion might give us clues about the nature of the underlying mechanisms that must be at work in the generation of the normal unity of phenomenal consciousness. The patterns of disruption seen at the phenomenal level may thus serve as important top-down constraints in the multilevel explanation of consciousness.

Gestalt Principles of Perceptual Organization

Our normal phenomenal world is made up of a large number of organized patterns of phenomenal experience. How does all that detailed organization arise? During the first part of the twentieth century, Gestalt psychologists discovered several "laws" or principles that the visual system uses to organize the content of visual awareness. Visual perception groups basic elements in the phenomenal visual field in such a way that those elements are experienced as *perceptual units* that naturally belong together. Without these grouping principles, there would be no coherent perceptual shapes or objects in visual awareness.

The grouping principles include the following (Palmer, 1999): *Proximity* or relative closeness: elements closer to each other relative to other elements tend to form a perceptual unit. *Similarity:* elements that share a common feature, such as color, size, or orientation, tend to form perceptual units relative to elements that do not share such features. *Common fate:* elements that move together tend to form perceptual units. The above principles concern the grouping of any kinds of simple elements; further principles have been formulated that primarily apply to linelike elements. *Symmetry* and *parallelism* group lines together, and *continuity* characterizes any linelike perceptual unit whose elements show smooth continuation. The principle of *closure* says that elements that form a closed figure tend to be grouped together (figure 12.1).

Thanks to these principles of perceptual organization, we are in our conscious visual perception surrounded by a world of coherent bundles of qualitative features: virtual objects (Gestalt windows). But could things be otherwise? Is it conceivable that the *organization* of qualitative features at the phenomenal level is lost, but not the qualitative features themselves? If the very existence of phenomenality was constituted by, or necessarily dependent on, perceptual organization, it would follow that if the organization is lost, then so is all phenomenal experience. That prediction does not seem to hold. Damage to the visual cortex can wipe out most of the organization of visual awareness at the phenomenal level, yet the basic qualitative visual features remain.

Apperceptive Agnosia: Visual Qualities Disorganized

Patients suffering from *apperceptive agnosia* have widespread brain damage in the occipital cortex and surrounding regions; a typical cause of the damage is carbon monoxide poisoning. The patients show preserved ability to detect even tiny differences in luminance and wavelength, and they can detect the movement of even small objects. They have a full visual field: they can detect these features in any part of the normal visual field. Hence they are not blind, wholly or even partially. They can recognize colors, name the colors of even small objects, and pick out colors on command (Zeki, 1992). By contrast, the patients typically fail in all tasks that require shape perception: they cannot name objects, written words or letters, or geometrical figures. They are unable to copy simple pictures, numbers, or letters and words. They may be able to infer or guess the identity of some object on the basis of cues from color, but that is an inference rather than a conscious visual percept. Nevertheless, the patients will immediately recognize an object through sense modalities other than vision: there is no general semantic or intellectual decline.

Although these patients still enjoy visual qualities, the disorganization of the content of visual awareness at the phenomenal level is so severe that the patients appear as helpless as if they were blind. The patients fail in the simplest forms of shape discrimination and do not seem to perceive objects as solid forms or even as surfaces in three dimensions (Farah, 1990).

It would seem that these patients must have lost a major part of the very fundamental organizing mechanisms that normally work beneath the phenomenal surface. Still, neither the phenomenal space—the subjective visual field—that supports visual qualities nor the qualities of visual experience themselves have been lost. The mechanisms

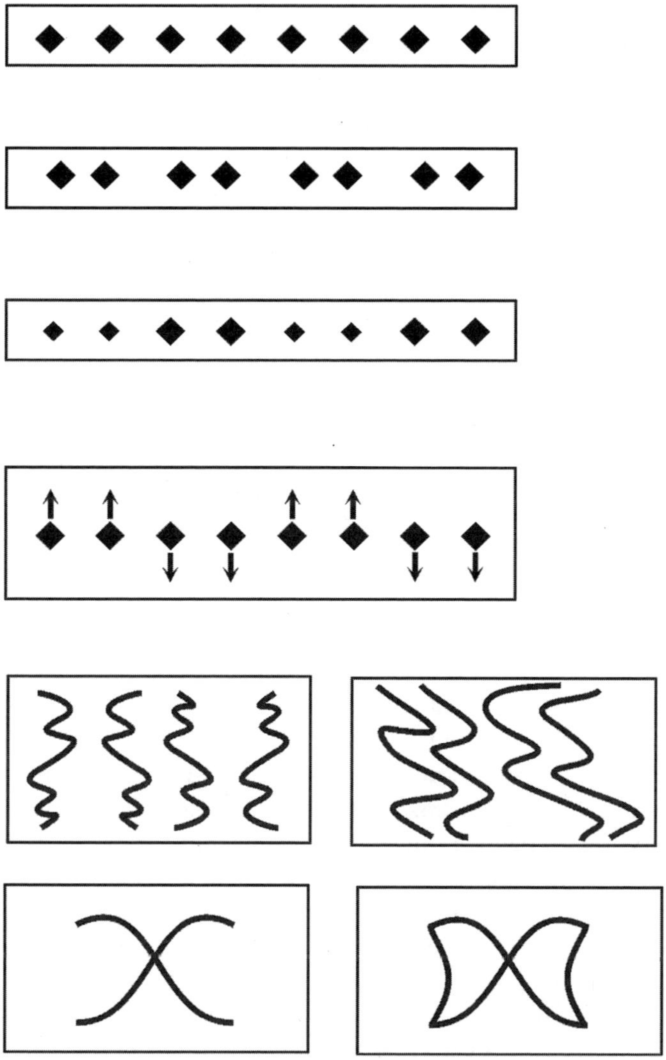

Figure 12.1
Gestalt grouping. Separate stimuli tend to be grouped (or bound) together to a perceptual unit when they are characterized by, for example, similarity, proximity, common fate, parallelism, or symmetry. (Modified from Palmer [1999], reproduced with permission of The MIT Press.)

that are gone seem to be the ones that implement the Gestalt principles of grouping. Therefore, the visual phenomenology of those patients is still qualitatively rich, but contains either none at all or only awfully restricted higher-level organization into perceptual units and objects. The binding of local regions to coherent Gestalt windows, or even to continous linelike elements or contours, has become impossible.

Qualities and Perceptual Organization

What are the theoretical implications of this remarkable dissociation between elementary phenomenal, qualitative experience per se, and the higher-level organization of those qualitative experiences? First, they show that whatever the lower-level cognitive and neural mechanisms of perceptual organization turn out to be, their proper functioning is not a *necessary* requirement for qualitative visual experience to occur. Second, the varieties of phenomenology worth having are those that show a high degree of organization. The patients are functionally blind: they cannot guide their behavior with the help of visual information. They have, moreover, lost much of the beauty of seeing, of having breathtaking visual experiences. They can still enjoy color qualities, but they cannot enjoy a scenic view, the face of a loved one, or the beauty of a painting, a photograph, or a film. They have lost much the same things that a truly blind person, lacking all visual qualia, has lost too.

The observation that chaotic qualities are rather worthless implies that the reason why phenomenal consciousness is so crucially important for us involves much more than the mere *presence* of qualitative features for the subject. What makes our typical human consciousness valuable, desirable, and astonishing is not only the capability to enjoy qualitative experiences, as opposed to being an unfeeling zombie, but the capacity to enjoy beautifully *organized* qualitative experiences. Qualitative features, wonderful inventions of nature as they are, do not in and of themselves make up the simulated realities where we live our subjective lives. It certainly is a miracle how physical matter organized itself such that any phenomenal features ever came to be, but a miracle of at least as much consequence is how nature invented mechanisms for *organizing* these features with such sophistication as to create an entire surrogate *world* in the brain.

The Continuum of Consciousness

The fact that chaotic qualities alone are quite pointless should be taken into account in philosophical discussions of consciousness. It is often taken for granted that conscious experience is a strictly *all-or-none* phenomenon. Such an uncompromising divide is part of what makes the explanatory gap seem so unbridgeable. On one side of the gap, there is the phenomenal world in all its majesty; on the other, there is the internal darkness of total zombiehood, or of blind, nonconscious neurophysiological processes. If consciousness is seen as an unanalyzable entity that admits no grades, no smooth continuum, then the gap will seem ever wider and deeper.

But perhaps the problem of consciousness will fragment into several different problems, hopefully more tractable ones than the original, when we notice that we are not dealing with one absolutely unanalyzable, undividable entity, consciousness, which is either totally present or totally absent. As soon as we acknowledge the *gradual nature* of the phenomenal world—that there may be experiential worlds that contain some rudimentary aspects of our own paradigmatic consciousness but lack several others—then the possibility is opened that perhaps the borderline between the phenomenal and the nonconscious is a gray area, involving a *smooth continuum* of several levels of organization. That would make it comparable to the gapless continuum in nature between the living and the nonliving.

I propose that the continuum from nonphenomenal levels to the full-blown phenomenal world can be outlined as follows: First, there is the unified spatial coordinate system or phenomenal space. It is necessary for any qualitative features to be present, but in itself it is not a qualitative feature (see chapter 9). It enables the higher levels of phenomenal organization to be realized, but it seems itself to be nothing that could be experienced as such, without the presence of at least some qualitative features within it. It resides at the very interface between the phenomenal and the nonphenomenal; in fact, it incorporates features of both domains.

This is a critical point when moving from the nonphenomenal domain to the phenomenal domain. The entities or properties at the interface of the two disparate realms are crucial for the explanation of consciousness. According to some pessimistic philosophical ideas, consciousness cannot be explained because the explanatorily relevant properties are accessible neither through introspection nor through neuroscience (McGinn, 1991). Thus, McGinn's view is that there is something there at the interface that is neither neural (objectively measurable) nor phenomenal (introspectively accessible), and precisely that hidden structure is crucial for the explanation of consciousness. By contrast, I suggest that the explanatorily relevant entities are *partially* accessible through *both* neuroscience and subjective experience, but not fully accessible through either alone. Phenomenal space, or the egocentric coordinate system, is intermediate between the conscious and the nonconscious, a crucial link between the phenomenal and the nonphenomenal realms. We can come to know it, and form conceptions of it, both through our own experience, and through accounts of the experience of others, and, at the end of the day, even through functional brain-imaging methods, though not necessarily the ones currently available.

Intermingled with phenomenal space there is the basic phenomenal level constituting the mere presence of spatially arranged qualitative features. This level may or may not be accompanied by higher-level phenomenal organization such as shapes (Gestalt windows) and virtual objects (semantic windows). The organized phenomenal entities reside at a still higher level which shows a part-whole relationship to the qualitative elements at the basic phenomenal level.

Deciphering consciousness in terms of multiple interconnected layers renders the phenomenon tractable. In terms of this continuum of levels, what has happened to patients with apperceptive agnosia? In brief, they still retain the basic phenomenal level of visual qualities, but have lost the higher levels of spatially organized bundles of qualitative features that form coherent perceptual objects.

Part Binding and Associative Agnosia

Patients suffering from *associative agnosia* were for a long time supposed to have intact visual perception of objects (i.e., intact Gestalt windows or percepts of objects) but the percepts were just supposed to be somehow *stripped of their meaning* (i.e., incapable of opening the respective semantic windows). This assumption was based on the fact that the patients can copy pictures of objects accurately, but they have no idea what the meticulously copied pictures mean. They can draw the picture, look at it, and not have any idea what the object depicted is. For outsiders, the picture is instantly recognizable as an accurate copy of the original picture (which the patient does not recognize either).

Careful studies have revealed that the patients do not in actual fact enjoy intact percepts, but they can still use shape information in a limited way. They can copy a picture *line by line,* but they *cannot see the picture as a whole* at any one time (Farah, 1990). Their ability to *copy* pictures is thus not adequate evidence of their being able to *see* (or visually experience) the pictures normally. The mechanisms of spatial grouping can bind together small bits and pieces of contour, sufficient for producing a piecemeal copy of a picture. But the visual *experience* that such patients have is still shattered in pieces, and they make lots of visual errors in the identification of objects around them. The most famous patient of this kind is the one reported by Oliver Sacks (1985): the patient who mistook his wife for a hat.

In the same vein, Marcel (1983) discusses patients characterized by the fragmentation of representations into their elements. Such a patient can be simultaneously aware of all features that are present in the visual stimulus field, but his visual system cannot put the features spatially together as objects. One patient with this type of agnosia described his phenomenal experience of vision as follows:

> . . . this confusion of lots of things, all of which were there, but did not seem to belong together . . . a lot of things which to any ordinary viewer would be parts of the same thing were parts of different things. . . . The effect was much more striking when a large number of objects were on the same table . . . it was not obvious what belonged to what . . . I should add that very often looking at pictures in daily papers for instance, especially if they were rather large pictures, I had to look at different bits and found it very difficult to combine them into a whole (Marcel, 1983, pp. 292–293).

A complete perceptual object is typically composed of several distinct parts, which in themselves are objects at a lower level of hierarchy (the wings and the body of a butterfly, for example). The parts must be correctly combined in visual awareness in order to make sense of the object—this is *part binding* (Treisman, 1996). In some cases of prosopagnosia (the inability to recognize faces), binding the parts of a face into a structured whole fails. One such patient explained that "I can see the eyes, nose and mouth quite clearly, but they just don't add up" (Pallis, 1955, p. 219, cited in Ellis & Young, 1988, p. 90).

It seems that there is a continuum rather than a sharp division between what traditionally have been called "apperceptive agnosia" and "associative agnosia." In the former, all mechanisms of spatial grouping have collapsed, and visual phenomenology totally lacks perceptual organization in terms of continuous lines, contours, or coherent shapes and objects. In the latter, some restricted binding is possible, but it often remains unstable and is prone to errors. For some patients, spatial grouping through the Gestalt principle of common fate is preserved, presumably because the neural mechanism of motion perception is separate from the mechanisms of other basic cues for shape (luminance contrast, texture, color). The patient described by Marcel could still use the mechanism of common fate to create coherent virtual objects out of the chaos: "[I]f a given person moved so that all parts of him went in one direction, that would . . . tend to make him into a single object" (Marcel, 1983, p. 292).

In associative agnosia *part binding* fails. The visual qualitative features cannot be organized across larger regions of phenomenal space in the subjective visual field. Yet, small-scale integration allowing the perception of single parts of objects may occur. Visual motion, which reaches the phenomenal level through a different path than the other grouping cues, can in some cases still organize perceptual elements into unitary wholes.

Feature Binding

The shape and contour of an object may be determined by several distinct elementary features such as color, texture, luminance, or coherent motion. The process by which these features are bound together in a single location in the phenomenal visual field, thus defining a coherent perceptual object, may be called *feature binding (or feature integration,* or *property binding)* (Treisman, 1996).

Thus, if you see a butterfly fluttering about in the meadow, what defines it as a visual object for you are the color and texture of the wings, its luminance, movement, and shape. All these disparate features coalesce into a single location where the coherent percept of the butterfly is bound together in your subjective visual field. You see the swallowtail as a single visual object, not the different visual features scattered all over the visual space without any coordination.

If we compare part binding and feature binding, one important difference between them is that in part binding the different parts of a single object do not occupy exactly the same location in the phenomenal coordinate system, but different, usually adjacent locations. Part binding requires a mechanism that unites several *adjacent* regions together into one larger region which defines the whole object. By contrast, feature binding concerns the different features of the same object. Those features must occupy the very *same* location in the phenomenal space to be features of one and the same object. These two types of binding might, therefore, be based on different kinds of mechanisms.

Feature integration fails when insufficient focal attention is paid to objects in the visual field. The failures lead to *illusory feature conjunctions.* They can be experimentally induced in the laboratory by presenting stimuli with different feature combinations, but not allowing enough time for serial focused attention to bind the properties appropriately. The subjects report seeing such combinations of color and form that never existed among the stimuli—the brain incorrectly "glues" a color and a form together in visual awareness (Treisman & Schmidt, 1982).

A neuropsychological disorder called *Balint's syndrome* is associated with increased frequency of feature binding errors. These patients have bilateral parietal damage and they usually suffer from simultanagnosia: they are able to perceive only one object at a time. However, although they can identify the single object they see, based on its defining shape, they do not necessarily see the object with all its features coherently bound together. On the contrary, they tend to miscombine with the shape they perceive other features, such as color, size, or motion that exist in the stimulus field as attributes of entirely separate objects! For instance, one patient, when shown a *red X* and *blue O,* often and confidently reported that *he saw the X as blue* or *the O as red.* For these patients, feature binding becomes a real binding problem in their everyday lives, as the multiple features in the visual stimulus field tend to combine inaccurately in visual consciousness, thus forming erratic conjunctions (L. C. Robertson, 1999, 2003).

Illusory conjunctions do raise some interesting questions as to what the relations are between the nonconscious mechanisms that modulate and organize the qualities at the phenomenal level, and the qualities themselves. When there are different colored forms in a stimulus display (a red X, a blue T, and a green O, for example), it is possible to visually experience a green T or a red O. In the stimulus display the letter O was constituted by pixels physically different in reflectance spectrum from the other letters. Yet, somewhere in the sensory system, between the proximal stimulus and the phenomenal level, the coding of the reflectance properties had to be separated from the coding of the form properties (although the form was physically defined by the reflectance differences). There had to be information about the form that was "colorless," and conversely, "formless" information about the color. Such pieces of information are obviously in a format dissimilar from the format in which the information surfaces at the phenomenal level. There it is impossible to have perfectly colorless forms or perfectly formless colors. The erroneous recombinations have to be determined at a stage prior to consciousness, because once at the phenomenal level, the color makes up the form, and the form is filled in by a color.

Illusory conjunctions are not constructed at the phenomenal level; they are only manifested there. If they were, we would be aware of formless colors chasing colorless forms (or vice versa) in visual awareness, trying to find the correct match and settle down. But nothing like that happens. On the contrary, subjects in the experiments are positive about seeing certain combinations of color and form, and reluctant to believe that such combinations were never among the stimuli.

Patient's with Balint's syndrome sometimes, however, report *unstable* feature bindings. One patient with Balint's syndrome frequently reported such problems in feature binding experiments in which multiple colored letters were presented:

> When I first look at it, it looks green and it changes real quick to red. I see both colors coming together. . . . When I look at it, it is an A. And sometimes I see like a shadow of it. . . . It looks like sometimes one letter is going into the other one. I get double identity. It kind of coincides. (L. Robertson, Treisman, Friedman-Hill, & Grabowecky, 1997, p. 307)

In Balint's syndrome, spatial representations defining the location of the features are damaged, and thus the brain does not know where each feature should go, and which features make up one object (more on Balint's syndrome in the next chapter).

Achromatopsia

It is possible to lose permanently the phenomenal feature of chromatic color while retaining shape perception and an organized but entirely achromatic inner world simulation (for a recent neuropsychological review, see Heywood & Cowey [1999]). In cases of complete cerebral achromatopsia the patient's model of the world simply loses all chromatic color: it becomes a black-and-white world; a virtual world painted only in shades of gray. The patient loses not only the ability to see colors in perception, to discriminate between isoluminant colors, and to match or name colors, but also the ability to *imagine* or *remember* what color qualities were like. Even dreams become entirely colorless.

Cerebral achromatopsia appears to be the perfect reverse of the philosophical thought experiment about the future neuroscientist Mary (Jackson, 1986). She is supposed to know *everything* about color perception that can be scientifically known in objective physical terms, but she has been confined to a black-and-white room all her life, until she is finally released one day. Then, for the first time in her life, she actually experiences colors. The question is, Did she thereby learn something new about colors that she did not know before? If she did, it is supposed to show that the complete objective-physicalist story of vision does not involve qualia, which must then be something nonphysical.

If there is something that Mary did not know about colors before her release, it appears to be *the very same thing that the patient with achromatopsia loses for good* at the onset of the dreadful condition. Thus, we can formulate the thought experiment anew:

Imagine that Mary's twin sister Maria also learned everything there is to know about color vision. She had been raised in a normal chromatic environment. But on the same day when Mary was released from her black-and-white laboratory, Maria became totally achromatopsic. Was there something about colors she therefore *did not know any longer*? If so, *what* was it that she lost?

A famous case of this sort of total loss of colors is described by Oliver Sacks (1995). This patient was a painter and therefore had an intimate relationship with colors, and knew them both experientially and intellectually better than most of us. But all that knowledge seems to have been lost through brain injury causing achromatopsia:

> It had gradually come upon him, during this time, that it was not merely colour perception and colour imagery that he lacked, but something deeper and difficult to define. He knew all about color, externally, intellectually, but he had lost the remembrance, the inner knowledge, of it that had been part of his very being. . . . It was as if his past, his chromatic past, had been taken away, as if the brain's knowledge of colour had been totally excised, leaving no trace, no inner evidence of its existence behind (p. 10)

> But black and white for him was a reality, all around him, 360 degrees, solid and three-dimensional, twenty-four hours a day. . . . neither "grey" nor "leaden" could begin to convey what his world was actually like. It was not "grey" that he experienced, he said, but perceptual qualities for which ordinary experience, ordinary language, had no equivalent. (p. 8)

Complete cerebral achromatopsia requires bilateral damage to a region in the extrastriate visual cortex in the lingual and fusiform gyri (area V4). But what happens if the critical location is damaged unilaterally? Does the patient lose half of the available chromatic qualities? That sounds like a perfectly reasonable hypothesis, given that the brain loses 50% of its machinery for the construction of color qualia. But the effect is not like that at all. Obviously, the brain is not organized in such a way as to construct some qualitative color dimensions in one hemisphere, and others in the other hemisphere. Rather, area V4 in each cerebral hemisphere contains the full palette of qualitative chromatic values, but the V4 in each hemisphere can only apply them to one half of the phenomenal visual field. Patients with hemiachromatopsia have only one half of the phenomenal visual field devoid of colors, while the other half appears normally colored (Zeki, 1992). Thus, whatever the mechanism for constructing qualitative colors at the phenomenal level is, each hemisphere alone is capable of carrying out the construction, but applying it only to one half of the phenomenal coordinate system. Each V4 therefore has access to only one half of the phenomenal visual field in the phenomenal coordinate system. The area V4 in the left hemisphere has access to the right side of the phenomenal field, and vice versa.

There are observations of patients who have dissociations between externally driven color *perception* and internally generated color *imagery;* it seems possible that one is preserved in the absence of the other (Shuren, Brott, Scheft, & Houston, 1996). In other words, there are some patients who cannot perceive any colors owing to damage to their visual cortex, but who nevertheless can employ colors in their visual mental imagery. Conversely, some patients can still see the real world in color, but are unable to generate any internal visual imagery in color. This curious dissociation could be explained by postulating two separate pathways that activate the phenomenal color system: the one a bottom-up pathway, the other a top-down pathway. If the mechanism for generating color qualities is in itself intact, but is disconnected from either source of activation, then color perception and imagery could be damaged independently of each other. But if the system generating the phenomenal color qualities itself is damaged, then colors disappear totally, from perception and imagery as well as dreams. This seems to be the case for Sack's patient described above.

The Mechanisms Involved in Phenomenal Color

Can anything be said about the mechanisms that construct the color qualities at the phenomenal level? A multilevel mechanistic model of the visual awareness of colors would have to include a description of the etiological pathways that causally modulate color experience at the phenomenal level. In visual perception, the causal chain leading to color at the phenomenal level in the brain starts outside the organism where there is electromagnetic radiation in the wavelength range of visible light. That physical energy hits the photoreceptor cells on the retina in the back of the eyes where the signal is transformed to graded electrophysiological potentials or spikes of neurons. This causes further electrophysiological events in the parvocellular layers in the lateral geniculate nucleus of the thalamus, where the cells transmit opponent-color signals or are wavelength sensitive, and the wavelength discriminative signals then cause further activity in the visual cortex.

Now it should be pointed out that all the processes along this etiological pathway are, first, completely *nonconscious, nonphenomenal,* and *uncolored* very likely up until the activation of V4. In other words, there is no phenomenal level of organization realized anywhere along this etiological pathway from the retina to V4. There is nothing there that could bear phenomenal color qualities. How do we know that? One good source of evidence comes from blindsight patients whose primary visual cortex is damaged. They do not experience any phenomenal colors in their blind visual fields, but nevertheless can still perform significantly better than chance in wavelength discrimination tasks (Cowey & Stoerig, 1992). The electrophysiological activity of the color-opponent coding cells (or wavelength discriminative cells) that probably supports the discriminative behavior of the blindsight patient is a completely nonconscious process and must not be identified with the subjective experience of phenomenal colors. It is part of the nonconscious etiological pathway that can modulate the phenomenal level, but the two must be strictly distinguished from each other. Wavelength similarity and discrimination judgments can be guided by implicit, nonconscious information.

At the phenomenal level we experience *six elementary colors.* They are the four unique chromatic hues: red, green, blue, and yellow, plus the two achromatic colors: black and white. They form the six qualitative reference points in the subjective or phenomenological color space. The elementarity, simplicity, or uniqueness of these phenomenal features refers to the fact that, for each of these color qualities, there exists *a "pure" form that contains no trace of any other color quality.* Hence unique yellow, for instance, is characterized subjectively by the color experience being *neither reddish nor greenish.* The elementary colors form opponent pairs so that two color qualities mutually exclude each other. No color is seen as both yellowish and bluish (or reddish and greenish) at the same time, whereas different varieties of purple are phenomenologically experienced as being composed of various degrees of blue and red mixed together.[1] The natural color system is a systematic arrangement of phenomenological hue experiences in a symmetrical color circle, scaled subjectively as proportions of the elementary hues (Valberg, 2001).

Subjects are capable of judging the amounts of elementary color qualities in their experiences of colored stimuli. This capability cannot be reduced to wavelength discrimination or to the activity of color-opponent cells in the retinal or thalamic level. However, the misleading use of color names to label cone opponent cells has led to the widespread misunderstanding that the neural basis of opponent colors would have been discovered already. Even textbooks often repeat the misconception that unique hue perception can be directly related to peripheral cone opponent processes. In fact, *no neurons have been found whose activity would code for the amounts of elementary colors in simple color sensations* (Valberg, 2001; Backhaus, 1998).

> Even if the elementary hues today are accepted as subjective references in phenomenal colour perception, it is necessary to emphasize that no opponent-cell correlations have been discovered. So far, *all attempts to determine the physiological nature of unique colors have failed.* (Valberg, 2001, p. 1650, italics added)

The elementary nature of unique color qualities provides yet another top-down constraint for the research program on consciousness. Whatever the lower-level mechanisms of phenomenal color qualities turn out to be, they will have to be able to support the six independent qualities as such; there will have to be *some* lower-level basis that explains why exactly *those* qualities are elementary and independent, why there are exactly this number of elementary color qualities, and why other colors (e.g., purple, orange) are compositional qualities, produced by combining the unique hues.

> We experience the six different elementary color sensations red, green, blue, yellow, black, and white, which constitute our color sensations, as six independent qualities. Since the electrical potentials of neurons are only one physical quality, even when superimposed from several neurons, the color sensations cannot be identical to the electrical excitations of neurons. (Backhaus, 1998, p. 382)

Backhaus's point seems to be that, in order for a microlevel theory to account for elementary color qualities, some underlying physical phenomenon will have to be found which contains six independent qualitative dimensions, and explains why some of them are mutually exclusive of each other (red-green, yellow-blue) and how certain others can be combined with each other in various degrees (blue-red, red-yellow).

Taken together, an exploration of the generation of color qualities has revealed several important facts that constrain the multilevel modeling of consciousness. First, there are several stages involving entirely nonconscious electrophysiological processes, coding for wavelength discrimination, that belong to the etiological pathway of color perception. Second, the phenomenal color space of human visual awareness involves six independent qualities, which constrains the potential underlying mechanisms. Third, blindsight and cerebral achromatopsia show that wavelength discrimination in the visual system is not sufficient for phenomenal color experiences, whereas the activity of an intact area V4 is necessary for them. Furthermore, the V4 in the right hemisphere provides all phenomenal colors but only to the left side of the phenomenal coordinate system, whereas the V4 in the left hemisphere takes care of the right side, respectively. Any model of phenomenal color experience should accommodate and explain these facts.

Phenomenal Motion in the Brain

The types of binding we have discussed so far exclude the temporal dimension and regard phenomenal objects as perceptual units frozen in time.The stationary visual experience of coherent objects involves the binding of different parts across different locations, or the binding of different attributes to the same location. When those binding mechanisms work properly, the result is the experience of a coherent Gestalt, whose parts and features belong together and form one holistic visual unit. But these phenomenal objects only suffice to build a motionless world. They are not sufficient for the construction of a fully *animated* visual world constituted by *dynamic* coherent objects.

Many visual objects around us are in motion: birds and butterflies fly by; cars and people move along the streets; tennis, badminton, and football are based on the perception of moving objects. What does the phenomenology of visual motion consist of? We see a moving coherent object as an entity that smoothly changes position over short periods of time. Perceived motion involves the experience that the very same object can be in different locations at different moments in time, in relation to other objects and to our bodies, but there is no discontinuity involved in this change of position; the change is gapless, smooth—the object slides across different locations in the phenomenal coordinate system—it shows perfect spatiotemporal continuity.

In fact, most contents of consciousness possess at least some short duration and an intrinsic temporal organization. Dainton (2000) describes the phenomenal passage thus:

. . . the flow or passage in experience is included in the phenomenal content of my experience. The total experience that results from my seeing a ball move between P_1 and P_2 does not consist of a stationary image of the ball at two different places. The content is *a ball moving.* (p. 176)

The perception of visual motion therefore requires a binding mechanism that works across the temporal domain and produces smooth changes in the relative location of a simulated virtual object in the phenomenal coordinate system. Such a mechanism appears to be separate from spatial grouping and part binding, for it can be lost without any loss of coherent but static virtual objects. The most famous case of a patient manifesting *cerebral akinetopsia* was reported by Zihl, von Cramon, and Mai (1983). The patient L.M. had bilateral damage to the middle temporal gyrus and the adjacent portion of the occipital gyri; this corresponds to the location of area MT which is selectively activated by moving visual stimuli (Heywood & Zihl, 1999). Her visual world was peculiarly devoid of perceived motion:

The visual disorder complained of by the patient was a loss of movement vision in all three dimensions. She had difficulty, for example, in pouring tea or coffee into a cup because the fluid appeared to be frozen, like a glacier. In addition, she could not stop pouring at the right time since she was unable to perceive the movement in the cup (or a pot) when the fluid rose. . . . In a room where more than two people were walking she felt very insecure and unwell, and usually left the room immediately, because "people were suddenly here or there but I have not seen them moving." . . . She could not cross the street because of her inability to judge the speed of a car, but she could identify the car itself without difficulty. "When I'm looking at the car first, it seems far away. But then, when I want to cross the road, suddenly the car is very near." She gradually learned to 'estimate' the distance of moving vehicles by means of the sound becoming louder (Zihl, von Cramon, & Mai, 1983, p. 315)

For this patient, there were only stationary visual objects which did not move, but appeared as suddenly jumping around. She could see the objects clearly at different distances and locations, but she had no idea what happened to them between these locations. For her, the objects did not move, they just jumped from one position to the next, but there was nothing in between (Heywood & Zihl, 1999).

The *binding of spatiotemporal continuity* fails in cerebral akinetopsia or motion blindness. Coherent virtual objects can normally change their relative position in the phenomenal space along continuous trajectories, and the phenomenal experience of a visual object in motion is the experience of its spatiotemporal continuity along such a trajectory. The patient with motion blindness cannot experience the spatiotemporally extended trajectories along which visually perceived virtual objects change their relative position because the specialized cortical mechanism that computes such trajectories for virtual objects is compromised. Objects become spatiotemporally discontinuous; they change their position without warning, suddenly. There is no sense of the trajectory along which the object smoothly slides.

Consequently, in akinetopsia there is nothing in visual experience that would allow *expectations* and *predictions* of the future position of objects. Our normal phenomenal experience of visual movement as a smooth trajectory allows instantaneous prediction of where a perceived entity is heading and where it will end up. We use these predictions all the time when dealing and interacting with moving objects, say in traffic or on the football field. Without the sense of visual motion, the virtual world is uncomfortably unpredictable, with virtual objects suddenly appearing in unexpected positions. When the visual world becomes unpredictable, interaction with the world becomes difficult and even dangerous, for it is impossible to determine whether one's own trajectory is going to collide with the trajectories of the other moving objects in the vicinity. It may be even difficult to determine which of the perceived objects are moving and which completely stationary.

The mechanism that malfunctions in cerebral akinetopsia is specific for the computation of spatiotemporal trajectories for *visual* objects. In other modalities (touch, audition) it is still possible to sense smooth continuity in the change of position or to be aware of the trajectory along which a virtual object changes its position. These preserved abilities cannot, however, take over the job of the visual function that has been lost.

Interestingly, it seems that the mechanism for the binding of spatiotemporal continuity can also be selectively spared when all other visual function is compromised. Riddoch (1917, quoted in Zeki, 1992) reported patients that could not describe the characteristics of the moving objects, but could sense and describe the pure sense of motion itself. They could not attribute shape or color to the motion, and they were totally blind to stationary objects. Therefore, Riddoch concluded that movement should be recognized as a special visual perception, separate from the perceptions of light, form, and color. Barbur, Watson, Frackowiak, and Zeki (1993) confirmed that in such a patient, motion signals reach area V5/MT without necessarily passing through area V1, thus activating the experience of pure motion, which was described by the patient *as if sensing a moving shadow crossing the visual field* (Beckers & Zeki, 1995).

I suggest that this special perception of pure motion is the experience of the smooth continuity of spatiotemporal trajectories within the phenomenal coordinate system. Our experience of visual motion is nothing but the sense of such a trajectory evolving within the phenomenal level of organization. To construct a visual (simulated) object in motion, the form and color and other local visual attributes must be bound together with the phenomenal trajectory.

Illusory Motion It is easy to create the experience of seeing an object moving in the subjective visual field even when no object in the external stimulus field is actually changing its physical position. If two lights near each other in the stimulus field alternate rapidly (~40 Hz) as to being on and off, "disembodied" motion is perceived between the

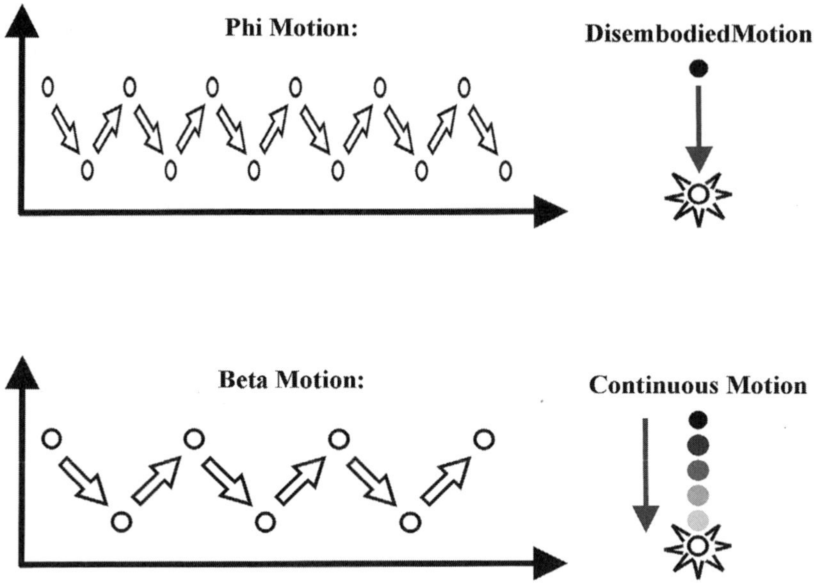

Figure 12.2
Apparent motion phenomena. Depending on the alternation rate of two stationary lights, different types of illusory motion are perceived. At high rates of alternation, disembodied motion of a single light without intermediate positions (phi motion) will be experienced. At lower rates of alternation, continuous motion of a single light without intermediate positions (beta motion) will be experienced. At sufficiently low rates, the illusion of movement disappears and sequential lighting up of two unmoving lights is experienced. (Modified from Palmer (1999), reproduced with permission of The MIT Press.)

two lights without the perception of any intermediate positions. This is called *phi motion.* If the rate is somewhat slower (~10 Hz), a single light appears to move continuously back and forth. This is called *beta motion.*[2] As it is easy to create phenomenal motion in the absence of real physical motion, much of the animation experienced in consciousness is actually based on illusory rather than real movement. All the motion we see in movies, TV, video tape or computer graphics is produced by presenting a rapid succession of discrete frames, each of which is entirely motionless (Palmer, 1999) (figure 12.2).

Interestingly, the patient who suffered from visual motion blindness was totally immune to apparent motion: she did not experience any illusion of motion in two-dot alternating displays where normal observers clearly and automatically see the dot moving. Under no combination of conditions did the patient report apparent movement. She always reported two independent light spots (Zihl et al., 1983). This further strengthens the view that the experience of visual motion is based on the same mechanism that is similarly sensitive to both real and illusory motion stimuli.

Hence, both the color and the motion we visually experience must be constructions of the brain, only appearing in the simulated world at the phenomenal level.

Superfluous Phenomenal Features: Synesthesia

Synesthesia is a relatively rare condition, occurring in about 1 in 2000 in the normal population (Baron-Cohen, Burt, Smith-Laittan, Harrison, & Bolton, 1996). A synesthetic individual, when one sense modality is stimulated, producing the appropriate phenomenal experience, invariably also experiences extraneous phenomenal features in another sense modality. For example, the perception of sounds can produce a simultaneous visual experience or colors, shapes, movement, patterns, or brightness. Within one individual the couplings of experiences between the senses always remain the same. The same sound always produces the same color. Different individuals with synesthesia have, however, different couplings of, say, sounds and colors. The synesthetic relationship usually operates only in one direction: sounds produce colors, but not vice versa (Cytowic, 1993).

The synesthetic phenomenal features are not necessarily bound to the same location in the phenomenal space as the sensation that produced it. Some synesthetic individuals who see letters coupled with colors report that the color fills the printed letter. Thus the letter is seen as if normal feature binding would apply to the illusory color. Others report that the color appears on an invisible screen located within arm's reach of their eyes, not in the letter itself. For some the color appears in the mind rather than outside the body (Grossenbacher & Lovelace, 2001).

These observations suggest that in synesthetic individuals the etiological pathway to consciousness includes additional feedforward branches from one sensory modality to another. The additional branches are idiosyncratic for each individual but remain stable, and they produce patterns of phenomenal qualities in an inappropriate sensory modality as if it had been directly stimulated.

For synesthetic persons, experiences at the phenomenal level include *richer patterns of phenomenal features* than for normal subjects, producing more complex, multimodality virtual objects. The multisensory experiences are not necessarily bound together into one location as a single virtual object, however, but are manifested as different but simultaneous sensory qualities in independent locations.

Synesthesia is often developmental and at least some forms of it may be genetically based (Grossenbacher & Lovelace, 2001). Hence synesthesia may be an indication of natural variation in the constitution of the phenomenal level in the human population. If the simulated phenomenal reality in the brain is a species-specific biological adaptation, there must be variation in its phenotypic manifestation. Natural selection would have operated on this variation during evolutionary history, and favored the most efficient phenomenal simulation of the world for each species in its ecological niche.

Summary

The purpose of this chapter was to exercise empirical phenomenology with regard to the unity and binding of visual objects, in particular the integration of form, color, and motion. We witnessed several surprising phenomena that disrupt the unity of visual consciousness: visual objects in consciousness may become disorganized or they may lose (or gain) specific features. Now that we have reviewed the data, we should try to find some cues in the data concerning the hidden mechanisms that determine *why* in these cases the phenomenal world is altered in precisely the ways it is.

First, different phenomenal features of visual objects seem to be produced independently of each other. The phenomenal world may miss the coherent form of objects but retain sensations of colors and motion (apperceptive agnosia); it may miss the qualities of chromatic colors but retain phenomenal objects with form and motion (achromatopsia); and it may miss the animation and temporal continuity of the visual world but retain coherent and colored but stationary objects (akinetopsia). This pattern suggests that the neural mechanisms underlying the different phenomenal features are likewise *functionally independent* of each other. For example, the fact that phenomenal colors cannot be produced does not stop the mechanisms of spatial grouping, part binding, visual motion, and feature binding from generating a fully animated phenomenal world with coherent but grayscale objects.

Moreover, the mechanisms of each phenomenal feature must have their own, *independent access route* to the shared phenomenal coordinate system. An alternative model of access to the phenomenal level, which can now be ruled out, would be linear and additive. According to such a model, first the object's form is determined, then its color, then its motion, and then its location, after which the object representation pops out at the phenomenal level. If any of these stages suffers from a breakdown, then the construction of the phenomenal object stops at that stage and *none* of the features of the stimulus object will be simulated at the phenomenal level. But that is not what happens. Instead, the mechanisms of different phenomenal features seem to operate autonomously and in parallel when contributing their outputs to phenomenal space.

The different mechanisms seem to *interact* only as they are *delivering* their own particular contributions to the phenomenal space. Form, color, and motion thus come to modulate the *same* location in phenomenal space in a coordinated manner. In the illusory or unstable feature bindings seen in Balint's syndrome, however, the coordination flounders as the location *where* the features belong (and *which* features belong there) remains uncertain. In the patient's brain, form and color information hence do not modulate the phenomenal space in a well-coordinated or stable manner, but combine the different features somewhat randomly. In synesthesia involving illusory color, the location of the color qualities may be independent of the location of the stimulus that triggered it, also showing a lack of coordinated interaction between the modalities.

Some observations about phenomenal colors offer further constraints about the potential mechanisms. The neural mechanism responsible for chromatic color seems to be located in area V4 in the visual cortex. Single-cell response properties of V4 neurons correlate with seen colors (phenomenal colors) rather than the wavelength composition of stimuli (Zeki, 1992). Yet it remains shrouded in mystery what lower-level mechanisms precisely could account for the four unique chromatic hues of red, green, yellow, and blue. Somehow their phenomenal uniqueness and the opponency pairs they form must be explained by their underlying mechanisms. Phenomenal uniqueness should be explained by the uniqueness of the physical basis, and the phenomenal opponency of red-green and blue-yellow by the physical impossibility of combining the constitutive (or the immediate etiological) mechanisms of red and green or blue and yellow. Area V4 appears to contain the mechanisms necessary and sufficient to modulate the phenomenal space in such a manner that phenomenal color qualities, incorporated in phenomenal space, are brought about.

Unilateral destruction of V4 creates a sharp division in the midline of phenomenal space, or the subjective visual field, so that one half of it is fully colored, the other entirely achromatic. Yet, the subjective visual world itself is still spatially unified. This curious situation brings out into the open the hidden seams of the phenomenal coordinate system. Somehow, in the normal case, the unity of phenomenal space reaches across the midline without any trace of a gap. Yet, as hemiachromatopsia and unilateral neglect (to be discussed in the next chapter) show, the underlying lower-level mechanisms must be spatially divided. One of the main fracture lines runs through the midline of the subjective visual field. The mechanisms of spatial integration resulting in a single unified phenomenal space remain a mystery.

Perhaps the most important theoretical lesson that was learned in the course of this chapter was, however, that qualities as such, without any organization, are barely worth having. Phenomenal consciousness involves a multilevel structure. Explaining consciousness involves explaining how the entire simulated *world* of phenomenal experience, and our *presence in* that world, is possible. Accounting for the bare presence of qualities is only a small part of the story; the other parts are no less significant and no less fascinating—but they may be more tractable.

13 Binding and Phenomenal Disunity II: Objects and Space

Simulated objects in phenomenal space have, in addition to their purely intrinsic visual features (form, color, motion), also immediately experienced features that *relate* them to other objects. The visual world we experience is a world of immediately *meaningful, familiar* objects, not a collection of unified but alien bundles of features. The simulated objects are immediately bound together with semantic-conceptual knowledge in semantic memory and thus related to the kinds of objects we already know something about. If semantic-conceptual binding fails, as it does in semantic dementia, then the objects of the world lose much of their rich meaningfulness.

The visual world we experience is also a world of *spatially located* and *spatially related* objects. In Balint's syndrome, spatial relations between objects are lost, as well as the visual space surrounding the object currently in focal awareness. In unilateral neglect, one half of the phenomenal space itself seems to be missing. In split brain, there appear to be *two independent phenomenal spaces* within the same brain, not directly in contact with each other. These strange disunities of phenomenal experience might again carry important messages concerning the organization and the underlying mechanisms of consciousness.

Opening Semantic Windows: Semantic-Conceptual Binding

A remarkable feature of objects in natural scenes is their immediate meaningfulness. As we serially scan our surroundings and shift our attention from one location to the next, not only do the elementary features of objects become bound into coherent entities but we instantaneously know what *kinds* of objects are present. Each separate object activates a coherent network of semantic knowledge. We not only see a coherent bundle of features ("Gestalt window"), we see it *as* a representative of a specific category of objects ("semantic window"). Consequently we are able to access an enormous amount of information about that kind of object.

This is not purely *visual* binding. Nothing changes in the pattern of visual qualia when the semantic window of a coherent bundle of features is opened. Furthermore, objects represented nonvisually can open semantic windows as well. If you have several objects in your pockets, semantic windows (such as "key," "coin," "handkerchief") are automatically opened when you explore the objects by touching but not seeing them.

To transform a Gestalt window to a meaningful virtual object requires *semantic-conceptual binding*. This form of binding allows us to experience the world around us as familiar and meaningful. In everyday perception, we take the meaningfulness of the surrounding world so much for granted that we find it difficult to even imagine losing it. However, semantic-conceptual binding is deficient in patients with *semantic dementia* (Saffran & Schwartz, 1994). Although a patient with semantic dementia typically has no visual problems, a visual shape or a coherent bundle of visual features (or the name of the object) presented to the patient fails to open the corresponding specific semantic window. The virtual world and its objects lose their meaningfulness and distinctive character as objects representative of specific kinds. Consequently, objects can be categorized by such patients only in terms of superordinate categories (e.g., fish, bird, insect), but all detailed knowledge of object-specific attributes is lost. The patients are unable to tell real from unreal objects if the former have been put together by combining the parts of different real objects, say the head of a mouse with the body of a lion.

One such patient (presented in the BBC program *Brain Story*) had lost all the other categories of animals apart from "cat" and "dog." He was shown pictures of different animals (such as a cow, duck, mouse, tiger), one by one, and asked, "What animal is that?" No matter which animal was shown to him, his answers were always either "a dog" or "a cat" (sometimes qualified with "small" or "big"). Yet, there was nothing wrong with his vision. He could see vividly the stripes of the tiger, but claimed that he had seen the same kind of dog recently. There were no other animals apart from dogs and cats that he seemed to know about. Any picture of an animal could open only one of the available semantic windows. It seems the categories that still remained in his semantic memory were the ones he had first learned in childhood and, therefore, the ones most deeply encoded and most resistant against the devastating deterioration of semantic knowledge going on in the temporal lobes of his brain.

If semantic knowledge is lost, semantic windows become coarse and cannot distinguish between the meaning of members in the same superordinate category. As you may remember, the classic (but incorrect) characterization of associative agnosia was that there are "intact percepts stripped of their meaning." In fact, this description seems to be much more accurate about semantic dementia than about associative agnosia.

Location Binding and the Space around Us

The contents of consciousness do not only include objects as coherent bundles of features, either static or moving along phenomenal trajectories. There is also the *space* around us: the space in which we feel that our body and all the perceived objects are embedded. We not only immediately see the shape and identity of an object, we are also aware of its position in relation to our own body and to other objects in the scene. This is *location binding* (Treisman, 1996). This ability is so profoundly built into the brain's simulation of the world that we may fail to appreciate its very existence.

Patients with dorsal simultanagnosia, or Balint's syndrome, however, have lost this ability, although they can still see single objects as coherent and meaningful bundles of features (Farah, 1990): part binding and semantic-conceptual binding are still functional in their brain. By contrast, as was discussed in the previous chapter, their feature binding is abnormal so that the features that are combined in a perceived shape frequently originate in separate stimulus objects, thus resulting in illusory conjunctions. But in addition to abnormal feature binding, the patients also suffer from a loss of spatial awareness outside their own bodies. They are functionally blind except for the perception of one object at a time in the visual scene (L. C. Robertson, 2003).

A patient with dorsal simultanagnosia might well be able to see a bird and even recognize it as a magpie, but he cannot point at it or describe where it is located in space. If shown more than one object at a time, a patient with simultanagnosia reports seeing only one. Awareness of objects other than the one currently perceived is lost. For such a patient, subjectively experienced visual space seems to collapse down to the space within the currently attended object, but the size of that space varies with the size of the object that defines it. An explicit representation of space is necessary for the accurate binding of features to objects and for the perception of multiple objects (L. Robertson et al., 1997). To be visually aware of only one object and nothing else besides effectively hides the relationships that the object bears to other objects in the environment.

It is difficult to imagine how the contents of consciousness appear for a patient with simultanagnosia. One does get the impression that it must be a single object–based tunnel vision. Still, the spatial scope of the tunnel is not fixed but flexible. It makes no difference whether the selected object is big or small, it does not matter how much visual space the object occupies: as long as it constitutes one perceptual Gestalt, it will be seen as a coherent whole by the simultanagnosic. But awareness of the spatial structure of the surrounding visual environment is completely lost. The subjective visual field seems to have lost its fieldlike, egocentric organization. There is no such visual field anymore for the patient. There is only a single semantic window open, and the spatial extent of the visual field covers exactly that window, nothing else. Visual awareness in Balint's syndrome equals one isolated semantic window at any one time.

The visual phenomenology in Balint's syndrome seems to have a connection to selective attention. Even in the normal case, visual selective attention is for the most part object-based: focal attention is directed to bundles of features at one location and the features in that location are then bound together to form one coherent whole. Although we can be *focally* aware of only *one* object at a time, focal attention is by no means equivalent to the *total* contents of visual consciousness. As you may remember, the theater-spotlight metaphor of consciousness identifies the contents of consciousness with the contents of focal attention. The metaphor seems to describe accurately the contents of visual consciousness in the simultanagnosic patient: visual awareness consists of a temporal sequence of spatially unrelated objects in the focus of attention. But that is a *pathological* condition, unlike our normal consciousness. If the theater-spotlight metaphor of consciousness would be accurate, then we would all be born with single-object tunnel vision—we would be innately simultanagnosic. Instead, we have an awareness of a wide visual space surrounding us, containing a multitude of objects. The mutual spatial relationships between different objects are entirely transparent to us in visual awareness. We just see instantly where each object is located in relation to other objects and our own body.

What has happened to the phenomenal space of a simultanagnosic? The disorder is confined to the visual modality; thus the phenomenal space has not disappeared completely The patient can still sense the space surrounding him through audition and touch. Bodily space is intact; the location of tactile sensations on the bodily surface can be correctly reported (L. C. Robertson, 1999). But since extrapersonal visual space does not exist anymore, the semantic windows at the phenomenal level can no longer be accurately located with respect to the body. In our normal visual field, our own bodies in relation to extrapersonal objects form an ever-present part of the visual phenomenal background. Any visual object we see is in some relation to that background. But for the simultanagnosic, there is no phenomenal background in the visual modality, thus no visual information about the relationship between the object in visual awareness, one's own body, and other objects.

Hemispatial Neglect and Phenomenal Space

Hemispatial neglect refers to a group of deficits where the patient's experience of spatially extended scenes and objects is limited to only one half of space, and the patient's actions may be similarily restricted toward stimuli in one half of space. The patients are incapable of exploring the space on that side and reporting stimuli that are presented there. Usually the damage is in the right posterior hemisphere, centering on the infero-posterior parietal region and the neglected space is the contralateral left side of space (Vallar, 1997; Farah, 2000).

In severe cases it is easy for external observers to notice that the patient is not conscious of the left side of space. If asked to copy a picture, the patient's drawing will depict only the right half of the original. If asked to cross out all letters printed on a paper, the patient will cross out only those on the right side. The neglect patient may eat food only from the right side of the plate (and complain that the portions are too small); he or she may dress only the right side of the body, or shave or make up on the right side of the face. One patient behaving exactly like this explained that "I look in the mirror and do all I see" (Sacks, 1985). The patients themselves do not experience any "missing space" as such. They are not aware of the fact that their phenomenal space is only one half of the space that it used to be, or that their contents of consciousness only represent one half of the external physical world. The missing half of the world is like a giant blind spot for the patients—they are unable to directly experience the "blindness" of the spot and therefore easily fail to appreciate its very existence, even when told about it.

There is great variation among neglect patients as to which aspects of spatial awareness have been compromised. All the various neglect symptoms share, however, the feature of *deficient reconstruction of some aspect of contralesional space,* whether perceptual, motor, imagined, or object-specific space.

Neglect Reveals Multiple Representations of Space

The large variety of symptoms and dissociations found in different patients reveals that the representation of space is not a simple matter in the brain. The disorder can affect only some part of space (extrapersonal, far space, or personal, near space); it can affect only perceptual or only motor functions or both; it can affect only visual perception or only visual imagery or both; or it can affect only some selective categories of perceptual objects (faces, words) (Vallar, 1998). These complexities of spatial deficits force us to abandon the intuitive idea that the unity of spatial perception is based on a single spatial system or unitary space map in the brain. Instead, spatial representation in the brain seems to have a modular structure such that different aspects of spatiality are handled by specialized representation mechanisms (Farah, 2000):

> Conscious space representation depends on the concomitant activity of a multiplicity of cortical (and subcortical) centers. Although it is by no means clear how this multiple system is coordinated, there is little doubt that the unity of space perception is not due to the activity of a unitary space map but results from the coordinated activity of several highly specialized sensorimotor circuits. (Rizzolatti, Riggio, & Sheliga, 1994, p. 238)

> The "internal representation" of space . . . or the "spatial frame of reference," far from being a single monolithic and supramodal system, should be conceived as having a highly multifaceted architecture, including multiple components or centres, which may be selectively affected by brain damage. (Vallar, 1998, p. 90)

At first glance, the fragmentation of spatial representation in the brain seems to threaten the very idea of a unified phenomenal space. How should we construe the relation between the unified phenomenal space that we normally experience and the multiple spatial maps found in the brain that seem to be in various ways affected in neglect?

The Disunified Mechanisms of Unified Phenomenal Space

I propose that the relationship between unified phenomenal space and the brain mechanisms of spatial representation is similar to the relationship between unified phenomenal objects and the brain mechanisms of object representation. The phenomenal unity in both cases lies at a higher level of organization than the neural mechanisms so far found in the brain. There is no doubt that we experience unified visual objects in consciousness, so the brain has to *somehow* bind together the different features of objects that are represented in different places in the brain. In the same vein, there is no doubt that we experience being immersed in a single spatially unified world, so *somehow* the brain has to bind together the distinct spatial maps representing different features or regions of space. The specialized spatial representations themselves reside at levels of organization below the phenomenal. We are not directly aware of them. If we were aware of them, our phenomenal experience of space would be piecemeal, each different region or aspect of phenomenally experienced space corresponding to a distinct neurally implemented spatial map. In that case the neglect patient's symptoms would not be at all surprising to us, as we would directly see that that is what must happen when particular spatial maps are destroyed. But by contrast the symptoms of neglect *are* deeply puzzling, even absurd, for us just because our normal phenomenal space appears to be an undivided, coherent whole.

The apparent conflict between one unified phenomenal space and the multitude of modular space maps in the brain resolves when put into the context of multilevel explanation. In a multilevel model of consciousness, there is room for both unity of phenomenal space and disunity of spatial representation. The distinct spatial maps at lower levels of organization contribute to the construction of the phenomenal space at a higher level of organization. Their contributions are in the normal case seamlessly bound together to create the phenomenal unity of the space surrounding us. The different ways in which this space may become distorted in spatial hemineglect simply reveals the isolated contributions of different specialized spatial maps.

The science of consciousness should aim at solving the *spatial binding problem.* That requires, first, identifying all the lower-level spatial maps that contribute to the phenomenal level, and second, describing how they interact so that the experience of one unified space arises at the phenomenal level. In order for us to experience phenomenal unity of space, there need not be any single area or circuit in the brain that reconstructs that space. It is probably the result of large-scale integration of the different maps in corticocortical and thalamocortical systems. The reason why the phenomenal unity of space has not been "found" in the brain, but the multiply distributed lower-level maps have been discovered, is that the measurements that have been applied are mostly highly localized and only reveal low levels of neurophysiological organization (say single-cell firing rates). Localized measurements reveal localized phenomena, but the phenomenal level is not an anatomically strictly localized phenomenon.

Space and Objects

When neglect patients are shown stimuli in the neglected perceptual field, they may be processed even to the level of meaning, but the stimulus information does not enter consciousness (see the discussion on implicit processing in chapter 22). Thus, neglect reveals that visually presented objects can still be fully processed in the brain, but outside of consciousness. Space seems to be fundamental to the subjective experience of the object to be generated. The representation of space is compromised, whereas object representations are relatively intact. This is sometimes dramatically revealed when objects or parts of objects actually residing in neglected space are perceived within the intact parts of phenomenal space (Ladavas, Berti, & Farne, 2000). The information depicting the object, if it is to enter consciousness at all, must be bound to an incorrect location in the available perceptual space.

Hemispatial neglect and simultanagnosia point in the same direction: the subjective experience of space and the subjective experience of objects in that space are created by distinct systems, both highly complex in themselves. An intact object perception system alone can at best support the perceptual space occupied by one object at a time. Where there is no phenomenal space, there can be no virtual objects or spatial relations between them either. If only one half of the space can be reconstructed, only one half of the objects belonging to that space can be perceived.

Hemispatial Neglect and Balint's Syndrome

If unilateral parietal damage wipes out the left half of visual objects and perceptual space, then bilateral damage of the same areas would be expected to wipe out all the rest, leaving the patient unable to become aware of visual objects at all. Yet, bilateral parietal damage (Balint's syndrome, simultanagnosia) does *not* wipe out both halves of visual objects. Instead, in Balint's syndrome whole objects are seen, though now the surrounding visual space has disappeared completely. Somehow the brain *gains* the left half of objects but loses *both* sides of background space.

The patients with Balint's syndrome thus seem to experience objects that are not embedded anywhere in particular in their phenomenal space, because there is no visual space outside the object to relate the seen object to anything else. This unexpected pattern might be seen as a threat to the views that phenomenal space is necessary for the perception of objects, and that space is more fundamental than the other features of objects.

When both parietal lobes are damaged, the object that is perceived is not spatially related to other objects, and the other objects drop from awareness. It is not that objects require perception of space to rise above the threshold of perceptual awareness—both features and objects can be perceived without spatial information provided by parietal input—but rather that awareness between features represented in different cortical feature maps and the spatial relations between objects requires explicit spatial information. (L. C. Robertson, 2003, p. 97)

So, perhaps conscious visual perception requires two different kinds of spatiality: one supports egocentric space and between-object relations in this space; the other supports the spatial relationships *among the parts of a single object.* Deouell (2002) makes an interesting proposal about the roles of these two different spatial representations. The egocentric space, based on posterior parietal mechanisms, supports awareness of the *mere existence* or the *mere presence* of sensory events. By contrast, the within-object representation, based on ventral stream mechanisms, supports the processing of the *identity* of the stimulus, but this processing is inherently implicit. Its results become conscious only if the subject becomes aware of the *presence* of the stimulus. The egocentric phenomenal space is fundamental to subjective experience—for the phenomenal *presence* of simulated objects in consciousness—the object representations cannot enter awareness unless the phenomenal space for them exists.

If this interpretation is accurate, then also patients with bilateral parietal damage should have difficulties in becoming aware of the mere presence of objects. As was mentioned in the previous chapter, the patients suffer from deficits of feature binding, which sometimes renders the objects they see rather unstable. At least the patient R.M. with Balint's syndrome, studied in detail by L. Robertson and colleagues (1997), seems to have been unaware of targets of most trials in one study (see Deouell, 2002). As there are only few patients with bilateral parietal damage reported in the literature, it remains to be determined to what extent bilateral parietal damage allows awareness of the mere presence of stimuli, and whether some patients lose it totally. Furthermore, it remains to be determined whether Balint's syndrome is even anatomically like "double neglect." The deficits do not appear to be centered on exactly the same parietal areas (L. C. Robertson, 2003). If that is the case, then there is a natural explanation for why bilateral parietal damage does not produce bilateral neglect.

Yet, if the phenomenological description is accurate, that the patients see objects but nothing else, then the visual space occupied by just one object and its features *must* be sufficient for phenomenal presence. The object is phenomenally present for the subject, but not present in any determinable visual location, because the phenomenal coordinate system constituting the phenomenal visual background has collapsed. Although bodily awareness remains intact, the contents of bodily and visual awareness cannot be spatially related with each other anymore. Certainly, the patient should be able to see parts of his own body if looking at them, but then he would not see any objects at the same time. And vice versa, when seeing an object, he would not see any part of his body or anything in the space between his body and the object. The crucial contribution of the phenomenal background is the *simultaneous* presence of the contents in the entire sphere of experience. Spatial relations between different phenomenal contents can only be directly present for the subject when the phenomenal contents themselves are simultaneously present.

It seems that the phenomenal coordinate system of the simultanagnosic patient is still capable of realizing, one by one, simulated objects of different sizes and shapes and in different locations in phenomenal space. Yet, the visual phenomenal background cannot be simulated anymore under any circumstances. When the visual phenomenal background is missing, the location of the single visual object becomes indeterminable, as the missing background cannot be experienced in any way, not even as just empty space surrounding the object. Phenomenal space as such still exists at the subphenomenal level, but it is only showing itself in the places where focal attention falls and allows simulation of a single object in the center of consciousness. In simultanagnosia, focal attention has become the only means through which visual qualities can still be realized in phenomenal space.[1]

Split Brain

The cases of unusual binding that we have discussed so far involve conspicuous changes in the patients' subjective experience and behavior due to various types of localized brain injury. Split brain is different. Split brain patients have undergone an operation in which the corpus callosum (and the anterior commissure) are sectioned. These structures normally allow the cortical hemispheres to communicate with each other. Thus, they should be involved in the high-level binding of cerebral activity into one coherent whole. Cutting the connections between the hemispheres might be expected to lead to drastic disunity of consciousness at the phenomenal level.

The patients who have undergone the operation, however, report that they do not feel their mind or consciousness has changed in any way after the operation. The patients are also quite normal in their everyday behavior. Still, there is something peculiar going on in their brains and minds, but the peculiarities can be teased out only in laboratory conditions. When visual stimuli are selectively projected to one visual field only (so that they end up in the contralateral visual cortex), then the left hemisphere reports (by verbal report or by pointing with the right hand) only those stimuli that were projected to that hemisphere. It denies having seen any of the stimuli projected to the right hemisphere. However, the patient's left hand (controlled by the right hemisphere) can point to a picture that matches what the right hemisphere has seen. If the patient is asked *why* his left hand pointed to the picture, his left (speaking) hemisphere will cook up some ad hoc story, but remains unaware of the true reason. The experience was not present in the left hemisphere's phenomenal sphere.

These results suggest that some form of the phenomenal level must be supported by each hemisphere independently of the other. In the left hemisphere there is a phenomenal level of organization in which semantic windows are generated in response to stimuli presented to the right visual field. The contents of the left hemisphere phenomenal level can become the objects of a full-fledged reflective, introspective consciousness. It produces judgments, categorizations, and verbal descriptions of its experiences. In the right hemisphere there also appears to be a phenomenal level of organization in which Gestalt and semantic windows are opened in response to stimuli projected to the left visual field. The right hemisphere has phenomenal experience that is not coconscious with simultaneous experiences in the left hemisphere. Left hemisphere reflective consciousness thus cannot take the right hemisphere phenomenal contents as objects of reflection. They do not exist for the left hemisphere–based reflective consciousness and are accordingly denied by it.

The right hemisphere possesses the phenomenal contents but it seems to have only very limited capacities of reflective consciousness (unless the patient has language abilities also in the right hemisphere). When two figures are presented simultaneously to the right hemisphere, it cannot judge whether the figures are same or different. In some patients, simple matching judgments can be made above chance, but many patients fail in such tasks. Patients who have language capacities in the right hemisphere can make many kinds of judgments concerning the stimuli, but regardless of that they cannot make simple inferences. Right hemisphere consciousness is thus phenomenal consciousness in the absence of reflective consciousness.

> . . . [The right hemisphere] seems to deal mainly with raw experience in an unembellished way. The left hemisphere, on the other hand, is constantly, almost reflexively, labeling experiences, making inferences as to cause, and carrying out a host of other cognitive activities. . . . The left hemisphere is busy *differentiating* the world whereas the right is simply *monitoring* the world. (Gazzaniga 1995b, p. 1398)

How do we know that there is phenomenal consciousness in the right hemisphere? One hypothesis that should be considered is that the right hemisphere responses are only implicit zombie responses rather than manifestations of phenomenal consciousness. This hypothesis is, however, not supported by the available evidence: the explicit behaviors manifested by the right hemisphere are quite different from the implicit, nonconsciously guided visuomotor actions in agnosic patients (see chapter 22 for details). Implicit action mostly consists in grasping and pointing to stimuli that are directly guiding the actions through implicit visuomotor representations. The right hemisphere can match one picture with another or draw or write something to express the phenomenal content that was present in its visual consciousness. The visuomotor zombie systems are not capable of such feats.

My interpretation of the split brain data is that both cerebral hemispheres support the phenomenal level of organization in an independent manner. As long as the split-brain patient is freely in sensorimotor interaction with his environment, the contents of phenomenal consciousness in the two hemispheres will mostly overlap. The phenomenal contents in the two hemispheres can be dissociated only in laboratory conditions by using lateralized stimuli. The experiments show that the left hemisphere has superior capacities of reflective consciousness: all the judging, differentiating, categorizing, and reporting of experience that goes with reflective consciousness is second nature to the left hemisphere. The right hemisphere by contrast has only very rudimentary capacities of reflective consciousness. Therefore, its phenomenal consciousness remains rather isolated. Perhaps right hemisphere consciousness is in some ways similar to our experiences during dreaming: vivid momentary phenomenal experience coupled with decreased capability for reflection, inference, critical thinking, volition, or sense of continuity of the self.

Summary

In our normal visual experiences, meaningful visual objects are embedded in a unified sphere of experience that defines the spatial background and relations between different objects and between ourselves and the objects. This typical structure of visuospatial consciousness is brought about by complex binding mechanisms that are hidden from direct experience. The neuropsychological syndromes we reviewed in this chapter expose the many bizarre ways in which the *un*binding of the phenomenal world may occur. Patients with *semantic dementia* preserve all the visual qualities of the phenomenal world, but the objects in their world become semantically impoverished. They live in a world where only a few simple categories of different things exist. The number of different semantic windows has dramatically decreased, so that, say, all four-legged animals have become either cats or dogs, or all flying animals either birds or bugs. They have not lost the experience of seeing, but they have lost much of the experience of *seeing-as*. The meaningfulness of the objects surrounding us is one basic source of information that must be bound together with the visual surface structure and features of objects to create the kind of phenomenal consciousness we normally enjoy.

Simultanagnosia creates a situation where phenomenal objects can still be seen and semantically interpreted, but the visual world of the patient consists at any one time of only a single, isolated semantic window. The phenomenal background has disappeared, and with it are gone the spatial relations between the object currently in focal consciousness and other objects. The disastrous effects of simultanagnosia on normal visually guided behavior—the patients are functionally blind—reveal the importance of the phenomenal background for our ability to successfully navigate in the world. Simultanagnosia furthermore raises questions about phenomenal space: what has happened to it? How can the patients experience a single spatially isolated object if phenomenal space is necessary for experience? The interpretation we ended up with suggests that phenomenal space still exists but can realize visual qualities only in the locations where focal attention falls. Visual qualities cannot come about outside of the attentional window, in the spatial background or the periphery of consciousness. For the simultanagnosic patient, attention is necessary for visual consciousness. But as simultanagnosia differs radically from our normal consciousness, it provides us with evidence that in the normal case, the contents of attention cannot be equal to the total contents of consciousness.

In hemispatial neglect, phenomenal consciousness seems to come in the form of half-objects and a half-world. The left side of phenomenal space and simulated objects has just disappeared. The patients themselves do not notice this, however. In neglect (unilateral posterior parietal damage), the brain allows the experience of only such objects (or object parts) that fall into the preserved side of space, although there is evidence that even the neglected stimuli are processed to a high level. This suggests that space is necessary for experience. In simultanagnosia (bilateral posterior parietal damage) experience of background space is gone, yet now the patient can see whole objects. As both types of patients usually have parietal damage, this raises some difficult theoretical questions. Why don't neglect patients see whole objects, too, so that one half of the object would be embedded in the background of normal visual space, whereas the other half would be hanging in "empty" space, without any background? Or why don't simultanagnosic patients lose visual awareness of *both* halves of objects?

These questions remain to be resolved. The phenomenology of vision in these patients offers important constraints on any theory trying to describe and explain the relationship between phenomenal space and the virtual objects in that space.

Finally, split-brain patients provide us with evidence of phenomenal spaces totally dissociable from each other. When the patients are presented lateralized stimuli, a situation comes about in which a simulated object in one hemisphere is not phenomenally present or coconscious with the phenomenal contents in the other hemisphere. Although both hemispheres appear capable of supporting their own, independent phenomenal level, only the left hemisphere seems capable of reflective consciousness.

These pathological cases suggest that the neural mechanisms of phenomenal unity are not localized in any single cortical area. Damage to different cortical regions deprives the subject of particular aspects of normal consciousness. Damage to occipitotemporal areas deprives the subject of the form, color, motion, or identity of phenomenal objects; damage to the posterior parietal cortex, from half or all of the phenomenal background space. Only separating the cerebral hemispheres from each other seems to create a situation where simultaneous experiences in the same brain no longer are experiences of the same subject.

14 Binding in Dreams

Empirical phenomenology studies the organization of consciousness by looking at altered experiences. In the previous two chapters we applied empirical phenomenology to the disunity of visual awareness in neuropsychological patients. We discovered what may happen to phenomenal unity when the underlying neural mechanisms are damaged. In this chapter we turn to another type of altered experience to explore the unity of phenomenal experience: dreaming. This approach combines the two model systems of consciousness science: visual awareness and the dreaming brain. We examine disunities in visual dream images: our experiences of objects, places, and persons in dreams. The dream data enrich and complement the data from neuropsychology. Dreaming reveals the limits of *reversible* phenomenal disunity in an entirely *intact,* nonpathological brain. By contrast, neuropsychological data reveal the nature of severe *irreversible damage* to the unifying mechanisms underlying consciousness.

The chapter starts by pointing out the theoretical connection between the concepts "dream bizarreness" and "binding." From there we begin our tour of the world of bizarre dream objects, places, and characters. The odd ways in which the brain combines information sources in dream images sheds light on the underlying principles of binding.

Binding and Dream Bizarreness

In the dream world we often experience unusual combinations of perceptual features forming novel, creative, even absolutely crazy or nonsensical wholes. We may encounter talking animals, dead relatives, spectacular fantasy characters, and distorted or metamorphosed persons and places. Although everyone is familiar with the oddities of dreaming, only recently has the idea been put forward that dream experience reveals how the binding mechanisms in the brain go awry during sleep.

In dreams the construction of simulated objects is not constrained by input from the sensory environment. The brain is left completely to its own devices. It seems that the brain cannot handle the internal simulation of external sensory input without flaws; nor does it always manage to construct appropriate Gestalt windows or connect them appropriately to semantic knowledge. The result is a phenomenon called *bizarreness:* places, objects, persons, and other dream contents that deviate in peculiar ways from their counterparts in waking life, or show unusual combinations of phenomenal features.

In dream research, "bizarreness" is, however, a broad and poorly defined notion. Often it has been understood to mean something like "very unlikely" or "physically impossible" events or entities depicted in the dream. Hobson (1988) distinguished three distinct forms of it: (1) incongruity or mismatching features of dream images, (2) uncertainty or explicit vagueness of dream images, and (3) discontinuity or sudden appearance, disappearance, or transformation of dream images. For example, bumping into a celebrity, say Madonna, in your own house would be a case of dream incongruity: there is a mismatch between the character and the place in which it appears. Meeting a person who is taken to be familiar in the dream but whose identity nevertheless remains oddly indeterminate would be an instance of vagueness. A person suddenly appearing out of nowhere or disappearing into thin air, or transforming into another person, would be a case of discontinuity.

Bizarreness has been mostly studied from a quantitative point of view: What is the frequency of bizarreness in dreams? What percentage of dream reports contain at least one bizarre feature? The answers to these questions depend a lot on the definition of, and criteria for, what counts as "bizarreness." In one study where the frequencies of bizarre features were quantified relative to the corresponding nonbizarre features (Revonsuo & Salmivalli, 1995), it was found that incongruity is a more common form of bizarreness than vagueness or discontinuity. Thinking and language were most often incongruous (the probability of inconguity being over 30% in these contents). For the features of dream objects, persons, and places, the probability of incongruity was about 15%. Discontinuity was most common in dream places. Overall, however, most features of dream content described in the dream reports in this study were found to be nonbizarre.

In consciousness research a more detailed qualitative analysis of bizarreness might be of value: How, exactly, are incongruous features combined in a dream? What kind of features get easily into incongruous combinations and which never do? We might discover theoretically significant facts about the normal composition and decomposition of the phenomenal level by observing the failures of coherency in the binding of the dream world.

Let's have a closer look at the curious virtual objects, places, and other dream contents that warp the structure of phenomenology during sleep. (The samples below are from the database of dreams reported in Revonsuo and Salmivalli, 1995.)

Part Binding in Dreams

As we left I noticed that the others had striped *umbrellas with the sheltering frame upside down.* I wondered what use could such things be put to, until somebody said that it's raining. (Subject 01)

This bizarre virtual object does have all the correct parts to it, but the parts are incorrectly related, resulting in an incongruous overall configuration. In this case the virtual object is made up of all the correct local features (folding frame, with a stick and handle). The Gestalt window receives the correct semantic interpretation as an umbrella; furthermore, the virtual object is even pragmatically appropriate—it is used in the dream to shelter the person holding it from the rain. It is just that the Gestalt window is in this case disfigured; apparently, the frame is rotated 180 degrees from its normal orientation. The binding of the correct parts into an appropriate whole configuration has failed. This suggests that as Gestalt windows are constructed below the phenomenal level, they are built up of (1) their respective parts, which have to be activated as separate visual features in (visual) semantic memory, and (2) a schema that defines the overall configuration of the parts. In the above example the parts or visual features have been activated, but the schema defining the spatial relations between the parts has not. The result is that the binding manages to produce unified objects (the umbrellas are perceived as such), but the internal constitution of those unified objects is inappropriate.

There was *a big oak* in the yard (as there really is), but in this dream there were *coconuts* in it. There were lots of them also in the ground. They were of all sizes, big and small. (Subject 11)

We were driving along a straight road, past a long row of white houses. In each of its separate yards there were dogs. In each yard, the dogs were only of one specific variety: on one veranda there were several bulldogs on leashes; some dogs were in doghouses, some were running free. I wondered about it and my father commented that there are lots of dogs in our city. *Some of the dogs had long legs, with hoofs. My father called them "pony-dogs."* (Subject 12)

These virtual objects are incongruous because the parts themselves are mismatching, although they are correctly related. Let's take the "pony-dogs" first. Obviously, they are built from the trunk of a dog, combined with the legs of a horse or a pony, or, at least, the dogs' paws are replaced by hoofs. How could a combination like this be created by the brain? Now, let us consider how the visual features of four-legged animals are likely to be stored in semantic memory. Think about the moose, deer, horse, dog, cat, and pig. They all have some visual features in common and some others not. The visual representation of any specific variety of four-legged animal then probably is a coherent combination of the different parts. If the parts and their mutual possible relations are encoded in a semantic network, each animal is brought about by a coherent pattern of activation in the network. When we see an unfamiliar animal for the first time, it probably is just one more variation on the same general theme, composed of a slightly different coherent pattern of features.

It is not difficult to imagine how a "pony-dog" comes about: in this dream there are lots of semantic windows open, depicting different kinds of dogs. Thus, there are lots of different kinds of corresponding activation patterns realized on the part of semantic memory coding the visual features of four-legged animals. However, in a part of the network that codes for the "legs" feature of visual representation of four-legged animals, an incorrect node coding for "hoofs" or "horse-legs" for some reason receives the greatest activation and becomes attached to the general scheme in the place where the legs should go. That semantic window, when it opens in consciousness, is a "pony-dog." Interestingly, the inappropriate feature is not *radically* inappropriate. A dog with elephant legs, chicken legs, or table legs would be far more radical; one with a hammer, a book, or a rhubarb as its leg would be completely outrageous. This tells us that the features that get inappropriately activated very probably still fit into the general picture, for with all likelihood the greatest activation goes to one of the neighboring nodes, coding for visually and semantically similar features.

The oak tree with coconuts is another excellent example of slightly dislocated binding. In this dream image, the visual form and the semantic activation engage in an interplay beneath the phenomenal surface of the dream. Obviously, an oak tree does have a certain kind of seed or fruit, namely the acorn. Now, in the semantic network coding for fruits and nuts (especially their visual features), the nodes <acorn> and <coconut> may be quite close to each other. All nuts are visually rather similar, considering their shape, color, and size. The activation pattern that is needed to create an oak with coconuts is not really that far-fetched at all. The coconuts, we are told, "were of all sizes, big and small," which suggests that the dream images of coconuts were not perfectly unambiguous. Coconuts are big for nuts, whereas acorns are quite small. That there were *small* coconuts around reveals that the representation of *size* of the nuts shows a full range between acorns and coconuts.

Failures of Semantic-Conceptual Binding in Dreams

In the next dream sample there is an interesting incongruity with regard to the virtual place:

> I was in some old house. The rooms were very neat, just cleaned up—it was as if I was at my grandmother's house, although the place did not greatly resemble it. (Subject 22)

It seems that the semantic interpretation given, and the associated feeling of familiarity, are so overwhelming that even a place that would be totally strange for us in waking life is regarded, without worrying about it too much, as a specific familiar place.

> I was at my grandmother's place. I had a dog, Topi, but in fact it was my cat Tipi. It was in the shape of a dog, but I thought that it was Tipi. (Subject 22)

Also in this case the unfamiliar dog that appears in the dream is, despite its appearance, interpreted as being the dreamer's real cat that has just taken the shape of a dog. This can be called *misidentification.* The particular place or object depicted is unfamiliar (and if encountered in real life would be experienced as unfamiliar) but in the dream nevertheless activates a certain familiar content in semantic memory, eliciting a feeling of familiarity and a false identification. Note that in these cases we are dealing with the familiarity and particularity of virtual objects or places, not their general semantic category or visual configuration. The house and the dog are perfectly good virtual objects; it is just that they are misinterpreted as being a *particular* house (which it evidently is not) and a *particular* animal (which the dog evidently is not, since it is regarded to be a cat from waking life). Similar bizarre forms of misidentification are often seen in neuropsychiatric patients (Halligan & Marshall, 1996).

In the next two cases the dream place is a curious mixture of different places:

Somehow I knew a bookshop owner and I needed something from the shop. He let me in the shop although it was Sunday. In addition to books, there were furniture, dishes, and all kinds of stuff for sale there . . . (Subject 03)

In this dream, the place "bookshop" contains merchandise not normally found in bookshops. The schema of "bookshop" seems to have been mixed with something like "department store."

Then we were as if in the city center in Turku, but the center looked like the center of my home town. (Subject 22)

The above is again a case of misidentification, this time of a specific place. Here the identity of the place remains indeterminate, for the dreamer cannot really judge whether the place is the one or the other. For some reason the map location activated during the dream is interpreting the current location of the self as the city of Turku, but the perceptual contents nevertheless correspond to the looks of an entirely different city. A visual representation of the dreamer's hometown is consequently misidentified as Turku. Geographical localization (where am I?) functions separately from the construction of the actual sensory content and from the interpretation of that content as a certain kind of place (city center).

Discontinuity as a Failure of Serial Binding

Discontinuity (or dream elements that unexpectedly appear, disappear, or are transformed) is a major form of dream bizarreness. Like incongruity, discontinuity of virtual objects and places can shed some light on the mechanisms that bring about the contents of the virtual world.

I was indoors with Monica and her cat. I felt something under my foot; there was a stone on the floor. When I looked on the floor again after a moment, I noticed that there was a small red pill there. After a while I saw another one, but bigger. Monica said that they are medicine for the cat and that they have to be picked up. I started to help her in doing so. At this point there were lots of pills on the floor, of different colors, big and small. When I was collecting them and putting them into a metallic box, they had turned into watercolors, and I had to figure out how to place them in their box so that they would be properly ordered colorwise. (Subject 13)

In the above example we have a whole series of discontinuities of virtual objects. Interestingly, it all starts when the dreamer senses something under her foot on the floor. This experience is a nice illustration of how the sense of touch and the virtual body exist in the dream, though not often explicitly mentioned. The tactile object under her foot is subsequently visually identified as a small stone, but after a while there is a small red pill instead in the same spatial location. The semantic window in that location of the virtual world was unstable and changed its features to an object of the same size, but different color and different category. Then more of the same sort of virtual objects start to appear, in different sizes and colors, as if the brain forgot to close the semantic windows but left them wide open. On the basis of the report it appears that the dreamer does not actually see how the new objects appear from thin air; they just are there when she looks back to the same place after attending elsewhere for a while. The multicolored pills undergo one further transformation: they become watercolors (circular, flat, multicolored "buttons"). All these transformations seem to flow from an unstable pattern of activation of visual features. This discontinuity does not seem to go along the lines of semantic categories (stone, medicine, paint), but rather along the lines of similarity of visual features (small, round, colored).

Discontinuity of virtual objects in dreams may be an indication that the brain has difficulties in tracking through time the phenomenal features that belong to a certain location if that location is not constantly attended to. The brain appears to "remember" that there ought to be *something* there that was quite small and roundish, and it makes the best guess it can to reproduce a similar virtual object every time the same location is attended. But since virtual objects do not exist when the dream self is not experiencing them, the activation patterns corresponding to a specific location (in the above dream, "on the floor") may have shifted, or even totally faded, as in the following example:

We were queuing for the salad bar. I took some cabbage and carrot, but then the cabbage had disappeared from my plate, so I took it again. (Subject 12)

The brain seems to have a better idea of *where* a virtual object should reside than *what* that object should be (location vs. identity). Dream objects that otherwise stay the same but just suddenly change their location do not seem to occur. The same virtual object does not jump around the virtual world abruptly changing its location; rather it changes identity or appearance, but stays where it was. Here may be an interesting parallel to the neural mechanisms of visual perception, which handle *where* and *what* information of visual objects separately. The unstable states seem to be located predominantly in the pathway and networks dealing with "what" information (the ventral stream), not "where" information (the dorsal stream). The result is a discontinuous virtual object in a continuous location.[1]

The next tale of phenomenal discontinuity is particularly fascinating:

I was walking along a wide passage. A red carpet was on the floor. On my right side there was a bookstore with very old-looking books in the window. In front of me the passage widened into a huge white room. Along the walls of the room there were flowers in big pots. I didn't recognize any of the varieties; even the colors were extraordinary. Many flowers had been shaped so that they looked like birds. One white flower was made into a swan. When I touched it, it felt like feathers. I walked further into the room. In front of my very eyes, the plants started to turn into stuffed birds. I walked to the birds and I touched them. They seemed lifeless, but suddenly one of the ducks winked an eye at me. I jumped back. The peaceful atmosphere of the garden had evaporated. I started to feel distressed. One of the birds turned into a bear that jumped out from beneath the leaves, showing its teeth. I turned around and started to run. (Subject 60)

So, here our virtual objects start out as multicolored flowers. Next, many of the flowers are noticed to be of the *shape* of birds. One flower is shaped like a swan, and when the dream self touches it, *the tactile sensation is that of touching feathers,* that is, the sensation of touching a *bird* rather than that of touching a *flower.* For some reason, subsequently the visual and other sensory features connected with the category of *birds* start to surface little by little. And in no time at all, the bird features completely overthrow the flower features in these virtual objects: the flowers *become* birds in front of the dreamer's very eyes! At first, they are *stuffed* birds, thus still retaining the feature of flowers as immobile and unreactive. But in the next moment, a stuffed, seemingly lifeless duck becomes alive: mobile and responsive.

As this dream vividly shows, virtual objects are quite malleable, but their transformations prefer to take routes where the underlying activation patterns slide smoothly across the networks of sensory and semantic features, instead of jumping abruptly from one type of object to an object belonging to a completely different or arbitrary category. Even in the above case, the animate objects (flowers and birds) did not transform into arbitrary inanimate artefacts such as tools or furniture or musical instruments; nor did the small inanimate objects in the above example (stones and pills) turn into animate objects.

Sometimes the discontinuities are quite unexpected and peculiar:

I am in a big kitchen, baking a blueberry pie. When I am mixing the dough, the mixer breaks. It won't work even after I shake it a little. So I take a screwdriver and open up the electric cord. I combine the wires and the mixer works again. I step aboard the mixer which now seems to be an automobile. I drive along a gray, smooth, floating road. (Subject 15)

Here a mixer turns into a car. It seems difficult to explain what could trigger such a change, for the two objects are quite far from each other semantically and visually. One possibility is that fixing the mixer with a screwdriver somehow primes the category of other mechanical devices which often have to be fixed, and the action conjures up the image of actually fixing a car. Strangely enough, the "road" along which the car is going seems to consist of the dough that the mixer was mixing a moment ago, so the context and environment have not changed totally.

I am with some friend at a department store. We are looking for lockers there, and the store suddenly turns into a swimming hall. In its own way, the place is also a hotel and at times a ship. Nevertheless, when we get out, there is no water nearby. (Subject 55)

Here the whole virtual place is discontinuous and unstable. The department store turns into a swimming hall, probably because the concept of "locker" is activated; lockers are what one typically finds in the dressing rooms of a swimming hall. Why is that very same place also "in its own way" a hotel and even a ship? We may speculate along the following lines: the only real places in the subject's environment with features from all of these simultaneously active representations are the big ferries sailing between Finland and Sweden. They have large tax-free shopping centers, some have saunas and swimming pools, and they are in many ways like big hotels. Perhaps the connection from the node "department store" to "swimming hall" through the triggering node "locker" primed to some extent the only node in the category of places that has features of both, and consequently the idea of the place as "hotel" and "ship" were sufficiently activated to become conscious, resulting in a place with very unstable and vague identity.

The Mechanisms of Bizarreness

Spreading activation in underlying semantic networks, then, has an intimate relationship to the semantic windows or virtual objects and places that we are directly aware of at the phenomenal level. This idea is also advocated by Reinsel, Antrobus, and Wollman (1992), and Fookson and Antrobus (1992). They argue that the disjointed, disconnected nature of dream imagery may reflect spreading activation in associative nets. Activation of the networks during REM sleep may be insufficient to fully support the same activation patterns typically activated in the waking state. Atypical patterns of activation in the networks may thus correspond to the production of dream images with improbable or bizarre features. These patterns of activation could be simulated in connectionist models. The simulation models would explain bizarreness as slight deviations in the overall energy pattern of a network, not exactly duplicating the pattern, as would be experienced in veridical perception.

In the light of our data, the discontinuities seem to be often driven from the top down (semantic levels) rather than from the bottom up (sensory levels): a stray association in semantic memory from one image or thought suddenly becomes incarnated as a concrete virtual object or place, so that the previous object simply turns into the new one, creating phenomenal discontinuity. This change seems to be, at least in many cases, semantically driven, not bottom up. There is a close interaction between the systems realizing the visual features of virtual objects and those realizing their semantic interpretation, and in dreams it is extremely difficult to say which came first. The semantic activation that spreads smoothly to nearby nodes seems to mold the windows that open into consciousness as virtual objects and places; therefore, we rarely see radical visual or semantic discrepancies between the original and the transformed object.

In agreement with this observation, Rittenhouse, Stickgold, and Hobson (1994) reported that in dream discontinuities, character and object transformations follow particular rules. In their study, the bizarre transformations of objects and characters appeared to be controlled by semantic constraints that require the transformed item to normally remain within its original category, object, or character. The only instance in which they observed an inanimate object transformed into an animate object was a fishing lure turning into a live fish. In our examples above, we noted flowers turning into stuffed birds turning into live birds, as if only gradual shifts in the visual and semantic features were possible at any one time.

The significant—and surprising—conclusion from the Rittenhouse et al. (1994) study was that many discontinuous dream images are, paradoxically, coherent. A dream object does not transform randomly into another object, but into an object that shares many semantic or associative features with the first. In the waking state such associations do not intrude into our consciousness, for they are unable to override the externally supplied sensory information.

Discontinuities in the dream setting, by contrast, were not found to be constrained in any detectable way by Rittenhouse et al. (1994). The theme and the place of the previous dream leave no traces behind after a sudden but complete discontinuity where the place changes, and no characters or objects or direct references to them are carried over from the original setting. It is as if the brain started a whole new dream story from scratch every now and then, and forgot all about what was going on a couple of seconds ago.

The discontinuities we have found in the home-based dream reports of students are sometimes quite surprising, but the associative links are, nevertheless, fairly easily deciphered.

> I am walking along a path in a forest with my mother. On the path there is growing thick hair, like human hair. I wondered about it aloud. My mother comments that many people grow such hair. At the same moment I notice that we are walking on top of a giant human, a man. (Subject 07)

In this dream, the transformation is radical, but still follows the paths of association. First, for some reason the grass on the path is not exactly as it should be: the semantic window that ought to represent "grass" has switched to a visually similar window with the content "hair." The dream self notices this oddity, and the reply from her mother tries to explain it away in a typical ad hoc manner. This time, however, the mother's words function as a powerful suggestion. Since the hair does not fit the overall context, and the mother suggests one where it would fit, the context immediately changes to the suggested one, although this again involves radically bizarre assumptions: the postulation of a giant on top of which the dream self is strolling.

Discontinuities of virtual objects reveal that the semantic level and the purely perceptual level of Gestalt windows are in constant interaction during the generation and maintenance of virtual objects. Changes that take place at the semantic level, hidden from the phenomenal surface, can change the interpretation of the Gestalt window at the phenomenal level, or even modulate the structure of the Gestalt windows to make them congruent with the activation at the semantic level. Therefore, we could say that virtual objects have a phenomenal surface to them, but that their roots go deeply into the networks of stored semantic knowledge. There is a tight connection to the semantic-conceptual "deep" level, and this connection appears to be a two-way information channel, where semantic and perceptual information constantly interact.

This two-level conception of virtual objects could guide empirical research in attempts to find the neural constituents of virtual objects in the brain. It delineates what exactly such research might look for—it presents top-down constraints to the search for the lower-level mechanisms. To look for the virtual objects that constitute the contents of coherent visual experience in the brain is, therefore, to look for structurally defined entities at one level (Gestalt windows at the phenomenal surface) that incorporate a two-way information channel to semantic-conceptual knowledge (the roots of the semantic window). Hence virtual objects are probably construed in specific neural activation patterns, mostly based on information in the ventral occipitotemporal stream. Furthermore, a third level of binding is required before the visual-semantic activation patterns become a part of consciousness: location binding. The Gestalt and semantic windows must interact with the dorsally based spatial information and be bound into a location in the phenomenal coordinate system.

The search for the neural constituents of virtual objects thus should look for high-level neural entities that have these three features: (1) a phenomenal, structured surface (Gestalt window); (2) an underlying semantic window (a two-way information channel); and (3) the Gestalt window related to a particular location within a larger spatial coordinate system (location binding). This kind of a neural entity requires complex interactions between the ventral and dorsal streams.

Binding and the Unity of Human Characters in Dreams

To get a more systematic grip on the different types of binding anomalies in dreams, we conducted a study on one specific but prominent type of phenomenal element in dreams: dream people, or the representation of human characters in dreams (Revonsuo & Tarkko, 2002). Previous studies reveal that on average, two to three animate characters in addition to the dream self appear in every dream. Most of these characters are other human beings, whereas animal characters make up only about 5%. In less than 5% of dream reports the dream self appears alone (for normative findings, see Domhoff, 1996; Strauch & Meier, 1996). Human characters constitute the third most frequently described elements in dream reports, outnumbered only by objects and action (Revonsuo & Salmivalli, 1995). A fair proportion of dream people include bizarre features: in 15% of human characters in dream reports incongruity is described; in 7% vagueness; and in 4%, discontinuity (Revonsuo & Salmivalli, 1995).

So when creating the phenomenal representations of human characters in dreams, the brain often combines information sources in peculiar ways which are then experienced as the bizarre features of these characters. In order to get an empirical grip on the mechanisms underlying the construction of such representations, more detailed phenomenological descriptions and analyses of bizarreness are required. In the study by Revonsuo and Tarkko (2002) we first developed a scale that contains definitional criteria for different types of dream bizarreness, distinguished from each other on the basis of the kind of binding that is disrupted. The main division was made between *internal bizarreness* and *contextual bizarreness.*

Contextual bizarreness concerns the relation of the character representation to the surrounding dream world: Does the virtual person appear in a virtual place where she might conceivably appear in the waking world? Does she engage in activities that are probable for her in the waking world? Internal bizarreness, by contrast, concerns the *intrinsic* form and content of the phenomenal representation, regardless of the context in which this representation happens to appear.

The intrinsic features of the virtual person include at least the following: (1) The structural composition and outlook of the visual representation: What does the person look like? Is there anything wrong with the spatial grouping and feature integration of the representation? (2) The emotional component signaling the familiarity or unfamiliarity of the person: Is there an appropriate feeling of familiarity connected with the person? (3) The long-term memory representations activated by the perception of the person: What information is attached to the virtual person? What kind of a semantic window does the Gestalt window of the person open? (4) The temporal continuity of the virtual person: How does the person appear in, disappear from, or transform during the dream?

The results revealed that about half (53%) of the 568 human dream characters that were studied included at least one bizarre feature. This relatively high proportion of bizarre characters is partly explained by the fact that bizarreness of action and speech, which are among the most common types of bizarreness (Revonsuo & Salmivalli, 1995), were classified as bizarre features of the dream character who realized them. Conversely, this result means that about half of the persons we meet in our dreams are *completely* in accordance with the expectations of our waking perceptual world. On average, the dreaming brain manages to keep all the various information sources coherently bound together in one out of two dream characters constructed during dreaming.

Binding anomalies were much more frequent at the level of *relating* the representations of human characters to other representations (contextual bizarreness) than at the level of the *internal features* of human characters (internal bizarreness). Sixty-three percent of bizarre features found in human dream characters concerned the relation of the character to other representations within the dream world (surrounding world, action, speech) whereas only 37% concerned the internal features of the representation itself (structure and outlook, familiarity, semantic knowledge, temporal continuity). All the categories of contextual bizarreness were more frequent than any of the categories of internal bizarreness. This result shows that binding aberrations are particularly likely to happen at the relatively global level of phenomenal representation where different types of semantic windows should be interrelated to form a coherent perceptual environment.[2]

Generating a globally unified phenomenal (dream) world thus seems to be the most demanding task for the cognitive and neural mechanisms underlying the phenomenal level. If global (contextual) and local (internal) binding are different kinds of processes for the brain, then their respective neural mechanisms should also be distinct.

Next we consider some dreams where human characters manifest various forms of bizarreness.

I was walking in the campus when I noticed Janis Joplin and her husband (I just had a feeling it was her husband; Janis Joplin had short red hair, but her face was like the real JJ). I heard Janis say to her husband that she was going to die real soon. Her husband said to her that people are often wrong about the future. (Suddenly they were gone and my girlfriend switched places with JJ and I did the same with JJ's husband). My girlfriend (at least I think it was her) said that she knew she is going to die soon. (Subject 20, a 23-year-old man; a translated and abbreviated dream report)

Here we have lots of interesting binding errors. The representation of Janis Joplin in this dream is bizarre in many ways: her outlook, especially her hair, is different from what the real JJ used to look like: there is an incongruence between the actual Gestalt window and the one stored in memory about the visual outlook of JJ. Furthermore, the dream self does not remember that JJ had been dead for more than 20 years at the time when this dream occurred; the semantic window to access the stored knowledge about JJ is not completely open. JJ also appears in a place (the campus of the University of Turku) where she most certainly has never been: this constitutes contextual bizarreness. The interpretation that the man is JJ's husband also has no factual basis: the dreamer "just had a feeling" that that is who it is. On top of it all, suddenly JJ disappears and the dreamer's girlfriend takes her place while the dreamer himself continues where JJ's husband left off; in fact, they continue the same conversation that was initiated by JJ and her husband!

If the dreamer had seen the same persons walking in the campus in the waking world, he would probably have interpreted the situation in a completely different way, perhaps along the following lines: "There's a young couple walking; the girl's face reminds me of Janis Joplin, but of course the real JJ is long since dead."

In the next example, there is incorrect feature binding of a dream character:

> I came to our student clubhouse with two friends. . . . I saw Kati (my classmate) sitting on the edge of the stage and sewing something. She was of a strange color: she was light green. (Subject 58, a 22-year-old woman)

In this dream, the complexion of a friend is changed to the most unlikely shade of light green. For some reason feature binding errors like the above are extremely rare in dreams. Perhaps their rarity is related to the "local" nature of binding required in feature integration.

One fairly common type of bizarreness in human dream characters is an inappropriate feeling of familiarity connected to a dream person. That is, a dream person who does not look like anybody we really know in the waking world is experienced or interpreted as familiar, as an acquaintance or a friend. The precise identity of these pseudo-familiar persons tends to remain rather vague or, alternatively, they are interpreted as specific persons such as relatives who really exist. The converse aberration, where a truly familiar person is not recognized as such but treated as a stranger, appears to be nonexistent in dreams.

> I entered a house with my father. I was walking around the house when I saw someone sitting by a table. I recognized this person; she was my grandmother (she didn't look like my grandmother and in real life my grandmother is dead). I went to her and gave her a hug. Beside another table I saw my mother and also gave her a hug (in real life my mother is dead). Further away there were people dancing. I was wondering if there were any other familiar people there. I thought that I could look for Jarkko, because he should be there because he was also dead (Jarkko is my classmate from years ago and in real life he is still alive). I found Jarkko, but his outlook was quite different from Jarkko's appearance in real life. (Subject 13, a 22-year-old woman)

In this dream we have a whole cavalcade of bizarre persons. There is the grandmother who does not look like the real grandmother, but who nevertheless is treated as she. Somehow the dream self does realize that the people she met in the house are in reality dead, which makes her believe that she is in a place where only dead people can be found. For some reason she then incorrectly remembers that a friend of hers is dead although he is not. And then she treats a person who looks like somebody else as that person. So here the connections between the Gestalt windows of the persons and the corresponding semantic windows are thoroughly muddled.

In fact, it seems that in quite many dreams, *several* bizarre persons tend to appear in a row rather than at random intervals. Thus, it may be that some physiological factor at the underlying neural levels of organization temporarily disturbs the organization of the semantic windows relating to dream persons, which easily leads to clusters of bizarre dream characters appearing within the same dream.

At least the following types of semantic distortions of persons are repeatedly found in dreams. First, there are cases of missing semantic knowledge—a sort of selective "amnesia" for some important piece of information. For example, some old friend or relative is encountered in the dream as if nothing had happened, although during wakefulness it is very well known that the person has moved away or died, and meeting him or her would be extremely unlikely or outright impossible. If such a person were nevertheless actually encountered in the waking world, we would have a hard time believing our eyes, because the first thing we would remember about the person would be that he is dead, or lives very far away and simply cannot be where he appears.

A second type of semantic distortion is the case of false pieces of semantic knowledge that we would immediately reject during waking. For example, a close relative or friend in the dream may suddenly have a profession that she has nothing to do with in the real world. Even more far-fetched are cases of impostor relatives: persons we have never met in the real world but whom we accept as our "sister" or "brother" or "cousin" or "uncle" in the dream. We know perfectly well that we do not really have such relatives: there should be no basis in semantic memory for such a peculiar semantic interpretation of the strangers we meet in our dreams. Nevertheless, impostor relatives appear regularly in dream reports (although not with a very high frequency). False knowledge and impostor relatives could be classified as cases of "confabulation."

In conclusion, as far as semantic memory is concerned, we tend to be both amnesic and confabulatory in our dreams. Furthermore, during dreaming we seem to have no insight into these memory deficits; we are unable to reflect upon the credibility of our interpretations in the light of previous knowledge and rational judgment. We accept false and distorted semantic interpretations without questioning, no matter how implausible they may be. Hobson (1997) suggests that our mental status during dreaming, characterized by memory disorders, confabulation, and lack of insight, can be classified as a specific type of madness: delirium. According to him, this state is caused by a chemical imbalance in the brain's neuromodulatory control systems: a loss of aminergic inhibition and a reciprocal gain in cholinergic excitation.

I would rather suggest that bizarre dream images and delusions should be primarily described and explained at the phenomenal, cognitive, and electrophysiological levels rather than to the neurochemical level. Neurochemical levels are probably several steps below the phenomenal level, whereas electrophysiological levels underlie it more directly. Still, in the final multilevel model of the constitutive mechanisms of dream images, the neurochemical levels will also have to be included.

Summary

The dreaming brain reveals how the phenomenal level is put together even in the absence of sensory input. Phenomenal features are bound to locations in simulated space;

object parts are bound together to construct integrated simulated objects; objects and persons are recognized and identified as *particular* objects and persons; they are temporally continuous and embedded in the overall spatial context of the phenomenal world. All the different varieties of binding that are required to create a coherent dream world may flounder, at least every once in a while. But some fail much more often than others. Specialized modules produce the Gestalt windows, the phenomenal surrogates of objects, almost flawlessly. Most dream objects look no different from their counterparts during waking perception. The dreaming brain has more difficulties in opening appropriate, coherent semantic windows. The knowledge about the dreamed objects and persons that the brain accesses (or confabulates) and which we fully buy during dreaming, is often suspect in the light of the knowledge we have about the same things in the waking state.

The most difficult task for the dreaming brain appears to be to relate several *different* simulated objects with each other, to form the *global* unity of the dream world. Any single specialized module does not seem to "know" very well what the other modules contribute to the phenomenal level at the same time; therefore, the overall unity quite often flounders, resulting in peculiar combinations of objects, persons, and places. It also seems to be a difficult task for the dreaming brain to keep track of the contents of consciousness across time: the simulated objects tend to appear, disappear, or transform magically during the course of the dream.

The dream world, although perhaps not all that flawlessly bound together, nevertheless manifests remarkable degrees of unity and consistency. The anomalies of binding are relatively small aberrations on the surface of a system that is largely well-organized as a simulated world. Despite the fact that many theories dismiss dreaming as simply nonfunctional, chaotic noise produced by REM neurophysiology, in actual fact the phenomenal content of dreams is not utterly chaotic, random, or fundamentally distorted. Dreaming shows a high level of organization and therefore may also serve important functions (see chapter 24). There is a world of difference between pathological distortions of consciousness caused by brain injury and the physiologically normal state of dreaming. But both sources of evidence, as different kinds of altered states of consciousness, are indispensable when we try to understand how the brain puts together the inner simulated reality: the phenomenal level of organization in the brain.

15 Cognitive Mechanisms of Phenomenal Unity

In the preceding chapters, binding and the unity of consciousness were primarily considered at the level of description most important for consciousness science: the phenomenal level. The dreaming brain and the damaged brain served there as sources of data about the hidden structures that integrate consciousness. Description of the phenomenal level as such is, of course, only the first step. After that we need to connect the phenomenal level to the underlying mechanisms. As we learned in chapter 11, there are two different kinds of levels at which the mechanisms may be described: the cognitive and the neural levels. The cognitive level of description uses the conceptual framework of cognitive science, and thus describes binding and unity in terms of information processing, computation, and representation. The cognitive level is not a biological level of organization in the brain, but an abstract way of describing any levels of organization in terms of their input-output functions.

The concepts "phenomenal consciousness" and "unity of consciousness" are not something to be found as such in cognitive science. For cognitive science the binding problem appears in a different guise. The information-processing mechanisms that receive and process sensory input are believed to be modular (Fodor, 1983). That is, stimulus information from a single object, say a bird that flies by, singing, is received through multiple sensory channels. The different features of the stimulus (shape, color, motion, size, location, sound) are handled by separate processing modules, in parallel, in the human cognitive architecture. The brain computes multiple sources of information over multiple channels simultaneously. Yet, at the level of higher cognitive processes—in the focus of attention, in working memory, in long-term memory, in our interactions with objects—the cognitive system treats a perceptual object as *a single unified package of information.* The binding problem for the cognitive levels of description thus is: How do the independent modules coordinate their outputs to create the unity of representation at the higher cognitive levels?

Selective attention is the cognitive process that seems to play a crucial role in bringing the unity of perceptual representations about. In visual perception, only the information in the focus of attention seems to be integrated to compose the unified perceptual objects of conscious experience. As attention and conscious perception thus engage in an intimate interplay in phenomenal experience, their exact relationship remains controversial. According to a widely held view in cognitive science, attention is the sole gateway to consciousness. Attentional selection operates already at a preconscious level and only the results of selection reach perceptual consciousness. The contents of selective attention thus exhaust the contents of subjective visual experience. This view of attention is related to the theater-spotlight metaphor of consciousness. A competing model postulates that consciousness is independent of attentional selection: there are contents of subjective visual experience also outside the focus of attention.

In this chapter, we explore cognitive theories and phenomena where the interaction between selective attention and visual consciousness is clearly manifested: the feature integration theory of attention, change blindness, inattentional blindness, and iconic memory. On the basis of these data, we will try to figure out what the relationship is between attention and consciousness.

Feature Integration Theory

There are several cognitive theories that in some way or another touch the cognitive binding problem. The one most relevant in the present context is Anne Treisman's feature integration theory. It is basically a model describing how we (visually) perceive the objects in the focus of awareness. Its initial assumption is, in accordance with the modularity hypothesis, that elementary sensory features (e.g., color and orientation) are coded automatically, preattentively, in parallel, and without focal attention in a number of specialized modules. Each module forms a *feature map* for the dimensions of the features it codes (say the color module constructs a map of the different dimensions of color).

Detection of *single* features takes place preattentively, and in parallel. This can be demonstrated with the attentional pop-out effect. Imagine that you have in front of you a large display with hundreds of small letters. Now, either all of them are green, or among them there are a few that are red. Your task is to decide as fast as possible whether there are any red stimuli present in the display, and if so, to point out their locations. If there are any red letters present, you need no special effort to find them. They simply "pop out" immediately from the mostly green background. You become immediately aware of the presence and location of "redness here" or "redness over there" or "no redness present." This result has been interpreted as showing that color is processed preattentively, in parallel with the other features. Another way of interpreting the pop-out effect is to say that it reflects global attention to the scene as a whole. A discrepant object is consequently seen as a *break* in the global structure of the array (Treisman, 1996).

By contrast, *conjunctions* of features are processed serially. In order to find an object defined by a conjunction (binding) of elementary features—a certain color combined with a certain form—say a unique *red circle* among many *green circles* and *red squares,* one must focally attend to one target at a time. Focusing attention on a particular location in the master map of locations retrieves and combines (or binds) whichever features currently are active at that location, creating a temporary *object file.* The contents of this object file can then be compared to stored representations in visual long-term memory to recognize the object. However, if features combine *without* focused attention, on their own, incorrect combinations or *illusory conjunctions* will occur. Treisman summarizes her theory as follows:

> According to feature integration theory, a scalable "window of attention" scans a "master map" of locations, selecting the features currently active in corresponding locations of various specialized feature maps, and suppressing those in other locations to prevent erroneous binding. The selected features are assembled to form an "object token" and are compared to stored representations to identify the object. (Treisman, 1996, p. 172)

Note that conceptually this level of description is completely different from both the phenomenal level and the neural level. However, attempts to connect the cognitive-level feature integration theory with the neural level are already underway. The hypothesis has been put forward that the master map of locations may be realized as a *parietal spatial map.* This map is localized in the posterior parietal lobes or at least necessarily depends on their normal functioning. The map mediates the explicit localization of objects in the visual scene, the individuation of separate objects from each other, and the binding of features through selective attention (Treisman, 1996).

Patients suffering from Balint's syndrome have bilateral posterior parietal damage (see chapters 12 and 13). They suffer from the complete disruption of spatial vision and severe difficulties in visual feature binding. This constellation of visuospatial and attentional deficits has been interpreted as caused by the disruption of the "master map of locations" residing in the parietal areas (L. C. Robertson, 2003).

The cognitive concepts of the feature integration theory do not mention consciousness as such. Thus, it is the job of the science of consciousness to figure out how these concepts relate to the phenomenal level of description. In the following I suggest one possible way of connecting the phenomenal level to the cognitive level. (For Treisman's own account of consciousness, see Treisman 2003.)

"Object Tokens" as Virtual Objects

There seems to be a natural connection between the cognitive and the phenomenal levels of description. Some theoretical ideas in the feature integration theory can be directly connected to the phenomenal level of description.

One noteworthy concept in Treisman's theory is variously called "temporary object representations" or "object files" or "object tokens." Some features attributed to the "object tokens" are not unlike the features of "virtual objects" at the phenomenal level. In feature integration, the elementary sensory features are "assembled" to form an "object token" which "mediates" the perception of objects.

According to Treisman, the temporary object tokens "must be capable of activating any motor program to allow the flexible choice of any arbitrary response to any perceived object" (Treisman, 1996, p. 172). "[T]heir output can be used to control the motor systems that generate action towards perceived objects, and to mediate conscious experience of perceived objects" (Treisman, 1994, p. 309). In an overview of the binding problem in 1999, Treisman considers the most crucial question to be: How is the output of the binding process interpreted and used by later stages? "[T]he outputs must be readable by whatever systems encode memories, determine choices, or select motor responses" (Treisman, 1999, p. 110).

The features of object tokens are similar to features typically assigned to the contents of consciousness. Contents of consciousness allow flexible voluntary choices among a multitude of potential courses of action, and contents of consciousness can be coded into explicit long-term memory. It is explicitly recognized in several models and theories of consciousness that voluntary action can *only* be mediated by conscious experience. Furthermore, "action toward *perceived* objects" seems to be something that can only be determined at the phenomenal level, for perceived objects that are present in subjective experience must reside at the phenomenal level.

I suggest the following identifications between the phenomenal level of description and the feature integration theory (the cognitive level of description). The entities identified as "object tokens" in feature integration theory are, if described at the phenomenal level, identical to the entities referred to by "virtual objects" or "simulated objects" in the world simulation metaphor of consciousness. That is to say that *both terms refer to the subjectively perceived objects* all around us in conscious phenomenal experience. The construct referred to as "the master map of locations" in feature integration theory is identical to those parts of the phenomenal coordinate system that are involved in the realization of egocentric visual space. *Both terms refer to the system in the brain that constructs experiential visual space:* the space in which visual experiences occur. Both terms also refer to the system lost in Balint's syndrome, resulting in visual consciousness of single objects only, without any visual background space.

These identifications lead us to the conclusion that, despite appearances to the contrary, cognitive psychology *does* theorize about the contents of consciousness at the phenomenal level. It is just camouflaged in the disguise of a cognitivist vocabulary of "information processing," "representation," "files," and "maps" rather than phenomenal experiences. Those concepts are derived directly from the computer metaphor of the mind. But this cognitivist language, when properly interpreted, reveals that cognitive psychologists have been forced to postulate theoretical entities that resemble phenomenal objects and virtual space.

Consciousness and Attention

In cognitive science "attention" has been the concept that comes closest to "consciousness" (or "awareness"). Often "attention," "awareness," and "consciousness" are treated as referring to more or less the same thing, although their precise relation is rarely explicated. However, it seems that the prevailing view in the cognitive neuroscience of consciousness includes the following claims:

1. Attention is a necessary prerequisite of consciousness.
2. The contents of consciousness are equal to or fully determined by the contents of selective attention.

For example, Dehaene and Naccache (2001) propose that the first claim is a major empirical observation that *any* theory of consciousness should incorporate. Baars (1997) seems to accept the second claim when he says that selective attention is the *process* of selection and consciousness is the *result* of the selection, the output produced by the process of selection.

As we observed earlier (in chapters 2 and 5), this idea of the relationship between attention and consciousness is the cornerstone of the theater-spotlight metaphor of consciousness. Why is this way of thinking about consciousness so widespread in cognitive neuroscience? It seems that the popularity of the theater-spotlight metaphor is partly based on empirical evidence from neuropsychology and visual attention and partly based on an ambiguity of what exactly is meant by "consciousness" in claims such as (1) and (2) above. To sort out how we should construe the attention-consciousness relationship, we will first review some of the evidence that seems to support the theater-spotlight metaphor. Then we will see how the same evidence might be interpreted in the light of the world-simulation metaphor. A clearer picture of the attention-consciousness relationship finally emerges when we explicitly separate several different notions of consciousness from each other (along the lines discussed in chapter 2). Thus, it turns out that the claim "attention is necessary for consciousness" is true under one reading of "consciousness," but false under another.

No Consciousness without Attention?

The theater-spotlight metaphor, if true, implies that there can be no consciousness where there is no attention. That is an empirically testable statement and should be backed up by convincing evidence. At least three sources of evidence are often cited as backing the idea that attention is necessary for consciousness: hemispatial neglect, change blindness, and inattentional blindness.

Hemispatial neglect (see chapter 13) is in many neuropsychological theories construed as an impairment of *spatial attention.* Consequently, the behavior of the patients is explained by the failure and reluctance to turn their *attention* to the contralateral space. According to this line of thought, the lack of awareness of the stimuli in one side of space is a *consequence* of the lack of attention to that space. If only attention could be allocated to that space, then awareness of the stimuli in that space would follow. This idea is corroborated by the fact that neglect may temporarily improve if the patient is trained to attend to the left side of space (Umiltá, 2001). The *lack of awareness* of stimuli in the left side of space is therefore caused and explained by the *preceding lack of attention* to that side of space.

A directly contrary way of construing what is going on in neglect is to say that the lack of awareness of one side of space causes the failure to attend to objects in that space. If the patient's sphere of phenomenal experience does not automatically include any "left side of space" as a part of the phenomenal background in his consciousness, then it is mighty difficult for the patient to (voluntarily) direct any attention to such space (or to any objects in such space).

What exactly is supposed to happen when attention "selects" something for more detailed processing? Could this selection operate on representations outside of consciousness? To answer these questions, we need a more detailed picture of the mechanisms of attention. Many theories see the mechanisms of attention in the following way. Preattentive perceptual representations compete for their access to higher-level processing. Some higher-level processes can *bias* the competition among preattentive representations so that the level of activation in specific representations surpasses the level of activation in other, competing representations. The mechanisms that selectively impose the bias on particular representations to the exclusion of others are the mechanisms of selective attention. The representations that receive the "extra" activation become bound together as coherent simulated objects. They can consequently be subjected to higher-level cognitive operations in refective consciousness and working memory.

The higher-level processes can select representations and bias their activation only if the representations are accessible to selection and biasing. To be accessible, a lower-level representation must first have reached an adequate stage—otherwise the representation is invisible or inaccessible to the selection mechanisms. Now there is solid evidence for the existence of implicit, nonconscious representations of neglected stimuli in the ventral visual stream (Driver & Vuilleumier, 2001). If those representations already exist anyway, why are the higher-level attentional processes unable to bias them so that they could enter consciousness? In other words, why are those undeniable object representations inaccessible to the mechanisms of selective attention? I propose that, in order to be accessible to the attentional biasing processes, *the representations have to be first related to phenomenal space.* If they are *not* phenomenally present for the brain, then they *do not exist* for the mechanisms that could select and bias them. Therefore, in this view it turns out that phenomenal presence—consciousness—is necessary for the adequate allocation of attention.[1]

Furthermore, there is evidence that, in healthy subjects, attention can to some extent modulate performance in the absence of awareness of stimuli (Simons, 2000; Koivisto & Revonsuo, 2004). Even so, attention without awareness does not allow us to modify behavior and select new goals in the same way that conscious experience of the stimuli allows. Thus, attention alone, in the absence of consciousness, would not be of much help for the neglect patient even if a nonconscious form of attention could be directed to the stimuli in the neglected hemifield. Attention alone is not equal to or sufficient for consciousness.

Recent electrophysiological studies in our lab provide direct evidence of the independence of visual awareness and attention. In these studies, an electrophysiological response called visual awareness negativity (VAN) has been used as an index of visual consciousness in normal human observers. In one study (Koivisto, Revonsuo, & Lehtonen, in press), VAN proved to be independent of the scope of attention (that is, it made no difference to VAN whether attention was focused on the global or the local level of the stimulus). In another study (Koivisto, Revonsuo, & Salminen, 2005), VAN proved to be independent of selective attention and to arise earlier than the electrophysiological effects of attentional selection ("selection negativity") do. That is, it made no difference to VAN whether the stimulus was a target or a nontarget; the EEG response to subjectively seeing the stimulus was similar in both cases. The effects of attention arise only after the effects of awareness have already become significant. Thus, these studies on the objective electrophysiological responses to awareness and attention support the view that subjective experience of a stimulus starts earlier than and is independent of the attentional selection of the same stimulus.

Change Blindness

Imagine that for a couple of seconds or so you see a photograph depicting some complex scenery, say some people in front of historical buildings and monuments, with trees, flowers, and grass in the background. You seem to have a momentary visual experience of the landscape with all its colors and details. After the picture disappears, a bright white background is flashed for a fraction of a second, after which the same picture reappears. You are told that there is some fairly big difference between the first and the second pictures. Would you be able to see the difference? Most people believe they would, but in actual fact it is extremely difficult to notice if one tree, building, person, shadow, cloud, or some other object has disappeared, shifted its location, or been inserted. This astonishing failure to detect even large changes in successive visual displays is called *change blindness* (CB).

To notice a change, one has to locate attention *exactly* on the object that is changing. Normally our visual system follows the transient cues that draw attention to the location of change and thus we automatically detect the change. If between the two pictures there is no mask (such as the white flash), then it would be a piece of cake for our visual system to notice the difference. We simply become immediately aware of how a building, person, or tree disappears or appears in the picture, because the location of the change reveals itself. But when the location of the change is masked from selective attention, we are just flabbergasted when told that a large change has occurred in the picture. For us it looks like the same picture, and it may take several trials before one can finally detect the change. Once one has detected the change, it is difficult *not* to see it every time the pictures change—now it really looks conspicuous.

Inattentional Blindness

Imagine that you are given the following task: A cross is presented briefly on a computer screen. Your task is to decide which is longer: the vertical or the horizontal line. You perform this task obediently for a few trials. Then after one trial you are unexpectedly asked by the experimenter whether you saw anything *else* appear on the screen during the previous trial. During the last trial, an additional object was displayed somewhere near the cross for several hundred milliseconds, but it may well be that when you are asked about it, you have no idea that there was anything else there besides the cross itself (Mack & Rock, 1998). This failure to report unexpected stimuli, irrelevant to the primary task but appearing in the same display with the target stimuli, has been called *inattentional blindness* (IB). Depending on the visual and semantic features and the precise location of the unexpected stimulus, IB is found in 25 to 75 % of subjects. IB-like phenomena also occur in more natural visual environments. As a famous experiment devised by Daniel Simons shows, when we are focusing our attention intensively on a basketball that is being passed from player to player, we may even fail to notice that someone in a gorilla suit is walking across the court!

Conflicting Interpretations of Change Blindness and Inattentional Blindness

How should these surprising failures to report what appear to be clearly visible stimuli (IB) or conspicuous changes in stimuli (CB) be interpreted? There are two conflicting ways to interpret them. The first identifies the contents of consciousness with the contents of selective attention; the second points to failures in visual memory rather than to the poverty of visual phenomenology.

The first interpretation of CB and IB proposes that we are not aware of *anything* beyond the spotlight of focal attention. That is to say that *there is no visual consciousness outside the focus of attention.* The most radical version of this view states that there *is* no phenomenal field outside the spotlight of attention. No type of form of consciousness extends beyond attention.

A less radical variety of this view states that there is a phenomenal background field surrounding the spotlight of attention. However, regions of the background field that are not currently visited or sampled by attention are not being modulated or refreshed by the corresponding regions of the stimulus field. Thus, if anything happens in the background stimulus field that does not immediately capture attention, the corresponding phenomenal field will not be updated, and therefore the new stimulus does not modulate the phenomenal level in any way.

According to both of the above interpretations, CB and IB are cases of true *blindness,* in that they involve total absence of visual phenomenology of the critical stimulus features. The "blindness" interpretation has been advocated by some of the researchers who originally discovered these phenomena (e.g., Mack & Rock, 1998). (However, it is not entirely clear which of the two alternatives of the blindness interpretation they advocate.)

A competing interpretation says that the regions in the visual field where the change took place (CB) or where the unexpected stimuli appeared (IB) do briefly modulate phenomenal consciousness. The phenomenal content of the modulation, however, is not selected for further conscious processing in reflective consciousness. Therefore it totally disappears from memory before it can be reported. We cannot retain in memory a detailed internal copy of the entire visual scene once it is gone.

This view suggests that we are momentarily conscious of all the stimuli across the entire visual field. But the presence of the visually rich field of phenomenal consciousness lasts only for a few hundred milliseconds. Then it disappears without leaving any traces of its existence behind. We rapidly forget everything there was, apart from those few items or features that attention has selected for further conscious processing and transported to working memory.

Iconic Memory and the Interplay between Attention and Consciousness

In cognitive psychology, the concept of "iconic memory" refers to a brief storage of visual information. There are several noteworthy properties of this storage (Palmer, 1999):

- its contents are extremely *rich:* it can hold practically complete visual information for a very short time (about 1 second).
- it holds information about the location, color, size, and shape of visual objects, but it does *not* contain information about the *category* or the *meaning* of the objects.
- it involves "visible persistence" or a *phenomenal trace* of the stimulus that has already physically disappeared.
- its contents *decay rapidly* and only a small part of them can be verbally reported before the contents become fully erased. Yet, for a brief duration, *any* part of the contents is in principle accessible for reporting. Where attention is directed before decay, there the contents can be reported (Sperling, 1960).

Iconic memory has been studied by briefly showing subjects a visual display with rich information (e.g., several rows and columns of letters). After the display has disappeared, the subjects are able to report only about four or five letters, although they *claim to have seen all of them.* When a cue indicating the row of letters they should report is given immediately *after* the stimulus has disappeared, subjects can report letters from any row at all. This shows that *all* of the information *was briefly available* for selective attention and report.

These observations suggest that the total contents of iconic memory (the contents of the phenomenal trace) match the contents of momentary phenomenal consciousness in vision. Furthermore, the contents of the reportable part of iconic memory match the contents of selective attention and reflective consciousness. The experiments establish that there is more in the phenomenal visual field at any moment than what can be reported or attended to. Yet, also the nonreportable contents are part of the contents of consciousness: they are phenomenally present for the subject. Reportablity is a conservative criterion of phenomenal consciousness and may lead to an underestimation of the richness and wideness of phenomenal experience.

According to the world-simulation metaphor, the interplay between selective attention and consciousness thus involves two levels of consciousness: phenomenal and reflective. In the visual modality, the contents of momentary phenomenal consciousness roughly match the rich contents of iconic memory. Selective attention operates on those phenomenal contents, integrates and binds them, and then transfers some of them to reflective consciousness.

By contrast, according to the theater-spotlight metaphor, attention selects among nonconscious (nonphenomenal) representations—only the results of selection are conscious. Baars (1997) compares this process to selecting the TV channel we want to watch: first there is the selective act, then the selected program is displayed on the screen.

I would argue that a more appropriate comparison is the kind of selection we make when there are several low-resolution thumbnail photographs on the computer screen, and we select among them the one we wish to see in detail, opening the link to the large, high-resolution version of the same picture. The crucial point is that when we select, the alternatives among which we select are *already visible* on the screen in some form. Accordingly, when selective attention operates, it chooses a content that already exists at the phenomenal level in some preliminary form, at some location. By biasing the level of activation to the chosen representation (or location), selective attention thus creates the coherent high-resolution version of the same object.

The world-simulation metaphor of consciousness is in harmony with the explanation of CB and IB according to which even the unreported visual stimuli cause a fleeting phenomenal trace, briefly present at the phenomenal level.[2] In CB, however, the intervening flash erases the contents of iconic memory totally. By the time of the second picture, there is no detailed image in storage (only the few items transferred to reflective consciousness) to which the seen picture could be compared to decide whether and where a change may have taken place. Furthermore, the *detection* of the change is a judgment that has to be made in reflective consciousness by comparing two different phenomenal contents that are never present in consciousness at the same time.

Lamme (2003) defends this interpretation of CB. He argues that momentary phenomenal consciousness leaves a trace in iconic memory. The trace can be recovered in some experimental settings, thus showing that there must have been a fleeting phenomenal awareness that left the trace. Lamme (2003) reports a CB experiment in which a cue reveals the relevant location where the change is going to take place. The cue is presented immediately *after* the first stimulus has disappeared but before the next (changed) stimulus appears. Such cueing *completely removes change blindness.* This is convincing evidence that for a fleeting moment the first stimulus is available in its entirety in iconic memory. Selective attention can still recover from iconic memory whichever item or feature in whichever part of the stimulus.

Does the same logic also aply to IB? We conducted an experiment to test this question (Koivisto, Revonsuo, Hyönä, Bergman, & Kallio, submitted). The *inattentional blindness hypothesis* states that the undetected stimuli never reach phenomenal consciousness in the first place. Failure of detection is an indication of true blindness; there is no visual phenomenology, no phenomenal trace caused by the stimulus. The *inattentional amnesia hypothesis* states that there is a brief phenomenal trace of the unexpected stimulus, but its representation in iconic memory degrades rapidly. It is no longer available for reflective consciousness and introspective verbal reports by the time the experimenter asks whether any new stimulus was detected. According to this interpretation, failure to report the stimulus is a failure to transform the information from iconic memory to a more long-lasting form in reflective consciousness, not a sign of the absence of phenomenal consciousness.

To directly contrast these two hypotheses, we presented a cue at the location in which the unexpected stimulus had appeared just a few milliseconds ago. We varied the delay of the cue from instantaneous to 1500 ms. The results showed that a cue given immediately or after a very brief delay helped to reduce IB significantly: now the subjects were much more likely to report the stimulus correctly than without the cue. However, a cue presented with a longer delay (1500 ms) was no longer effective. This pattern of results suggests that the unexpected stimulus is briefly represented in phenomenal consciousness and iconic memory, but all traces of it disappear within a few hundred milliseconds, after which it cannot be selected for reflective consciousness or reported anymore. If the results of this experiment hold in further studies of IB as well, then inattentional *blindness* may turn out to be inattentional *amnesia.*

Phenomenal Vision outside the Attentional Spotlight

The world-simulation metaphor, unlike the theater-spotlight metaphor, claims that visual phenomenology also exists *outside* of the focus of attention, and *before* attentional selection takes place. We have a subjective visual *field,* a spatial *expanse* of visual experience, and we see *something* in every part of this expanse. Precisely what is it that we see there? Our subjective, phenomenal visual field is structured through attention into two parts: the region of focal awareness and the surrounding regions of peripheral awareness. A paradigm example of phenomenal experience outside attention are the regions of the visual field where attention has not visited yet. Let us call them regions of *preattentive vision.* What kind of contents of consciousness inhabit those regions? What would visual consciousness be like if it consisted *only* of preattentive vision? It might be a more or less chaotic field of preattentive features: colors, line orientations, motion, and so forth, here and there and all around, forming a tangled texture of phenomenal features.

Still, that does not seem to be the case. Experimental evidence (Wolfe, 1999) shows that the preattentive field is not a uniform, undifferentiated field, but a scene that has been divided into subregions through some basic figure-ground segregation and grouping processes. These subregions consist of some sort of candidate objects that possess no global shape but bear preattentive features as attributes. The preattentive object representations are not sufficient to support object recognition. The preattentive scene is thus merely a collection of unrecognized objects in a rough spatial layout. There are no proper visual objects, but only *visual "stuff"* that is *loosely bundled* rather than tightly bound together:

> Thus, across the great bulk of the visual field, unrecognized objects are held together by the spatial organization of the early visual system. At later stages, a recognized object is held together by the explicit binding of the selected set of features. Working in tandem, these processes of bundling and binding deliver a coherent perceptual world. (Wolfe & Cave 1999, p. 16)

Attention moves across the field of visual stuff, selecting among the loose bundles or the candidate objects one by one. The one chosen enters the focus of attention. There, the loose bundling undergoes a transformation. It becomes a tightly bound "object file"—a coherent virtual or phenomenal object that can be recognized (i.e., that can open a semantic window). Evidence furthermore indicates that when the focus of attention *departs* from the virtual object, *it falls apart again,* rapidly receding back to the state where it was before attention arrived. It becomes again just a bundle of loosely related features without any global shape.

If we could freeze a momentary frame of visual consciousness depicting the whole visual field, or better still, observe a sequence of such frames in slow motion, what would we find there in the subjective visual field? First of all, there would be a phenomenal expanse full of preattentive bundles that hang around in loosely defined groups. Second, attention selects one bundle at a time, moving serially from bundle to bundle. Like some kind of magical magnifying lens, it settles on a bundle and a miracle happens: the preattentive features under the lens instantaneously organize themselves to form a unified global 3D shape, with all the features defining the object coherently bound together. A full-fledged virtual, phenomenal object is thus instantaneously reconstructed from a few pieces of disorganized visual-phenomenal stuff. But the life of an organized virtual object is short. As soon as the spotlight of attention departs, the virtual object is shattered into pieces once more, as if it had never existed in the first place. But in some other place to which the focus of attention has moved, another virtual object is being created for its short-lived existence.

Yet, not all of what was gained will necessarily be lost after every shift of attention. Under natural viewing conditions where the visual stimulus field is stable and the observer can control the rate of visual scanning, the visual system immediately constructs a schematic depiction of the spatial layout of a scene (Intraub, 1999). That scene persists across saccades and organizes the brief glimpses into an understandable global scene of multiple objects which all seem to be present at once. My guess is that, under natural viewing conditions, objects that have been attended to and recognized, although they fall apart again to the loose bundles of features in the periphery of vision, *the semantic windows opened during focused attention* on those virtual objects *still remain open.* Even when I do not focus on the visual stuff that appears outside the computer screen where I presently focus, I see the vague peripheral blurs *as* books or *as* papers or *as* tables and chairs, although their visual appearance is that of shapeless, vaguely defined blurs. Nevertheless, I have no doubts about the identity of the objects at the location of the blurs; a certain blur is seen as some specific object, not as a totally unrecognized bundle of features. There is a *semantic interpretation* attached to the blur; the semantic window is still open, although the Gestalt window has become badly disfigured. The semantic interpretation is probably supported by the schematic representation of the whole familiar scene. Even a mere visual blur is capable of *keeping the semantic window open,* although the same blur would *not be capable of opening it all by itself* when it appears for the first time.

In a nutshell, the relationship between attention and visual consciousness is *not* that the latter is entirely dependent on the former. Attention seems to be necessary only for visual awareness of *coherent* objects, but outside focal attention there is a whole field of phenomenal visual background, full of phenomenal visual stuff that is not organized into coherent visual objects. As was discussed in chapter 2, selective attention is necessary for *reflective* consciousness, because the objects of reflection (or the input for further conscious cognitive processing) must be first selected and focused upon from phenomenal consciousness to be taken as input for reflective consciousness.

Summary

The relationships between consciousness, attention, and binding have been explored. First we introduced the feature integration theory that explains how feature binding is supposed to work in vision. Although the theory uses only a cognitive vocabulary that does not explicitly mention consciousness, some of its theoretical constructs are tightly connected to the phenomenal level. We put forward the idea that the theory's "object files" are in fact the phenomenal objects of visual experience, and that the "master map of locations" has a close relation to visual phenomenal space.

Then we turned to the more general question of the relationship between attention and consciousness. A widely spread view in cognitive psychology maintains that attention is necessary for consciousness. We studied the most compelling evidence cited in favor of this idea: neglect, change blindness, and inattentional blindness. A competing hypothesis of the relationship between attention and consciousness was put forward. According to it phenomenal consciousness is independent of attention. Attentional selection operates on the phenomenal contents of consciousness. After selection of the focus of attention the selected phenomenal items become the contents of reflective consciousness. Only then do they become accessible to verbal reporting. Evidence for this latter view was found from experimental work on iconic memory. Also, the evidence from neglect, change blindness, and inattentional blindness can be explained from this point of view in a satisfactory manner.

We closed the chapter by giving an evidence-based description of the phenomenal contents and dynamics of visual consciousness. There is a constant interplay between the preattentive phenomenal background, selective attention and the focus of consciousness, and the coherently bound visual information transferred to reflective consciousness. Coherent visual objects are created when focused attention falls on them, but they dissolve back into loose bundles of preattentive features as soon as attention departs. The phenomenology of visual consciousness, however, delivers a coherent, familiar, and meaningful world for us. That phenomenology can be accounted for by the aforementioned mechanisms. The incoherent bundles of preattentive features can be experienced only as vague parts of the phenomenal background before being attended. When attended they become coherent virtual objects. After attention has departed they dissolve back to a bundle of features, but even so they seem to keep their semantic windows open. That creates for us the feeling that we are at all times surrounded by a world of coherent meaningful objects, even when we do not necessarily focus on those objects or see them as tightly bound entities. Whenever we focus on them, they instantaneously become coherent and meaningful; and after we have focused on them even once, they tend to remain meaningful for us even if they become just blurry figures in the phenomenal background.

16 Neural Mechanisms of Binding

The challenge for neuroscience is to explain how the brain brings together all the sensory information that originated in one stimulus. Somehow the brain has to construct integrated neural representations that mediate between the unified external stimuli and the internal surrogates of those stimuli—the unified percepts directly present in consciousness. Neuroscientists search for appropriate *neural codes* in the brain that could combine the stimulus information from multiple input channels, distributed all over the cortex. Grandmother cell coding, population coding, and temporal coding are the three major theories that have been put forward to solve the neural binding problem. Of these alternatives, the temporal coding hypothesis looks most promising for the science of consciousness. In temporal coding, individual neurons bind together to form unified wholes by transiently *synchronizing* their firings in a shared rhythm. Consequently, it has been speculated that large-scale synchronicity around 40 Hz, or in the gamma band (20–80 Hz), might be the neural basis of the unity of consciousness. We will explore the theoretical basis behind this idea and review some of the empirical studies that lend support to it. The results so far suggest that whenever we have a coherent visual object present for us in consciousness, high-frequency synchronization is involved in its construction at the neural levels.

Neural Coding

In neuroscience, the binding problem is closely connected to the fundamental theoretical problem of *neural coding*. The neural representation of a coherent stimulus has to be carried by some kind of neural "code." A neural code that represents the physical features of the stimulus in an integrated manner could solve the binding problem for neuroscience.

However, this view sees binding as stimulus-related rather than consciousness-related (see chapter 11). The "coherent object" coded by the brain is taken to be an external stimulus object with a multitude of physical features. The coding of those many features in the different sensory channels of the brain should somehow be coordinated and integrated so that the brain refers all the features to the same stimulus object.

The whole idea of a "neural code" is embedded in a representationalist philosophical framework (but as pointed out in chapter 8, representationalism involves philosophical commitments that make it a questionable theory of consciousness). Therefore, in neural coding, there is the *content* or *object* of the representation somewhere outside the brain, and an internal neural *vehicle* of the representation in the brain. The stimulus object out there in the external world constitutes the information content carried by the code. Whatever neural process *reliably covaries with* the presence of the object is the internal neural code of the representation.

Grandmother Cells

Neuroscientists have proposed several different candidates for serving as the neural code. The oldest idea is known as the cardinal cell or *grandmother cell* coding strategy. According to this doctrine, the firing of a single cell signals exclusively a single event. Each neuron at a lower stage of representation responds by modulating its rate of firing to a single elementary feature of a stimulus (say, a certain color, shape, motion). This is a *rate code.* In such a coding system, binding is achieved by convergence from a group of lower-order neurons to a single higher-order neuron. In a higher-order neuron an increase in the rate of firing signals the copresence of several particular elementary features. For example, when the lower-order neurons for the features "yellow," "oblong," and "curved" project to a single higher-order neuron, causing it to increase its rate of firing, then the presence of a banana as a unified object in the stimulus field is being coded and signaled by the higher-order neuron.

This strictly hierarchical coding strategy is generally agreed to be inappropriate to account for human perception (see, e.g., Singer, 1994; Fotheringhame & Young, 1997; Gray, 1999), because there are not enough neurons for every distinct perceptual whole we see during our lifetime. Thus, grandmother cell coding does not seem to be able to solve the stimulus-related binding problem.

Single-cell rate coding does not look like a promising solution to consciousness-related binding either. It is difficult to see how a single neuron or its firing rate could constitute a coherent simulated object at the phenomenal level of organization. There are no structural or functional properties in a single neuron that could account for the experiential differences between different kinds of simulated objects at the phenomenal level. A butterfly looks entirely different from a blueberry. When consciously perceiving such things, if each of the surrogate objects in visual consciousness were based on the firing of one single devoted cell, how is it that their visual appearance—the combination of form, color, part-whole relationships, 3D structures as we experience them in phenomenal visual awareness—can be so very different?

The standard representationalist answer is that the representational *vehicles* do not *resemble* their *content* in any way, and the actual objects are out there. But a butterfly and a blueberry look very different also if visually experienced in the absence of the respective physical stimuli, say during dreaming. How could the visual structure and organization of each phenomenal dream image be brought about by just switching the firing rates of the single cells "coding for" each of those objects? There is *no explanatory relation* between the firing rate of one cell as opposed to that of another that could explain why one of them produces the visual experience of, say, a yellow swallowtail flying by and the other, that of a small, round, dark-blue berry.

Top-down phenomenological constraints must be taken seriously by any theory that attempts to explicate the lower-level mechanisms of perceptual experience. Differences between experiences at the phenomenal level must be based on corresponding differences at lower levels of organization inside the brain, not on differences outside the brain. Otherwise, no explanatory relation between the lower and higher levels could be established.

Population Coding

A more plausible idea of neural coding is called "population coding" or "assembly coding." The basic idea here is that the representation of a stimulus consists of a *pattern of activity* in a large group of neurons. Each distinct object is represented by a distinct pattern of activity, distributed across a population of neurons rather than by convergence to a single higher-order neuron. This provides the system with a much higher representational capacity than grandmother cell coding does, because in assembly coding a single neuron can at different times participate in many different representations.

A critical question for assembly coding is, How do the neurons coding an object actually become connected to form the integrated assembly? What are the *mechanisms* that connect the distributed neurons to a functionally unified assembly? The traditional answer to this is that the neurons forming an assembly have *reciprocal connections,* and the responses between the components of the assembly become stronger. The "strength" of the responses is determined by the rate of firing (rate code).

It is at least conceivable that complex patterns of activity in neural populations might structurally correspond to the patterns of phenomenal experience. The activation patterns could in principle resemble or be isomorphic with the surrogate objects in consciousness. Thus, unlike grandmother cell coding, population coding might establish an explanatory relationship between neural microlevel phenomena and the contents of the higher phenomenal level.

The main problem with population coding by the rate of firing is the "superposition problem": How to code for more than one stimulus entity at a time? How to tell apart the assembly related to one object from another simultaneously responding to another object? (Singer, 1994). The content of visual consciousness has more to it than just one isolated object at a time. If all the brain can do when several objects are present is to increase the rate of firing for all features currently present, then all the features are combined to form one complex object rather than a scene consisting of several independent objects. If rate coding in neural populations is insufficient to tell different objects apart from each other, then it cannot be the general solution to the binding problem.

Temporal Binding

In order to solve this problem, the notion of *temporal coding* has been introduced. The idea here is that one specific cell assembly is distinguished from others by the *synchronicity* of firing in all the members belonging to the same assembly. Different but simultaneously active assemblies can be distinguished from each other by the *timing* of their activity (rather than the *level* of activity). Synchronous activity may furthermore constitute a *recurrent regular pattern* or *oscillatory rhythm.* An oscillatory rhythm shows a characteristic frequency of simultaneous neuronal discharges of, say, forty cycles per second, or 40 Hz.

In the beginning of the 1990s the hypothesis of temporal coding started to receive empirical support from animal studies. Wolfgang Singer, one of the main architects of the theory of temporal coding, presented several predictions that may be derived from the temporal coding hypothesis and empirically tested (Singer, 1994, p. 208):

1. Spatially segregated neurons should synchronize their responses if activated by features that can be grouped together to form one perceptual unit.
2. Synchronization should be frequent among neurons within a particular cortical area but it should also occur across cortical areas.
3. The probability that neurons synchronize their responses both within a particular area and across areas should reflect some of the Gestalt criteria used for perceptual grouping.
4. Individual cells must be able to rapidly change the partners with which they synchronize their responses if stimulus configurations change and require new associations.
5. If more than one object is present in a scene, several assemblies should form.
6. Synchronization probability should at least in part depend on the functional architecture of reciprocal corticocortical connections and should change if this architecture is modified. Specifically, the disruption of synchronization should impair visual perception.

A fair amount of empirical support has been found for these predictions in animal studies (for a review, see Singer and Gray [1995]). In most of the experiments, cats and monkeys have been used as subjects. In many (though not all) experiments the animals have been anesthetized during the measurements of neural synchrony. Their visual system has been stimulated with light bars (simple linelike stimuli) that have been oriented optimally with regard to the neurons' response preferences. Such stimuli have been moved across the visual stimulus field and thus across the receptive fields of the neurons whose responses were recorded.

In these experiments, multiunit activity or local field potentials from groups of neurons in the visual cortex (especially V1) have typically been recorded. Synchronization of neural activity has been found to oscillate around 35 to 45 Hz in response to the unified stimulus. The synchronization is observable among adjacent cells in the same visual area, between spatially segregated cell groups within the same visual area, between groups in different visual areas, and even between groups of cells located in visual areas of the two different hemispheres. The most effective stimulus configuration to induce synchronization is a single linearly moving contour. When the contour is broken into two separate coherently moving bars, synchronization becomes weaker. When the two bars start to move independently of each other, no significant temporal correlation between neural activity in different locations is observed. Thus, Gestalt features of the stimulus strongly modulate synchronization.

Singer (1994) suggests that synchronization reflects Gestalt criteria for perceptual grouping (proximity, similarity, continuity, common fate). Furthermore, there is evidence that neural connections on which patterns of synchrony depend are intracortical and can be disrupted. First, if the corpus callosum is cut, synchronization between cells in the different hemispheres disappears. Second, the misalignment of eyes during early development is associated with disruption of synchronization (Roelfsema, Engel, König, & Singer, 1996).

Gestalts in the Brain: Binding and Synchronizing Connections

Singer's group has suggested that the neural mechanisms of synchronization are primarily mediated by intracortical (i.e., corticocortical) connections. They have put forth a theoretical model of such *synchronizing connections* (Roelfsema et al., 1996, Roelfsema & Singer, 1998). The architecture of these hypothetical connections incarnates the Gestalt criteria for perceptual grouping. All the neurons linked together by the synchronizing connections form a neuronal matrix in which vast numbers of various patterns of synchronized activity can potentially be realized. Actual patterns in this matrix are hypothesized to develop in the following way: First, (visual) input automatically coactivates *all* the cells that respond to *any* of the features or combinations of features currently present in the stimulus field. This coactivation means that all those cells increase their firing rate (as in ordinary population coding). As they do this, the intracortical synchronizing connections of the same neurons get activated as well. The pattern of activated intracortical synchronizing connections forms the *interaction skeleton.* Hence, the firing rate of the currently active neurons selects first all the *possible* links along which synchronization may later spread.

Next, to segregate different perceptual objects from each other, there must be some neuronal *tag* that spreads to all and only such units that respond to the *same* object or the *same* perceptual whole. Imagine that you are looking at different objects on a table: a plate, a banana, a blueberry, for example. To define which parts of the visual field define these coherent image regions, the tag that spreads in the matrix uses the Gestalt principles as cues. Thus, the label that identifies the relevant group of neurons spreads according to cues such as good continuity, proximity, symmetry, and similarity (figures 16.1 and 16.2).

Neuronal synchronization could function as the spreading tag. Synchronization spreads to all those neurons in the interaction skeleton that are both *independently activated* and *directly connected by Gestalt cues.* Therefore, each independent, internally coherent cluster of synchronization that emerges in this process represents one single perceptual whole and defines a coherent image region.

Local synchronization is easily achieved because the perceptual grouping criterion of *proximity* is strongly reflected in the architecture of the synchronizing connections. However, for the perceptual whole to hang together not only locally but globally, the effective spread of synchronization to neurons not directly connected with every other one in the same pattern is necessary as well. This could be achieved by employing a regular firing pattern such as oscillations within a narrow frequency band. A regularly oscillating rhythm is essential for global synchronization between all the elements of the whole.

Global synchronization can be established thanks to the *transitivity* of synchronization even across several synaptic connections. If each pair of two adjacent, directly connected cells are firing in synchrony with the same regular frequency, then necessarily *all* the neurons participating in the same pattern do, even ones distant from each other in the interaction skeleton. This transitivity of synchronization is proposed to account for the nonlocal Gestalt grouping criteria. It could create the connectedness between separated elements of the same contour or separate features of the same object (Roelfsema et al., 1996)

The above description is primarily a theory of bottom-up binding during sensory input processing. However, top-down influences also have a role in establishing perceptual wholes. In Singer's (1994) theory, attention is seen as an internal, top-down synchronization mechanism that is needed especially to organize complex feature combinations. Attended percepts differ from nonattended ones in that the responses of neurons coding for the attended percept are strongly synchronized with each other. Although the representation of the perceptual whole itself is realized in *intracortical* connections (the interaction skeleton and the synchronizing connections), the *attentional modulation* of synchronization may be realized through subcortical connections such as *thalamocortical interactions.*

A

B

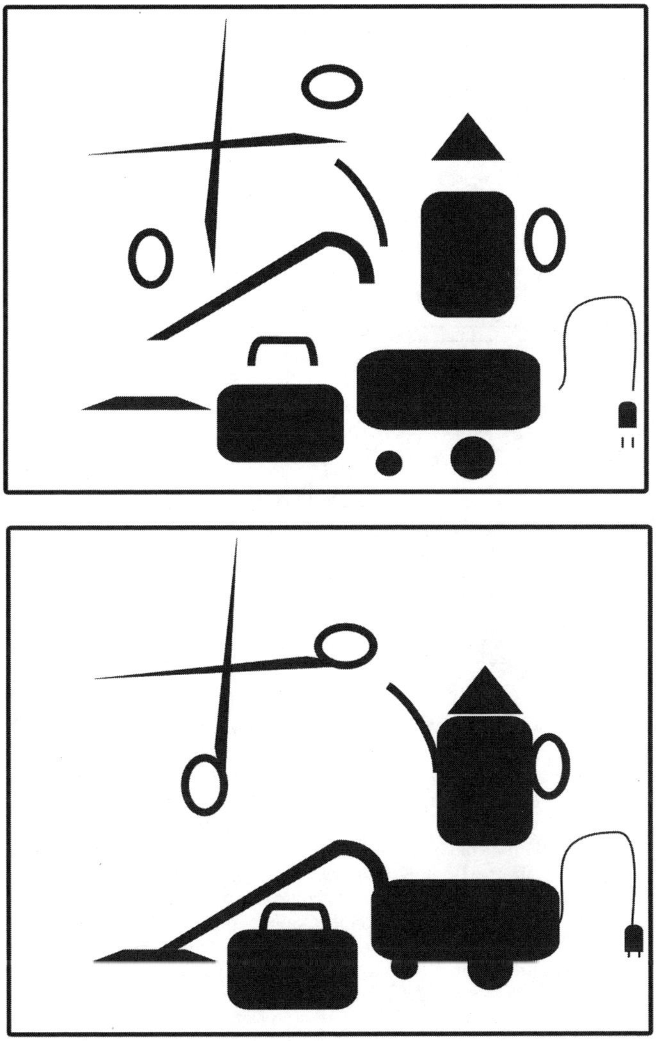

Figure 16.1
Object recognition and connectedness detection. Object recognition is greatly facilitated by detecting the connectedness of separate image regions. In (A), parts of objects are not connected, which makes it difficult to perceive the parts as bound together into coherent familiar objects. In (B), the parts are connected, which renders the objects immediately recognizable coherent wholes. (Modified from Roelfsema, P. R., & Singer, W. [1998]. Detecting connectedness. *Cerebral Cortex,* 8, 385–396, by permission of Oxford University Press.)

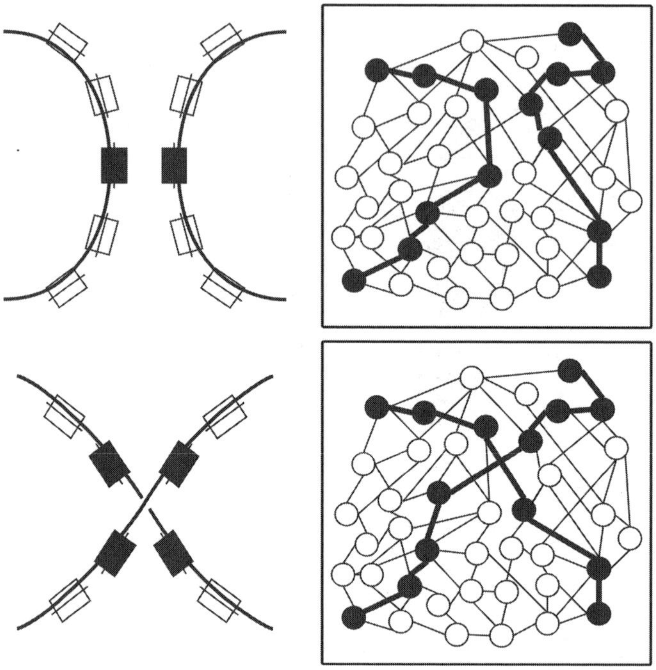

Figure 16.2
Coherent patterns of connectivity and synchronicity in a neural network. A small local difference in the pattern of connectivity can lead to a large difference at the level of the whole perceptual unit. The patterns on the left depict the local difference between two figures: the upper constitutes closure (the patterns defined by the lines do not intersect), the lower pattern depicts continuity (the lines cross and continue after that) The patterns on the right are depictions of how synchronicity in a neural network could realize this perceptual difference. Synchronous activity defines a coherent pattern of activity in the network. Note that the pattern of activity in the neural system is depicted as approximately *isomorphic* with the perceptual whole that will appear in conscious experience. Thus this neural mechanism might provide us with an explanatory relationship between phenomenal contents at the phenomenal level and electrophysiological patterns at the neural levels. Exactly such relationships are required to construct a genuine explanation of consciousness-related binding or a lower-level constitutive explanation of the patterns of phenomenal properties found at the phenomenal level. (Modified from Roelfsema, Engel, König, & Singer [1996]. Reproduced with kind permission of The MIT Press.)

This view is compatible with the idea that attention is a biasing mechanism (see chapter 15). The spotlight of attention may involve a mechanism for strengthening the synchronicity (and also for increasing the firing rate) of the subset of neurons that are involved with the same perceptual object. Thus, attention biases the relevant types of activity in the neural mechanisms of object representations in such a way that a more detailed perceptual representation of the selected content is created in focal awareness. Furthermore, scalp-recorded gamma oscillations have been found to correlate not only with coherent objects but also with spatial attention, suggesting that attention and conscious perception might share a similar neural mechanism (Tallon-Baudry 2003).

Consciousness and Neural Synchronicity

Is Singer's theory about stimulus-related binding or consciousness-related binding? Does he say anything explicitly about consciousness? In 1994, he said fairly little:

> . . . it is possible that access to the level of processing where representations reach consciousness is gated by coherence. It may be that the only activation patterns that reach the threshold of conscious awareness are those that are sufficiently organized or coherent. (Singer, 1994, p. 101)

Later, however, some developments took place on this front. Fries, Roelfsema, Engel, König, and Singer (1997) provided evidence for the hypothesis that coherent patterns of neural activity are necessary for consciousness. They showed that in binocular rivalry, power in the gamma band increases for the neurons representing the dominant (conscious) stimulus, but decreases for the ones representing the suppressed (unconscious) stimulus.

Engel et al. (1999) argue that appropriate synchronization may be one of the *necessary* connections for awareness. However, it does not appear to be a *sufficient* condition. Cortical synchronization can be observed even in anesthetized animals—in fact, a substantial proportion of the empirical studies on neural synchronization have used anesthetized animals as subjects. Certainly, they were not visually aware of the stimuli when synchronization was observed in their visual cortex. Thus, in those cases at least, the synchronization was only stimulus-related and completely dissociated from visual awareness (but it is not just an artifact caused by the anesthesia itself, because the synchronization phenomena become even more pronounced when the animals are awake [Singer, 1999]).

Engel and Singer (2001) have formulated even more specific (and more speculative) ideas about the relationship between neural synchrony and consciousness. They propose that there are four processes (arousal, segmentation, selection, working memory) that may together form the neural correlate of awareness, and that the neural mechanisms of each of these processes involves neural synchrony.

First, *arousal* is characterized by an enhanced precision of neuronal synchrony and a shift to high oscillation frequencies. Arousal seems to be a necessary condition of awareness, since in states of very low arousal (e.g., NREM slow-wave sleep) there are hardly any contents of consciousness. Thus, Engel and Singer (2001) suggest that neural synchronization could be the underlying mechanism for the *state* of being conscious as opposed to being unconscious.

Second, phenomenal consciousness is always *organized,* which requires the segmentation of different objects from each other and the background. Synchrony could function as the neural mechanism of this process. So they suggest that the higher-level organization of the phenomenal level could also be accounted for by neural synchronization.

Third, if only a subset of all input information is *selected* to awareness, synchronization could act as a signature of those representations that will be made globally available in the system. Fourth, synchronization may transiently *stabilize* neural states so that the information can be held temporarily in a *working memory* mechanism. Hence, they suggest that synchronization could be the mechanism of (the contents of) selective attention and reflective consciousness.

Engel and Singer (2001) further speculate that temporal binding may establish patterns of large-scale coherence, so that even cross-modality binding becomes possible. Finally, their overall view of the neural basis of consciousness is a hierarchy of neural assemblies bound together by neural interactions in different frequency bands. The microlevel entities in this hierarchy are incorporated in global models of the world and the self.

All in all, Engel and Singer (2001) propose that synchronization is the neural mechanism of *all* the major aspects of consciousness: the state of being conscious, the organization and unity of the world simulation in consciousness, and the higher-order forms of reflective consciousness. The hypothesis is bold and speculative, but at least it is empirically testable.

Theories about Neural Synchronization

The brief history of relating consciousness to neural synchrony goes back to the classic paper of Crick and Koch (1990). They were the first to explicitly suggest a connection between neural level binding through synchronization and the phenomenal level unity of perceived objects in visual consciousness:

> We suggest that one of the functions of consciousness is to present the result of various underlying computations and that this involves an attentional mechanism that temporarily binds the relevant neurons together by synchronizing their spikes in 40 Hz oscillations. . . . objects for which the binding problem has been solved are placed into working memory. (p. 272)

Crick and Koch emphasize the role of attention in generating coherent contents of awareness, but otherwise their theory is quite consistent with that of Singer. (However, they have changed some of their ideas since 1990; see Crick & Koch [2003].)

Rodolfo Llinás (Llinás & Ribary, 1994) proposes that 40 Hz oscillations subserving temporal binding are generated in thalamocortical loops. One type of loop is created between the specific sensory nuclei in the thalamus and the corresponding sensory cortices, which project back to the specific nuclei. Another type of loop resides between thalamic nonspecific intralaminar nuclei and layer I cortical cells projecting back through layer V. This model of thalamocortical interaction may be directly related to two different types of binding. The *specific thalamocortical loop* is assumed to be responsible for the binding of distributed sensory fragments into single *coherent objects* of awareness (spatial grouping and feature integration). The *nonspecific thalamocortical loop* is assumed to provide the overall context or functional *conscious state* where the individual objects of awareness are related to each other within one globally coherent representation. Thus, they seem to suggest that it binds all the single objects into the overall phenomenal space. Consistent with this model, lesions of specific thalamic nuclei abolish modality-specific contents of consciousness, whereas lesions of nonspecific thalamus (especially the intralaminar nuclei) abolish the global background state of consciousness, resulting in coma. The *interaction* of these two thalamocortical loops through synchronous oscillatory activity around 40 Hz is hypothesized to take care of the binding of perceptual content into a single coherent experience (Llinás & Paré, 1991, 1996; Llinás, Ribary, Contreras, & Pedroarera, 1998, Llinás, 2001).

Llinás's theory deviates from Singer's in that it emphasizes *thalamocortical* connections as the source of synchronization whereas Singer's theory sees *intracortical* connections as the primary source and realizer of synchronization and binding. It is not entirely clear how dissimilar these views are in the final analysis, for both of them assign at least some role to both intracortical and thalamocortical connections.

Human Studies on Binding and Synchronization

Much of the empirical evidence supporting the synchronization hypothesis has been based on invasive microelectrode studies of animal subjects. But we do not know for sure what a cat or a monkey visually experiences in these experiments. In studies using human observers, the brain's electrophysiological responses have been recorded with noninvasive macroelectrodes, typically scalp EEG. Although they pick the average signals from massive populations of neurons, the results are mostly in harmony with the animal studies.

Lutzenberger, Pulvermueller, Elbert, and Birbaumer (1995) showed coherently moving bars to human subjects, and detected increased 40 Hz power over the occipital lobe in response to the stimulation. Although this experiment is nicely in concert with Singer's findings in animals, it is primarily evidence for stimulus-related synchronization, not necessarily consciousness-related. Busch, Debener, Kranczioch, Engel, and Herrmann (2004) have found further evidence that the gamma-band response in human EEG reflects stimulus-related features in early visual areas, such as stimulus size.

In order to reveal consciousness-related synchronization, illusory figures that do not contain physical coherence should be used. In this spirit Tallon, Bertrand, Bouchet, and Pernier (1995) and Tallon-Baudry, Bertrand, Delpuech, and Pernier (1996) showed real and illusory coherent triangles to subjects and detected a 40 Hz EEG component around 300 ms post stimulus to both types of stimuli. Tallon-Baudry, Bertrand, Delpuech, and Pernier (1997) reported similar findings when the subjects had to detect a hidden object in a picture (they used the famous black-and-white picture including a hidden Dalmatian dog as the stimulus). Naive subjects did not detect the dog; for them, the image consisted of meaningless, seemingly random black-and-white regions. The induced gamma response around 280 ms was weak. However, once the subjects were trained to see the hidden stimulus, a much larger induced gamma response was observed. This was true whether or not the hidden dog was actually present in the stimulus! This surprising finding may reflect the top-down activation of the image of the dog, because now the subjects had an internal mental image of what they were looking for in the stimuli (Tallon-Baudry & Bertrand, 1999). The researchers suggest that the induced 40 Hz response reflects assembly coding activated either from the bottom up or from the top down (or perhaps both).

My own group conducted an experiment on binocular fusion in human vision that may to some extent illuminate the issue of whether 40 Hz synchronization is consciousness-related or not (Revonsuo et al., 1997). The stimulus we used was a random-dot autostereogram which (without binocular fusion) looks like an incoherent collection of random dots without any obvious patterns or perceptual grouping. After binocular fusion, the very same stimulus looks like a symmetric 3D shape with a clear object-like shape: it forms a global coherent Gestalt. The hypothesis that 40 Hz synchronization is associated with the binding of visual percepts into coherent wholes was tested by measuring scalp EEG in a task in which the subjects perceived this stimulus in one condition as an incoherent collection of random dots and in another condition as a coherent, symmetric 3D Gestalt.

Continuous viewing of the same stimulus in the incoherent vs. coherent condition was not associated with significant differences in 40 Hz synchronization (quantified as a relative change in 36–44 Hz band power between the two conditions). Thus, although there is a radical *phenomenological* difference in visual awareness between these two stable views of the stimulus, no corresponding difference in 40 Hz band power was detected. The same was true of lower frequency bands at 8 to 13 Hz and 13 to 20 Hz.

Next, we tested whether the perceptual *construction* of the coherent (but illusory) Gestalt is accompanied by transient 40 Hz synchronization. The subjects free-fused the random-dot stereogram and pushed a button as soon as they saw the 3D Gestalt clearly. In the control condition, they fused a similar-looking stimulus from which no unified percept emerged. An increase in 40 Hz power (relative to the control condition) was observed at occipital and right posterior electrode sites in a time window 500 to 300 ms before visual awareness of the coherent percept was reported. No corresponding changes in band power were observed at the lower frequencies we analyzed (8–13 Hz, 13–20 Hz). Hence 40 Hz synchronization seems to participate in the construction of the unified percept, but not in the continuous viewing of the same stimulus once it has been constructed and persists in visual awareness. This result suggests that 40 Hz synchronization does not directly correlate with the phenomenal content of visual awareness per se, but with the *construction* of such content immediately preceding its emergence into visual awareness. This lends support to the thesis advanced by Singer (1994) and

Engel et al. (1999), that temporal binding is a prerequisite of the access of information to phenomenal consciousness.

The relationship between the synchronicity recorded with invasive microelectrodes and the scalp EEG oscillations remains to be determined. In any case, a neural assembly would have to be quite large to generate a signal that reaches the scalp. Thus, scalp-recorded gamma synchronicity is more likely to reflect large-scale synchrony between different cortical areas than local synchrony within a single area (Tallon-Baudry, 2003).

Further evidence from human studies is accumulating (e.g., see Tononi, Srinivasan, Russell, & Edelman, 1998; Rodriguez, George, Lachaux, Martinerie, Renault, & Varela, 1999; Tallon-Baudry, 2003), suggesting that gamma-band synchronization is correlated with the conscious visual perception of coherent objects. The hypothesis that neural synchronization is the mechanism of binding at the neural levels of organization therefore looks more and more plausible. However, the issue is far from settled yet. Several open questions remain: If there are so many different kinds of binding (spatial grouping, feature binding, part binding, location binding, etc.), could neural synchronization be the mechanism for *all* of them, or is it restricted only to basic spatial grouping? In any case, that is the only type of binding that most of the studies have looked into.

The bold hypothesis presented by Engel and Singer (2001), however, suggests that neural synchrony in different frequency bands could account for the many different varieties of binding that must be accomplished to create the unified phenomenal consciousness that we experience. The empirical plausibility of that hypothesis remains to be evaluated in the light of further evidence.

During its brief history the study of the neural mechanisms of phenomenal unity has generated empirically plausible hypotheses and preliminary models that deserve serious consideration. Ultimately, this research can be seen as a part of the larger project of the search for the neural correlates and the biological constituents of consciousness. That is a fascinating but somewhat confusing area of empirical research and philosophical speculation. It involves an *explanatory gap* between the subjective world of consciousness and the objectively measurable world of neuroscience. We explore that fascinating topic in part V.

Summary

The temporal coding hypothesis was found to be the most promising candidate to account for consciousness-related binding. Neural assemblies defined by the temporal simultaneity of firing might be capable of the rapid and flexible construction of the unified objects we experience in visual consciousness. Empirical evidence from animal studies using multiunit recordings and from human studies using scalp recordings support the view that unified visual wholes are constructed with the help of synchronized neural oscillations in the gamma band. The exact picture of what is going on in the brain when this happens is still rather misty. The theories relating consciousness to neural synchronicity have speculated that major aspects of consciousness (phenomenal consciousness, selective attention, feature integration, simulation of a world and a self) may all be based on neural synchronicity. While these are fascinating hypotheses, they remain to be empirically tested.

V A Bridge across the Explanatory Gap

The explanatory gap between subjective consciousness and objective neuroscience has been regarded as the most difficult challenge for the science of consciousness. But if we take the multilevel framework of the biological sciences seriously, then the explanatory gap will be seen in a different light. The gap is created by missing levels of description in our current understanding of the brain. Whether the gap can be bridged will depend on the current state and future development of cognitive neuroscience.

17 The Explanatory Gap

The worldview of science implies that nature forms one unified continuum. Although physical, chemical, and biological entities differ from each other in many ways, they are nevertheless parts of a single smooth continuum in the natural order. The more complex phenomena are ontologically based on the simpler, more fundamental phenomena, without any gaps or radical discontinuities.

An explanatory gap presents a radical breach in this worldview, an inexplicable break in the continuum of the natural order. For example, at one time in the history of science, a deep gap prevailed between living organisms and nonliving physical substance. It seemed inconceivable that the two wholly unlike realms could be parts of a single continuum. Consequently, the breach in the human *understanding* of the natural world was projected back to the *world* itself.

Now science has gotten rid of the gap between the living and the nonliving realms. A profound gap, however, remains at the interface between the phenomenal and the biological worlds. On the one hand they seem to lie on the same continuum, interfacing somewhere in the neurobiology of the brain. On the other hand, the phenomenal world we find in our conscious experience is so radically dissimilar from the neurobiological world we find in the brain that any continuum leading from one realm to the other is hard to imagine.

In this chapter we first clarify the nature of the explanatory gap in the multilevel framework of explanation. Our observations reveal that explanatory gaps are created whenever science remains ignorant of several levels of organization between different types of phenomena. Many of the gaps in the history of science have already disappeared; perhaps the manner in which science successfully dealt with them would be an advisable strategy with regard to the present explanatory gap as well.

The Explanatory Gap and the Theory Reduction Model

In philosophy, the explanatory gap between consciousness and neuroscience is seen as a gap in the lawlike statements that connect the subjective psychological realm with the objective neurophysiological realm. Elsewhere in the physical sciences, lawlike identity statements such as "heat is the motion of molecules" do not leave any gaps. We now understand why the concept of "heat" refers to the same thing as "the motion of molecules." The identity statement is fully explanatory.

Psychophysical identity statements, by contrast, seem unintelligible. It seems we cannot even *imagine* any psychophysical identity statements that might be explanatory. Any statement linking a term referring to qualitative experience (say "seeing green") with any term referring to a neurophysiological property (say "firing of z-neurons") leaves a gap. We simply have no idea why or how a psychophysical identity statement *could* be true. Even if neuroscience would have established that the firing of z-neurons is invariably coupled with seeing green—even if we knew that the identity statement just *must* be true—the knowledge of the perfect correlation would not offer us any explanation as to *why* or *how* the coupling occurs.

The notion of "explanatory gap" was originally introduced by J. Levine (1983; see also J. Levine 2001). According to Levine, an explanatory gap looms large as long as the explanandum has not been made *intelligible*—as long as the connection between the two phenomena given in the identity statement is arbitrary, just a nonintelligible brute fact. In the case of identity statements connecting the phenomenal and the neural this surely seems to be the case. We have no explanation why "seeing green" should be identical to "firing of z-neurons," or to any other neurophysiological property. If such an identity statement is accepted, it must be accepted as a brute fact or as a fundamental law. Fundamental, inexplicable brute facts are, however, not expected to appear in science outside the domain of physics.

In philosophy of mind, the conception of an explanatory gap is derived directly from influential ideas in the philosophy of science: the *theory reduction model,* also called the *deductive-nomological* or *D-N explanation* (see chapter 1). According to these approaches to explanation, scientific knowledge consists of sets of sentences (theories and laws). Reductive explanation implies that the vocabularies of two distinct theories are merged into one by formulating bridge laws and identity statements. These intertheoretical laws explicitly connect the terms of the old theory with the terms of the new and more comprehensive theory.

The philosophical discussion concerning the explanatory gap should be seen against this background. The psychophysical identity statements are *attempts to formulate bridge laws* across the explanatory gap between the neurophysiological and the phenomenal/psychological domains. If it is taken for granted that the only way to explain consciousness is to find the suitable psychophysical bridge laws, then it is no wonder that the discussion focuses on the possibilities of finding such laws (or on showing that such laws cannot be found, or that even if found they are unintelligible brute facts, and so on).

J. Levine is well aware that the discussion about the explanatory gap is based on accepting a certain framework of explanation:

> One might object at this point that my position presumes something like the deductive-nomological account of explanation, an account that is certainly controversial. In fact, I quite openly endorse the view that explanations involve showing how the explanandum follows from the explanans. I believe that the deductive-nomological model, in analysing explanation in terms of exhibiting a necessary connection between explanans and explanandum, is certainly on the right track. (J. Levine 1993, p. 130)

Quite independently of any problems related to consciousness, a handful of philosophers of science have come to the conclusion that the D-N model of explanation is inappropriate for the biological and cognitive sciences.

> However, the problem with the theory reduction model is deeper. In many contexts, especially those encountered in biology and psychology, knowledge that is to be integrated does not reside in laws stated as universal conditionals. Indeed, the linguistic representation of knowledge in terms of laws is largely inappropriate within these domains. (Bechtel & Richardson, 1992, p. 260)

Instead of universal laws and linguistic representation of explanatory knowledge, explanations in the biological sciences come in the form of *multilevel mechanistic models* (discussed in chapter 1). If the theory reduction model and D-N explanation are inappropriate models of scientific explanation for biology in general, they are not likely to work when we try to understand the relation between brain and consciousness. If multilevel explanation is the proper philosophical background for explaining consciousness, then the explanatory gap should be redefined in a way consistent with the multilevel framework.

Explanatory Gaps and Multilevel Explanation

There is a natural way to understand how explanatory gaps may be created within the multilevel framework of the biological sciences. A multilevel biological model might ignore some levels of organization simply because they have not been discovered yet. If the levels of description in the model thus simply jump across several levels of organization in nature, then the model will display *radical discontinuity* between the properties of the lower-level parts and the properties of the higher-level whole (Bechtel & Richardson, 1992). If at any particular point in the history of science there should be restricted access to and limited knowledge of certain levels of organization in nature, it is unavoidable to jump across the levels of organization about which nothing is known. Genuine explanatory gaps have been created in this way a number of times in the history of science. The hypothesis I advance is that *the explanatory gap between consciousness and brain is created in precisely that way.*

We shall take a brief historical tour to show that something like this has happened in the history of science many times before. At the end of the nineteenth century there were two profound explanatory gaps in the scientific understanding of the natural world: the first between physics and chemistry, the second between chemistry and biology. Perhaps we could learn something from them.

Historical Explanatory Gaps: The Gap between Physics and Chemistry

The gap at the interface of the physical and the chemical domains was based on the difficulties in understanding chemical bonding in physical terms. The atomic theory of matter, first clearly formulated by John Dalton at the beginning of the nineteenth century, was by and large accepted in the scientific community by the turn of the century. According to Dalton's theory, different elements are composed of different kinds of atoms, and chemical compounds are made of molecules, each different compound composed of a fixed number of atoms of certain elements. At that time, atoms were still very hypothetical entities and some chemists resisted the whole concept, until Einstein's paper in 1905. Einstein provided a simple explanation of a well-known phenomenon in terms of the motions of atoms. The phenomenon in question is readily observable with the help of a microscope: it is called "Brownian motion" and it is visible in tiny particles of pollen in a drop of water. Although the reality of atoms was thus established, there was still very little understanding of the internal microstructure of atoms. Consequently, not even remotely plausible microexplanations of chemical bonding existed.

This situation led many to advance the view that the laws of chemical bonding—which elements have the power to bond with which others—have to be taken as "brute facts" of nature, accepted with "natural piety" (McLaughlin, 1992, p. 55). A similar attitude has resurfaced in the current theorizing on consciousness. Some philosophers (e.g., Colin McGinn, 1991) have argued that the principles connecting conscious phenomena with neural phenomena are perfectly natural, but forever out of the reach of human understanding.

Another reaction to the physicochemical explanatory gap sometimes encountered among chemists was the postulation of new fundamental chemical forces. Such primitive natural forces were thought to be on a par with Newtonian gravity, not explicable in terms of any underlying mechanisms. This move has a close modern counterpart, too. According to some philosophers, the phenomenal features of consciousness have to be taken as fundamental in neuroscience, just the way electromagnetic forces and gravity are taken as fundamental in physics. Mirroring the historical cases, the connections between phenomenal and physical properties are supposed to be governed by a set of new fundamental laws, psychophysical laws (Chalmers, 1996). Presumably, those laws would have to be swallowed with similar "natural piety," like the supposedly fundamental laws of chemical bonding.

The explanatory gap between physics and chemistry dissolved with the advent of Bohr's model of the internal structure of atoms and the groundbreaking theory of the periodic table of elements. Bohr's theory managed to explain the periodicity and the properties of the chemical elements in terms of the electrons at the outermost shell of the atom. Bohr's theory of the mechanisms of chemical bonding described the nature of *a previously unknown microlevel of physical organization.* That level could immediately be connected with the already detailed descriptions of the higher level of chemical organization and the regularities that obtained at the level of chemical phenomena.

Historical Explanatory Gaps: The Gap between Chemistry and Biology

Paradigmatic bits of dead matter, such as stones, are at the mercy of external forces. They do not do much on their own, they stay still unless pushed by external forces, they may wear or decay, but they never develop or reproduce. By contrast, paradigmatic living entities such as mammals are warm, growing, developing, self-reproducing, autonomously mobile, and interact in many ways with their environment. How could the latter be composed of nothing but the former? Earlier generations of scientists and philosophers must have felt the same kind of astonishment in the face of this question as we experience when pondering the relationship between consciousness and brain. Thus, they felt that something extraordinary must be added to dead matter in order to make it alive. Biological theories that "solve" the problem in this manner are varieties of vitalism.

Broad (1925) distinguished two versions of vitalism: "substantial vitalism" and "emergent vitalism." The former postulated a special substance (called "entelechy" by some advocates of the view) that needed to be added to nonliving matter to make it alive. This view is an obvious counterpart of Cartesian (substance) dualism as a theory of consciousness. Broad himself advocated emergent vitalism, according to which living entities are entirely composed of nonliving matter, but there are properties specific to entities of a higher order, properties that Broad called "ultimate characteristics." For Broad, chemical bonding would count as an ultimate characteristic of the chemical order, and the power of reproduction as an ultimate characteristic of the vital order (McLaughlin, 1992).

In emergent vitalism, biological processes are not reducible to chemical processes, for biological processes were thought to involve motions influenced by fundamental vital forces that cannot be analyzed in terms of lower-level processes. This view is the counterpart of emergent materialism and property dualism of current mind-body theories. Not surprisingly, this kind of view includes the plea to fundamental, inexplicable forces, appearing at the higher levels of organization. The postulated fundamental forces are entities whose emergence is not intelligible even in the light of perfect knowledge of all the lower levels of organization involved. By contrast, in multilevel explanation, when all the levels can be perfectly described by a multilevel model, the emergence of phenomena at the higher levels of organization becomes intelligible.

The explanatory gap between the living and the nonliving disappeared in a matter of a few decades around the middle of the twentieth century. Obviously, the gaps were generated by the epistemic situation in which the theorists found themselves. There never were any *ontological* gaps in nature. Although at one time a number of brilliant people imagined nature that way, none of those fundamental entities or forces or primitive brute facts of nature ever existed, nor were they eventually needed in the explanations. The gaps were gaps in the knowledge of the relevant facts coupled with a lack of corresponding models and theories. And what were the relevant facts about? They were, above all, *facts describing previously unknown and even unimaginable levels of organization in nature.*

Broad (1925) presented a thought experiment concerning the possibility of an explanation of chemical bonding. It demonstrates the unimaginability of an explanation before the relevant empirical facts are discovered. He invites us to imagine a mathematical archangel who has no mathematical or perceptual limitations.

> A mathematical archangel, gifted with the further power of perceiving the microscopic structure of atoms as easily as we can perceive hay-stacks, could no more predict the behavior of silver or of chlorine or the properties of silver-chloride without having observed samples of those substances than we can at present. (pp. 70–71)

As McLaughlin (1992, p. 88) notes, Broad's point is that even a being who could literally *see* the subatomic structure of chemical elements would have no idea how the elements would affect each other chemically. Analogous conceivability arguments flourish today in the philosophical literature on consciousness. There is the widely known case of Mary (Jackson, 1986). She is depicted as "the neuroscientific archangel," brought up in a black-and-white environment, who knows *everything physical there is to know* about how visual perception works in the brain. She has never seen colors, though, and when she steps out from her achromatic laboratory, she learns something new about visual perception, namely what colors look like. Thus, Jackson's argument is that even perfect physical knowledge of the brain does not include knowledge of phenomenal consciousness. Someone like Mary may have a complete description of the physical aspects of the brain without having any accompanying understanding of phenomenal consciousness.

In essence, what we are trying to imagine in these thought experiments is the brain *in its entirety,* a perfect account of all the levels of organization and their mutual interconnections in the brain. Even though we are assumed to be able to accomplish that miraculous feat, we are still supposed to fail in seeing how consciousness could be involved in that picture, exactly as Broad's archangel failed to see how chemical properties would follow from microphysical ones.

Of course, the close resemblance of the historical cases to the modern ones is no absolute proof to the effect that the problem of consciousness is at bottom no different from the problem of chemical bonding. But it certainly makes one wonder what the true source of the present-day explanatory gap is. It seems that whenever science has no account readily available of the relationship between dissimilar levels of organization, scientists and philosophers easily resort to envisioning the relationship as a uniquely special case. Thus, either the relationship is viewed as in principle unaccountable or at least as requiring the postulation of entirely new fundamental forces or laws. But once the explanatory gaps have been removed by further research, it is quickly forgotten how baffled everybody once was.

The gap between biology and chemistry was due to ignorance of a whole range of extremely complex levels of organization: ignorance of the structure and function of macromolecules, the organization of complex biochemical pathways, the structure of genetic material, the structure and function of various cell organelles, and so on. The explanatory gap in biology was created by trying to relate sets of phenomena that actually do lie along the same gapless natural continuum but which were separated by several levels of organization, unknown and unimaginable at the time. The adherents of emergent chemical or vitalistic forces simply happened to be situated in an epistemically unfortunate position. There were no methods available to even start investigating the relevant levels of organization in nature that eventually had to be revealed in order to render the phenomena intelligible.

Lessons to Be Learned from Explanatory Gaps

In view of the problem of consciousness, what are the lessons we might learn from the history of various explanatory gaps and the typical reactions to them? First, at any given time scientists and philosophers tend to underestimate the power of future discoveries in explaining phenomena currently inexplicable, and they overestimate the powers of imagining the nature of the things that, on the whole, are scientifically discoverable or explicable. They are reluctant to admit that there may be facts about the natural world that are currently unimaginable for them, but discoverable at some point in the future, and that will possibly be considered entirely obvious after that.

Second, the methodology available for conducting empirical research strongly constrains the discoveries that science is capable of making at any particular time. Many absolutely fundamental discoveries in the biological sciences would have been impossible without the development of new methods. The rapid development of basic neuroscience and the neuron doctrine would not have been possible without the development of more sophisticated microscopes and tissue staining methods developed in the late nineteenth century. In the case of cell biology, many fundamental discoveries were made after World War II at the level of the internal structure of the cell and its subsystems, thanks to the development of the electron microscope. It has a resolution about 100 times finer than even the best light microscopes. The new research instruments may be based on technology that was unimaginable only a few decades earlier.

Third, the explanatory gaps in the history of science were *not* dissolved by constructing philosophical knockdown arguments or thought experiments. Instead, they evaporated as new empirical methods were developed, new data were collected, and new levels of organization were discovered. Finally, novel levels of theoretical description made the phenomena intelligible. Thought experiments and imaginative metaphors may be fruitful when they are utilized to envision new avenues that actual experimental research might take, but they will likely be worthless if they are used as evidence to show what can never be discovered or understood. In the absence of the relevant empirical facts, we simply cannot imagine or foresee the perfect future science regarding *any* phenomenon. It is all too easy to *say,* "Imagine the world's best neuroscientist who has perfect knowledge of the brain." But unfortunately, perfect knowledge cannot be imagined on the basis of ignorance.

Fourth, even if some aspects of the relationship between consciousness and brain were to escape our understanding for ever, and the explanatory gap were to become our final fate, we would not be justified in making *that* conclusion until there is absolutely *nothing* more to learn about the brain. At the moment, neuroscience is light-years away from even a modest understanding of the brain. As long as we ourselves are in such an epistemically unfortunate position, we should resist making deep ontological conclusions.

Finally, perhaps we should take the historical gaps, especially the ways in which they were made to disappear, as a hint: The existence of an explanatory gap between neuroscience and consciousness indicates that *there are multiple levels of organization in the brain that are unknown to current neuroscience.*

Summary

If there are levels of organization in nature not captured by the empirical methods and theoretical models presently available in science, then there will appear to be a radical discontinuity between different domains of scientific knowledge. The explanatory gap in the conceptual structure of scientific theories is subsequently projected back to nature, creating the illusion that there is a corresponding *ontological* discontinuity in the hierarchical organization of nature itself.

The philosophical reaction to explanatory gaps appears to be similar regardless of where the gap in scientific knowledge happens to be situated: typically, inexplicable emergent properties and novel fundamental laws are proposed to appear mysteriously at higher levels of organization in nature. The emergent features and the fundamental laws governing their behavior are supposed to remain unaccountable even if absolutely *everything* will, one fine day, be known about the lower levels.

The historical lesson concerning explanatory gaps should be taken seriously. Perhaps the present gap between consciousness and neuroscience is just another case of radical discontinuity in the available levels of description, not a metaphysical breach in the very constitution of Mother Nature herself.

18 Beyond the Neural Correlates of Consciousness

The biological approach adopted in this book assumes that consciousness is a level of organization in the brain. According to this approach, the explanatory gap is simply due to our incomplete understanding of the higher levels of neural organization. Hence, even our best neuroscientific models and theories of the brain do not, as yet, include the phenomenal level. At present, we do not know how to connect the phenomenal to the neurobiological. Obviously, working toward such a connection is the prime empirical challenge for the science of consciousness. Somehow we should figure out how the phenomenal level of organization is related to the lower levels of organization in the brain. In the framework of multilevel biological explanation this is the search for the *constitutive* explanation.

In the cognitive neuroscience of consciousness this mission is called the search for the *neural correlates of consciousness* (NCC) in the brain. Yet, there seems to be no overall theoretical account of the scope and limits of this enterprise. Miscellaneous results are cited in the literature, when this or that measurement has been found to show *some* sort of relationship with *some* aspect of consciousness. Every now and then these results are hailed as if the problem of consciousness had been altogether solved. Still, the overall picture that various results provide does not seem to yield a neatly converging theoretical story of the nature and location of consciousness in the brain. Just about every conceivable part or activity of the brain has, in some experiment, been named as an NCC.

This somewhat confusing situation reflects the lack of a proper background theory that would guide the experimental approach. A research program on consciousness should offer adequate guiding principles so that neuroscientists would acquire a fairly clear idea of *what* they are searching for in the brain. When this idea emerges, they should furthermore figure out what the available brain measurements are likely to reveal about such a phenomenon, if anything. In this and the following chapters we analyze these questions in the light of the biological approach to consciousness.[1]

How to Find the Phenomenal Level in the Brain?

If consciousness is a real biological phenomenon, it should be possible to specify how exactly it is related to other biological phenomena in the brain, especially to the ones that have been already empirically discovered and described in the neurosciences. Figuring out what those relations are is to seek the *constitutive explanation* of consciousness. In general, constitutive (or downward-looking) explanations describe the *lower-level mechanisms* of the phenomenon (see also chapter 1).

The brain is a complex system involving a hierarchy of mechanisms. Different levels in the hierarchy involve biological entities and patterns of activity at different spatiotemporal grains and scales. The *hierarchical* structure of the system implies that the activities of entities at the lower levels are *component patterns* in the more inclusive higher-level patterns of activity (Craver, 2001). If the phenomenal level is a higher level of neurobiological organization, its constitutive explanation ought to refer to lower-level patterns of activity that compose the phenomenal contents of consciousness.

There are two possible routes to connect the phenomenal level with the lower levels. First, we begin at the higher level and from there move down toward the immediately underlying levels. *Top-down constraints* are determined by the characteristics of the phenomenal level itself. When we know the features of the higher phenomenal level, we can infer what sort of lower-level mechanisms could possibly support them, and conversely, what can be ruled out as potential mechanisms. Second, we may begin at the levels of single neurons and move upward toward higher levels that support complex, multimodal, unified clusters of neural activity. *Bottom-up constraints* approach the phenomenal level from that direction. When these two independent sets of constraints are connected at some level of spatiotemporal grain and complexity, we will be closing in on the neural constituents of consciousness.

Defining the "Neural Correlates of Consciousness" (NCC)

One of the major goals in the cognitive neuroscience of consciousness is to discover the NCC. That is deemed a crucial step in explaining the relationship between consciousness and the brain. But what kind of relationship are we talking about? Knowing that the activity of a brain area correlates with consciousness surely tells us something, but will this knowledge help us to explain consciousness? To figure out the answers we need a clear idea of correlation as a relationship.

When two types of phenomena correlate, they show a mutual relationship such that when there is a change in one type of phenomenon, there will be a change in the other type of phenomenon. The type of change and the nature of the relationship may vary considerably. There may be a linear change in the magnitude of the phenomena, or a nonlinear state change, or anything in between. The mutual relationship may be positive or negative: a greater or smaller magnitude of one phenomenon may covary with a greater or smaller magnitude of the other phenomenon. The relationship may be weak or strong. If it is strong, then all changes in one phenomenon may be mirrored as changes of comparable relative magnitude in the other phenomenon. If weak, then only some changes are mirrored as changes in the other phenomenon, or the magnitudes of the changes may not be closely mirrored.

To count as a *correlate* of consciousness it is sufficient for a phenomenon to have almost *any* sort of regular, measurable relationship with almost *any* aspect of consciousness. If NCC is defined in this loose manner, then the set of NCC is potentially enormous. Therefore, Chalmers (2000) has made an attempt to narrow down the set of interesting NCC by characterizing the *direct* NCC as the *minimal* system whose states are sufficient for the corresponding conscious state. He furthermore suggests that the NCC for the *background state* of consciousness (e.g., wakefulness, sleep, dreaming) should be differentiated from the NCC of specific *contents* of consciousness; these may be entirely different neural systems. He argues moreover that the core of NCC research is to find the cortical areas whose neural activity correlates with and predicts specific contents of consciousness.

Will Discovery of Neural Correlates Explain Consciousness?

According to Chalmers (2000), the primary goal of the cognitive neuroscience of consciousness is to determine the neural activities that *correlate with* the *specific contents* of consciousness. There are, however, some problems with this. It appears that the relationship defined by correlation is too weak to count as an explanation of consciousness. Furthermore, it remains unclear what the notion "contents of consciousness" refers to here.

As discussed in chapter 2, the term "content" may refer either to the *representational* content or the *phenomenal* content of consciousness. It seems that Chalmers (2000) has "representational content" in mind:

> We have seen that an NCC here will be a neural representational system whose contents are correlated with the contents of consciousness. To determine whether such a system is truly an NCC, then, we need methods that monitor the representational content of the system. (p. 33)

On the basis of this theoretical commitment, Chalmers argues that the most informative studies in NCC research are neuron-level (or single-cell) studies in monkeys (in the future perhaps also in humans). At the single-neuron level it is possible to *monitor representational content* in neural systems. Monitoring the representational content of single neurons means that it is possible to first determine the external object or feature to which the neuron responds (or what it "codes"). Next, one should check whether the neuron increases its firing rate when the same feature emerges to consciousness. In the ideal case the emergence to consciousness happens without any accompanying change in the physical stimulus, as in binocular rivalry.

There is one major problem with this approach to NCC research. If we follow this track, the task of finding the neural basis of consciousness in the brain seems to reduce to looking for and writing down lists of correlations between stimuli, single neuron firing rates, and verbally reported experiences. That is because representational content is nothing but correlative content: any kind of neural activity at any level of organization can "code" or "represent" any external stimulus feature or motor response (including verbal report), as long as it reliably correlates with it. Consequently, even a single neuron can be said to "code for" or "correlate with" or "have the representational content of," say, "banana" if its firing rate increases selectively for external physical bananas falling into its receptive field.

But when we want to *explain* the visual *experience* itself (i.e., its *phenomenal* content), correlation does not suffice. Suppose that we explain the subjective visual experience caused by presenting a banana as a visual stimulus (or a similar experience during dreaming about a banana). In this case, the explanandum consists of the patterns of phenomenal features at the phenomenal level of organization. At that level, there is a coherent oblong-shaped, phenomenally yellow Gestalt window that opens the semantic window for "banana."

To explain the pattern of phenomenal features present for the subject, simply citing the correlations between external bananas and neural activations (or even between the activations and verbal reports of banana experiences) is not going to be sufficient. Just by citing a list of such correlations, no *explanatory relationship* will have been generated between the organization at the phenomenal level that constitutes the banana experience and the neural activations that correlate with it.

Yet, the observed correlation may have predictive power. It may be possible to issue predictions such as "when neuron N^{1234} increases its firing rate over the limit of twenty per second, then the visual experience of a banana will appear in visual awareness during the next 1500 milliseconds." But note that correlative relationships and predictions like this give no clues, no explanation whatsoever, as to *why* they hold.

It is widely acknowledged in the philosophy of science that correlative relationships and predictions based on them do not suffice for genuine *explanations* of the respective phenomena. Many ancient cultures could predict various astronomical phenomena (sunrises, tides, solstices and equinoxes, solar eclipses, and so on) without any idea what the phenomena or the underlying theoretical principles in actual fact were:

> From the position and phase of the moon, pre-Newtonians could predict the behavior of the tides, but they had no explanation of them. Various kinds of correlations exist that provide excellent bases for prediction, but because no suitable causal relations exist (or are known), these correlations do not furnish explanations. (Salmon, 1989, p. 49)

Chalmers (2000) admits that finding the NCC as he defines it will not by itself yield an explanation of consciousness, or necessarily even be the key to understanding the processes underlying consciousness. He claims that if the goal of NCC research were set as high as that, then it would not be clear whether any NCC even exists or how to search for it. He prefers that the search for NCC be "theoretically neutral rather than theoretically loaded" (Chalmers, 2000, p. 37).

Chalmers's suggestion, however, seems to be committed to representationalism. That is far from a "theoretically neutral" approach. Representationalism as a theoretical basis for consciousness research includes many difficult problems (see chapter 8). Furthermore, it is inconsistent with biological realism. Treating consciousness as a representation guides empirical research toward identifying merely correlative, nonexplanatory relationships between the externally based *representational content* of consciousness and brain activity. Moreover, all such correlations are deemed equally important, because there is no requirement other than the correlation itself as to what would constitute a theoretically significant relationship between some neural process and the phenomenal level.

A purely correlative approach guarantees a safe haven for anyone who believes that consciousness cannot be really explained by referring to the brain. One can admit that in neuroscience, all the neural-phenomenal correlations will be found and mapped in detail, while at the same time one can deny that any genuine explanation of consciousness follows. The purely correlative approach offers a safe haven even for dualistic views, because correlation is a relationship that implies no *ontological* connections between the two kinds of phenomena that correlate. Two ontologically different substances or properties might show an empirical correlation. Even the activities or features of an immaterial soul might *correlate* with physical brain activity.

To wrap up this discussion: The discovery of the NCC does not necessarily lead to any explanation of consciousness. Nor does it rule out dualistic theories of consciousness. Therefore, the biological science of consciousness needs a stronger relationship with which to tie the phenomenal level to the brain.

The Constitutive Mechanisms of Phenomenal Content

According to biological realism, the primary target is to find neural phenomena in the brain that go *beyond* mere correlative relationships with consciousness. The relationship between the phenomenal level and the lower neural levels is not correlation, but hierarchical constitution. The phenomena at the lower neural levels *constitute* the higher phenomenal level. Thus, what neuroscience should be looking for, if it aims at discovering and explaining consciousness, are the *constitutive mechanisms of consciousness* (CMC), rather than just the NCC.

To explain the features at the phenomenal level is to explain the patterns, organization, and dynamics of subjective experience by referring to patterns, organization, and dynamics of biological phenomena lying immediately below the phenomenal level. Features at the lower levels thus bear an explanatory relationship to features at the phenomenal level. Unlike correlation, hierarchical constitution ties the two types of phenomena ontologically together. The higher-level phenomena not merely correlate with the lower-level ones but are ontologically dependent on them too.

The Discovery of Consciousness in the Brain

NCC research should primarily look for two types of phenomena in the brain: The phenomenal level of organization (consciousness itself) and the immediately lower levels of its constitutive mechanisms (the CMC). But how could biological phenomena at these levels of organization be found in the brain? A general strategy in the biological sciences is to acquire data from the relevant levels of organization. The data and the theoretical models based on the data are usually presented in a visualizable form. The visualization of phenomena and data has played a crucially important role in biological discoveries. Just consider the role of microscopy in the development of cytology. It would have been impossible to build a precise theoretical model of the cell without having access to visualization of the actual entities and their organization within the cell. Hence, the relevant levels of organization have to be first made accessible to observation, collection of data, and visualization of the phenomena of interest. Then follows the construction of an idealized model depicting the components of the system and the causal interactions that are involved in the generation of the observed phenomena.

At first glance it seems that cognitive neuroscience and functional brain imaging can certainly deliver the desired goods. After all, visualization of the brain in stunning 3D multicolored maps is one of the most conspicuous features of modern cognitive neuroscience: "brain mapping" (Toga & Mazziotta, 1996) appears to be a kind of combined microscopy and cartography of the mind-brain.

But the most crucial question for the biological research program is this: Do the currently available methods acquire data from and visualize phenomena at exactly *those* levels of biological organization where the phenomenal level and its constitutive mechanisms are realized? We return to the closer examination of this question in the next chapter.

Discovering consciousness in the brain will require that we are capable of constructing a multilevel theoretical model of the phenomenal level and its mechanisms. Only an explicit model based on the relevant empirical data would let us "see" (albeit indirectly) how consciousness resides in the brain. Developing the multilevel model requires that we have data originating from and depicting the relevant levels of biological organization. It will not be possible to reconstruct the structure and dynamics of those levels from the data if the signals collected by our research instruments originate at levels of organization that are nowhere close by them.

Empirical Criteria for the Discovery of the Phenomenal Level

No doubt the current and future methods of brain imaging produce awesome visualizations of various biological phenomena in the brain. But how do we decide which of those data are adequate for revealing the phenomenal level and the CMC in the brain? What would count as the *discovery* of the phenomenal level of organization in the brain? We need to be extremely careful here, for the danger is to slip on the side of either uncritical optimism about the capabilities of current neuroscientific methods ("And here we can see how consciousness beautifully lights up in this neuroimage") or on the opposite side of hopeless pessimism ("Even perfect neuroscience with a complete description and explanation of the brain will not tell us anything at all about consciousness").

There seems to be no shared criterion for what *counts as* the discovery of consciousness in the brain. If such criteria are not clearly and explicitly defined, no amount of data can decide the issue one way or another. For some, any empirically observed NCC will be sufficient; for others, no amount of NCC found in the brain would be sufficient. Fortunately, biological realism offers a way out of this cul-de-sac. If we accept that consciousness *literally* resides in the brain, then it follows that there must be *some* biological phenomenon in the brain that literally resembles or is similar to consciousness. Well, what phenomenon might that be? Of course, it is consciousness *itself.*

A particular experience is a specific pattern of phenomenal features at the phenomenal level of organization in the brain. Hence, to count as the discovery of the phenomenal level, the data we collect should reveal a level of organization in the brain that somehow *directly corresponds to our subjective phenomenology.* The data must in one way or another reveal the fact that there is a phenomenal world being constructed in the brain. Furthermore, the data should reveal what kind of bundles and patterns of phenomenal features are present at this level, and how they are spatiotemporally organized. The data should allow at least some sort of reconstruction of a model that includes the structure, organization, and content of the phenomenal level: *the world experienced by the subject.*

That is what *discovering consciousness in the brain* means: purely brain-based data that allow the construction of a model of the subject's phenomenal world.

In information-theoretic terms, the brain measurement adequate for the discovery of consciousness should constitute an information channel between the phenomenal level (as the object of the measurement) and the neuroscientist (as the subject doing the measurement). Physically, the research instrument serves as the information channel. When data are being registered, entities and activities at the phenomenal level should serve directly as the *input domain* of the information channel. The sensors pick signals directly originating from the phenomenal level. The outputs of the instrument convey the signals to the researcher. The data structures registered and stored by the measuring instrument (curves, maps, activation patterns, and what-have-you) constitute the *output domain* of the information channel. They are the only things directly accessible to the researchers. If they do not transmit any information about the state and the contents of the phenomenal level, then nothing does.

A measurement that fulfils these criteria would transmit information directly about the phenomenal level of organization. Such data would allow the reconstruction of a model of the phenomenal level (as it was experienced by the subject during the brain measurement).

The model of the phenomenal level would, of course, have to be entirely based on the data acquired from actual brain measurements rather than inferred from some external sources. It should be possible in principle to construct a model of the phenomenal level from the brain data without collecting any introspective verbal reports from the subject or without the researchers peeking at the stimuli presented to the subject. That is, without resorting to observation of the representational content or the behavioral consequences of the state.

Resorting to the representational content is, however, all too easy. The researchers simply place themselves in the subject's position (say, they look at the same stimuli) and then they reflect upon their own experience ("OK, so *this* is what the subject experiences when he reports seeing the stimulus"). They would of course get a reasonably good idea of the subject's visual consciousness in this way, because they infer the experience of the subject on the basis of their own experience. But that inference takes place independently of any brain-based data. The inference is based on the subjective experience of what happens in their *own* brain in the same situation, not on what can be *objectively measured* from the subject's brain. If they then find any neural activity in the subject's brain that correlates with the presence of the stimulus, they can surely establish correlations between experiences and brain activity, but not necessarily any understanding of what the exact relationship between the experience and the brain activity might be.

The only way to distinguish the phenomenon itself from the myriads of its correlates is the fact that the CMC is the only NCC found in the brain that fully explains *why the phenomenal world of the subject is in one configuration rather than another.* A certain configuration of the CMC supports, constitutes, or realizes a certain configuration at the higher, phenomenal level. A detailed description of the state of the CMC should thus allow us to reconstruct the state of the phenomenal level of organization. In that way it is possible to create genuine understanding of how specific neural states constitute the phenomenal level, and why some other neural activities only show correlations with it.

The Dream Catcher Test

As the name suggests, our model system, the dreaming brain, plays a central role in the dream catcher test. This test defines the criteria for what would count as the *genuine discovery* of the phenomenal level in the brain. As long as no research instrument can pass the dream catcher test, consciousness remains hidden from objective, third-person science. Before the test is passed, only correlations between neural activity and consciousness have been established—and mere correlation explains nothing, nor does it definitely rule out any philosophical theories about consciousness.

But once this test is passed, it will be possible to go beyond mere correlations. A multilevel model of consciousness, based on constitutive rather than purely correlative relationships, will become feasible (however, it is the theoretical *model* of consciousness rather than the empirical measurements as such that go beyond the correlations). We return to the model-building task later. For now, we shall just define the criteria for the discovery of consciousness in the brain.

The dream catcher test requires two groups of researchers: let us call them the brain team and the dream team. The brain team possesses the latest research instruments to collect data from the living human brain. The members of the team believe that their instruments are capable of revealing the phenomenal level in the brain. To test the accuracy of their statement, the brain team will be allowed to register from the conscious human brain whatever signals they see fit. They may collect as complete a database as possible about the biological phenomena that occur in the brain.

The only restriction is that they are allowed to take the measurements *only when the subject is in REM sleep.* This restriction ensures that the subject's phenomenal world cannot be inferred from the external physical stimuli that surround the subject. Neither can it be inferred, at least not in any detail, from the previously established correlations between neural activity and representational content. In other words, the researchers are totally blind as to the phenomenal content of the subject during the measurement.

If monitoring the external correlations to stimuli were allowed, the result would not suffice for the discovery of the phenomenal level. In that case the results would be based on indirect inferences like this: neurons N^1–N^{1234} in ______ (fill in your favorite brain area) exhibit a complex, selective pattern of firing whenever the organism is in place X (or perceives object Z). Accordingly, whenever the same pattern appears during REM sleep, the subject is dreaming about being in place X (or seeing object Z).

Based on the correlational data alone, no multilevel model can be constructed, showing *how* exactly the observed electrophysiological pattern constitutes the corresponding pattern of phenomenal features at the phenomenal level. There is no compelling theoretical reason to believe that the observed pattern *directly* participates in the construction of the phenomenal level of organization.

Thus, if we want to secure, beyond the shadow of a doubt, that passing the test will require the discovery of the phenomenal level in the brain, the brain research team must manage to complete its task without resorting to *any* information about the representational content of brain states. That is, without any information as to what the physical stimuli or the peripheral sensory activations were, and without any access to the subject's introspective reports.

After the brain team has collected its data and left the laboratory, the dream team enters. It is allowed to use whatever means it sees fit to collect as complete a database as possible about the phenomenal dreams experienced by the subject. The dreamer is awakened at the same moment when the brain team finishes its collection of data. The dream team may then interview the subject immediately after she wakes up, or let her write and draw, and so on, to get as complete a description as possible about the phenomenal level of organization in the brain when the subject's brain was in REM sleep.

The task for both teams is to construct, from the different sources of data available for each team, a full-scale, multimodality 3D computer animation of the dream events that unfolded just prior to awakening the subject, and exactly as they were experienced by the subject. Both teams work independently, without knowing anything about each other's work. The resulting dream models will portray—in as much detail as possible, and as closely resembling the subject's original experience as possible—the dream setting, the objects, persons, and interactions present in the dream; and the temporal progression of the dream events.

Both teams collect data from a number of different subjects until they have completed, say, 100 dream models. The dream models constructed by the two teams are then sent to a team of judges who have no information available about the subjects or the experiment. The only information they have is that each animation in one database should be paired with one animation in the other database, on the basis of overall similarity. They are instructed to take one animation at a time from the dream database and to find the animation in the brain database that most closely resembles it. The judges' task is to match the dream models from the two teams correctly, solely on the basis of the information contained in them. They attempt to determine which two dream models in fact describe one and the same sequence of events at the phenomenal level of organization in the brain (i.e., one and the same dream).

When the judges consistently perform the matching task with better-than-chance accuracy, then the data acquired from the brain measurements alone have allowed a reasonably accurate reconstruction of the phenomenal level of organization. The patterns of brain data thus must have reflected the patterns, organization, and dynamics of phenomenal features at the phenomenal level in the brain. Therefore, the instruments and measurements that were used to acquire and process the data can, in this very strict sense, discover consciousness in the brain.

Conversely, as long as the data acquired by the methods of cognitive neuroscience give us no hints whatsoever about what is going on at the phenomenal level of organization we have not empirically discovered the CMC in the brain.

The *dream catcher test* is the Turing test of consciousness science. Once the methodology exists that is capable of passing the test, empirical consciousness science will have taken a quantum leap. Passing the test means that the pessimist philosophers who maintain that *no* amount of brain data can tell *anything* about consciousness have been decisively defeated. Moreover, philosophers who maintain that the contents of consciousness are externally based and therefore not to be found in the brain will also have to reconsider their views.

But as long as our empirical methodology is nowhere even near passing the test, the philosophical issues remain open. Of course, there is no *guarantee* that *any* method will *ever* be able to pass the test. If that turns out to be the case, then biological realism will be in difficulties. Before it is justified to reject biological realism, however, our research instruments should have revealed *all* the biological levels of organization in the brain. If even at that late point no traces whatsoever of phenomenal content have been detected, biological realism goes down the drain, then and there.

How far is the day when an attempt to pass the dream catcher test could seriously be made? Astonishing as it may be, it seems that a group of researchers claim they *already have* a dream catcher—for rats! At least the study by Louie and Wilson (2001) has been widely publicized as such a wonder. For example, *Newsweek* (5 February 2001) reported this study in a story entitled "What Rats Dream About":

> Do animals really dream? For all the evidence that they do—the twitching and growling of sleeping dogs, for example—nobody knew for sure. That's why scientists were so excited last week when a pair of Massachusetts Institute of Technology researchers studying the brain activity of sleeping rats reported that they could tell not only when the animals were dreaming but also what they were dreaming about—in the case of lab rats, running their maze . . . Indeed, the researchers report in the journal *Neuron,* they could tell precisely what part of the maze the rats dreamed they were in. (p. 51)

I return to this study in chapter 20. There, I evaluate whether we are warranted in believing that the above study truly revealed what the rats were dreaming about, and if so, whether the research instruments used in that study constitute a true dream catcher or not. Before we start to analyze the methods of current cognitive neuroscience as to their capability for discovering the CMC, we have to first get a rough idea what we are looking for in the brain. That task awaits us in the next chapter.

Summary

Neuroscience attempts to overcome the explanatory gap by searching for the neural basis of consciousness in the brain. To find the downward-looking constitutive explanation of consciousness implies that we will have to reach *beyond* the NCC. Mere correlation between two entities does not suffice as an explanatory relationship. In addition to correlations between conscious and neural phenomena, a microlevel of neurobiological organization should be identified in the brain that *directly mirrors* the structure, organization, and contents of the phenomenal level. A brain-sensing or -imaging method is required that retireves information directly concerning the phenomenal contents of consciousness.

But how do we know when (or whether) such a level has been discovered in the brain? How do we know that it has not been *already* discovered by the modern functional brain-imaging technology? To answer questions like these, the dream catcher test was devised as a criterion for the empirical discovery of the phenomenal level in the brain. Any brain measurement that passes that test necessarily allows the reconstruction of the subject's phenomenal world without resort to correlations of brain data with external stimulus objects. The dream catcher test sets strict empirical criteria for deciding whether or not a brain measurement has discovered the phenomenal level in the brain.

19 Closing in on the Mechanisms of Consciousness

When we search for the lower-level neural mechanisms of consciousness, we may close in on them from two directions: from the top down or from the bottom up. In the top-down strategy, we take into account all the information we have about the phenomenal level itself: its internal organization, its temporal dynamics, its unity, and so on. Next, we try to figure out what must be required from the underlying mechanisms to support such a higher level of organization. That is, we use *top-down constraints* to guide us to the neural sources of consciousness. In the bottom-up strategy, we analyze the higher levels of neural organization, already established in neuroscience. We try to figure out whether some of them could support the phenomenal level. Thus, we use *bottom-up constraints* to lead us upward from neurons to consciousness. At some levels, the top-down path and the bottom-up path should meet. Somewhere there lie the direct neural constituents of consciousness. In this chapter we follow those paths and formulate a speculative hypothesis about the mechanisms of the phenomenal level.[1]

The Top-Down Strategy: The Features of the Phenomenal Level as Constraints

Let us first consider the top-down strategy: What features of the phenomenal level could be used as constraints to define the neural mechanisms that directly constitute consciousness?

Although we are far from having a comprehensive description of the phenomenal level, some of its central features can already be outlined at this point. In the case of visual awareness there must be some sort of a spatial fieldlike structure. In the focus of attention, the phenomenal features of one object at a time are bound tightly together. The phenomenal contents in the focus of selective attention consequently make contact with a wide variety of other cognitive systems through reflective consciousness.[2]

By contrast, in parts of the subjective visual field outside the focus of attention there are more loosely bundled groups of features that constitute candidate objects and a schematic layout of the whole scene. If the stimulus suddenly disappears, this complex visual tapestry is retained in iconic memory for about 1 second, but then it evaporates without leaving any traces in long-term memory.

So, at least *visual* awareness has some sort of *dynamically changing center-periphery structure.* This structure forms the basis for the distinction between *phenomenal* (or *primary*) and *reflective* consciousness (see chapter 2). Probably a similar twofold structure applies to the phenomenal level in other sensory modalities as well.

Then there are the *temporal* features of the subjective visual field, which may be very revealing when we search for consciousness in the brain. The neural constituent of consciousness must be capable of changing its configuration very quickly, for the contents of phenomenal consciousness can change at a very rapid rate. Pictures of objects and scenes can be seen and understood with remarkably short stimulus durations. If we are shown images of different, unrelated objects or complex scenes with short stimulus duration (e.g., around 100 ms) we have no difficulties in seeing and recognizing the content of the image.

This can be easily demonstrated in the following way (Biederman, 1990): Turn on your TV with the sound off, close your eyes, and change channels. When you have no idea what channel or program is currently showing, blink your eyes as rapidly as possible to get the briefest possible glimpse of the screen. You will have no difficulty in immediately interpreting the image on the screen, although you will have never seen it before and had no idea in advance what it might depict. Also, formal experiments have confirmed that in a 100 ms exposure of a novel scene, people can usually interpret its meaning (Biederman, 1990).

Even if pictures are presented in a rapid sequence at about 100 to 300 ms per picture, we have the capacity to understand each brief glimpse momentarily, although we are not capable of remembering all of the glimpses later on:

> At presentation rates ranging from about 110 ms to 333 ms per picture, the subjective experience is a very interesting one of grasping and losing large amounts of information within moments. . . . Not only can viewers extract the gist of a picture under these extreme conditions, they can extrapolate the scene's layout and understand the view within the context of the larger, real-world scene from which it was culled. (Intraub, 1999, pp. 66–67)

This means that visual awareness can completely *reorganize* itself three to ten times per second. Even in normal everyday perception, the phenomenal level is constantly transforming its configuration at a time scale of a few hundred milliseconds. Consequently, the neural mechanisms of consciousness, whatever they may turn out to be, must be capable of a correspondingly rapid reorganization.[3]

The top-down strategy furthermore indicates that the phenomenal level must be *integrated* or *unified* so that different kinds of phenomenal features are somehow brought under one single spatiotemporal coordinate system. That coordinate system or phenomenal space is the basis for our experience, as Thomas Metzinger [1995a] would say, of being *one* self in *one* world.

The phenomenal level is capable of realizing an astronomical number of different patterns and bundles of phenomenal features, and different values and dimensions of qualities. The set of all possible combinations of different patterns is inconceivably large: every experience any individual has ever had must be realizable as a specific pattern of phenomenal qualities, and so are all the possible experiences that nobody has had as yet. The *combinatorial capacity* of the system must therefore be immense.

Taken together, it follows from the top-down constraints that the mechanisms of consciousness must possess at least:

1. integration into one overall coordinate system;
2. rapid temporal reorganization;
3. an internal center-surround structure, involving the interplay between phenomenal consciousness, selective attention, and reflective consciousness;
4. a vast combinatorial capacity.

Further top-down constraints can be found from the data on brain damage and altered states of consciousness (reviewed in chapters 12, 13, and 14). There we discovered that

5. different phenomenal features have *independent access* to the unified phenomenal space;
6. the existence of phenomenal space appears necessary for any experiences to come about;
7. phenomenal objects have a layered structure:

a. a phenomenal surface forming the *coherent Gestalt window* of visuospatial features; and

b. deep connections to semantic knowledge, turning the coherent Gestalt into a *meaningful semantic window*.

Any level of organization found in the brain that does not possess or directly support features like the above cannot be among the constitutive mechanisms of the phenomenal level (at least as far as visual consciousness is concerned).

The Bottom-Up Strategy: Defining the Neural Correlates of Consciousness

The opposing strategy is to go from the bottom up. The idea here is to measure, by using some brain-sensing or -imaging method, the changes at the neural levels of organization that take place simultaneously with a change in consciousness. Consciousness may be manipulated in two different ways. The *global state* of consciousness might change (the individual loses or regains consciousness, or enters a globally altered state). Alternatively, only some *specific content* of consciousness changes. That is, some information enters into or disappears from the phenomenal level or, more accurately, the realization of some pattern of phenomenal features either commences or ceases.

In any case, the idea is that the change at the phenomenal level has to be accompanied by corresponding changes at the lower levels of neural organization. Empirical measurements should reveal two points: first, the *anatomical location* of the neural populations whose activity changed; second, the *nature of the neurophysiological activity* that correlates with consciousness.

There are several competing hypotheses about the nature and location of the direct neural correlates of consciousness (NCC). In the following review, I again mostly concentrate on the model systems, visual awareness and the dreaming brain, and what they have revealed about the NCC. If we first consider the question about the anatomical location of the NCC, we see that there is very little agreement about it at present. Just about every distinct cortical lobe and area has been proposed by at least some researchers to be the seat of the NCC.

The Role of V1 in Visual Consciousness

Early sensory cortex has been argued to be the only site that contains detailed high-resolution information about primitive sensory features and, therefore, it must be part of the NCC. For example, Pollen (1999) argues for V1 to be the NCC for certain types of visual experience. By contrast, Crick and Koch (1995) argue that V1 is not part of the direct neural correlates of visual awareness. Extrastriate areas such as V4 might be, because Crick and Koch believe that links to frontal executive areas are a necessary part of NCC, and V1 lacks them.

Theories about the role of V1 in visual awareness can be divided into hierarchical models and interactive models. *Hierarchical models* propose that only higher-level extrastriate areas (visual areas beyond V1) are directly involved in the construction of visual awareness. Damage to V1 causes blindness simply because the flow of information to higher-level areas is disrupted. By contrast, *interactive models* propose that V1 participates directly in the construction of visual awareness by forming dynamic recurrent circuits with higher-level areas. The crucial contribution from V1 to visual awareness comes not when the initial sensory input first arrives at V1, but later when higher-order areas send feedback signals back to V1. Even in interactive models, V1 activity alone is *not sufficient* for visual awareness. In fact, it seems that the activity of no *single* visual area, be it occipital, temporal, parietal, or frontal, is *sufficient* for visual awareness (Tong, 2003).

It remains unclear, however, whether V1 is *necessary* for visual awareness. To resolve this disagreement, evidence provided by the dreaming brain should be considered: What happens to the subjective experience of visual dream imagery if the primary visual cortex is damaged? If V1 is truly necessary for subjective visual experience—if it is part of the constitutive mechanism for constructing the phenomenal level in vision—then V1 lesions (cortical blindness) should not only wipe out subjective visual perception but also all types of internally generated visual experience, such as dreaming.

The available evidence indicates, however, that this is not the case. Damage to primary visual cortex does *not* lead to cessation of visual dream imagery; only damage to extrastriate areas in medial occipitotemporal structures does so (Solms, 1997). Furthermore, positron emission tomography (PET) studies measuring regional metabolic activity in the brain have shown that during REM sleep V1 is deactivated, whereas extrastriate visual cortex is activated (Hobson et al., 2000).

Therefore, V1 cannot be absolutely necessary for subjective visual experience. Its direct contribution to the phenomenal level must be so meager that it makes no major difference to internally generated visual experiences like dreams. Therefore, it seems that the phenomenal visual field is not realized in V1, nor is its existence directly dependent on the activities in V1.

Extrastriate Visual Areas and the Microconsciousness Hypothesis

Zeki and Bartels (1999) believe that visual areas in extrastriate cortex contain multiple specialized modules, each one capable of creating some primitive phenomenal features of visual consciousness such as color (in V4) or motion (in V5). They say that each module is capable of generating its own little "microconsciousness": a restricted set of phenomenal features.

Their suggestion of multiple independent microconsciousnesses violates one of the top-down constraints discussed above: the constraint that the phenomenal level is fundamentally *unified* under one spatial, egocentric coordinate system.[3] If it were not, how could the phenomenal features of the microconsciousnesses be spatially related to each other? How could several different phenomenal features (color, shape, motion), generated by distinct microconsciousnesses, reside in one and the same virtual object in a single location in the phenomenal field?

Dainton's analysis is to the point in showing what would be left if the unity of experience was taken away:

> That this mode of unity is a crucial feature of experience as we know it is easily appreciated: remove this unity from a typical stream of consciousness and what would be left? At most a myriad instances of point-like quality, each so entirely isolated from the rest that, from the point of view of experience at least, they could as well exist in different universes. (Dainton, 2000, pp. 238–239).

We know that the phenomenal elements of our experiences do not exist in different universes, but form a global phenomenal whole instead. There must be *some* coordinate system under which the different phenomenal features are related to each other.

Thus, it seems that the microconsciousness hypothesis cannot be the whole story about the neural constituents of consciousness. Visual features must be spatially related to each other and to the phenomenal body image somehow—they are features of one integrated phenomenal world. It may be that highly specialized modules such as V4 and V5 do contribute specific contents of consciousness to the phenomenal level, in the sense that only their activities are capable of modulating specific patterns of qualitative features within phenomenal space. But the phenomenal qualities do not themselves reside in V4 or V5 in an isolated manner. Neither are they first created there as tiny isolated bits of phenomenology, and then transported elsewhere. The results of processing in V4 and V5 become parts of the phenomenal level of organization only when they interface with the overall phenomenal coordinate system.

The claim that there are several microconsciousnesses boils down to the empirical hypothesis that the phenomenal level is realized in different forms and in multiple locations in the brain. These microinstantiations of the phenomenal level are supposed to be in principle completely independent of, or isolated from, each other.

There is little evidence supporting the view that multiple microconsciousnesses exist (furthermore it is unclear what kind of experiences might count as evidence for their existence). An isolated cortical module such as V4 or V5 cannot realize the phenomenal level all by itself. Although V4 is probably necessary for phenomenal color and V5 for phenomenal motion, they are not sufficient for bringing about those phenomenal features. Instead, the minimal realization basis of the phenomenal level appears to require a fairly large neural space such as that of an entire cerebral hemisphere.

NCC in the Temporal Lobe

The striate and extrastriate occipital cortex are by no means the only cortical locations proposed as the seat of the NCC of visual awareness. Single-cell studies of binocular rivalry in monkeys (Sheinberg & Logothetis, 1997) provide us with evidence that most cells in the inferotemporal cortex modulate their activity in concert with changes in the content of visual awareness. Therefore, the temporal cortex has been regarded as a serious candidate for being the NCC of visual awareness.

In humans, neural activity in occipitotemporal areas along the ventral visual stream has been reported to correlate with subjective visual awareness in studies of visual hallucinations (ffytche, Howard, Brammer, David, Woodruff, & Williams, 1998), binocular rivalry of place and face stimuli (Kanwisher, 2001), and during REM sleep and dreaming (Schwartz & Maquet, 2002). Furthermore, damage to these areas leads to cessation of visual imagery in dreams (Solms, 1997).

In view of these empirical facts, it seems difficult to exclude ventral stream temporal cortex from the NCC. On the contrary, the contribution of ventral stream areas appears absolutely necessary for visual experience. Yet it is doubtful that temporal activity alone would be sufficient.

The Parietal Lobes and the "Central Representation"

In contrast to the above suggestions, Taylor (2001) argues for the inferior parietal lobe as the location of NCC. He tries to show that an area in the brain that is the NCC should be devoted to specific kinds of information processing, known to characterize phenomenal consciousness.

The features of conscious experience regarded by him as important are, first, the body-based inner perspective (or the perspectivalness of phenomenal consciousness); second, goal-directedness (as in voluntary, intentional actions); and third, attention (without which consciousness of an object is impossible). Taylor (2001) argues that these high-level features come together in the central representation, which is a combination of multimodal activations, including sensory and bodily information, future planning, and attentional selection of the currently most important information.

The central representation is spatial, or a set of spatial maps that either fuse into a continuous one or are somehow in register with each other. All this comes together in the inferior parietal lobe which supports the central representation, the ultimate NCC. The other parts of cortex (occipital, temporal, frontal) may be necessary for certain types of consciousness to occur, but they are not sufficient.

Evidence from the dreaming brain lends support to the idea that the inferior parietal contribution is necessary to the phenomenal coordinate system. Damage to inferior parietal areas, especially in the right hemisphere, is associated with a global cessation of dreaming in all sensory modalities (Solms, 1997). Spatial processing in the inferior parietal lobe thus seems a necessary ingredient of the phenomenal level, or at least for information to *enter* the phenomenal level. Without the involvement of these areas the brain cannot construct the space in which phenomenal features could be actualized.

Furthermore, there is evidence that the superior parietal lobe plays an important role in the construction of an internal representation of one's own body. A patient with damage to this area tended to lose awareness of her right limbs unless she was able to see them (Wolpert, Goodbody, & Husain, 1998). Wolpert et al. (p. 532) described the loss as "a failure to maintain an internal representation, common to both the sensory and motor systems, which is necessary for perception and action." Furthermore, Frith, Blakemore, and Wolpert (2000) regard such internal models in the parietal lobe as the basis of phantom limbs. This "internal representation" generated by the superior parietal lobe appears to be what I have described as "the virtual body," one of the most central ingredients of the world simulation in the brain.

Dorsal-Ventral Interaction: Necessary for Visual Consciousness?

At the phenomenal level, simulated objects and the virtual self are all placed in the context of phenomenal space. When it comes to visual objects, this requires interaction between the dorsal visual stream (which handles the spatial aspects of vision) and the ventral visual stream (which takes care of the objects and their features). Results from brain imaging in normals (Kanwisher, 2001) and neglect or extinction patients (Driver & Vuilleumier, 2001) suggest that visual processing both in the dorsal and the ventral streams remains outside consciousness unless there is *interaction* between the two streams. Therefore, the areas that link ventral and dorsal streams might be closely involved in the construction of the phenomenal level.

The strongest candidates for this interaction are temporoparietal areas, especially the (human) inferior parietal lobule and the (monkey) superior temporal sulcus (STS) (Heilman, Watson, & Valenstein, 2000).

Hippocampus as a Recipient of Conscious Input

S. Köhler and Moscovitch (1997) propose that the regions necessary for consciousness are those that project to the hippocampal formation and surrounding cortex. They reason in the following manner: Only those events that were consciously apprehended or perceived at the time of their occurrence can lead to subsequent conscious recollection. The hippocampus is necessary for conscious, explicit recollection; therefore the regions that support consciousness must project heavily to the hippocampus. The hippocampus requires "conscious input" for its operation and may therefore serve as a guide when tracing back toward the original neural substrate of consciousness.

However, connection to the hippocampus might not be *necessary* for some area to be involved in the construction of consciousness. As the experiments on iconic memory and change blindness show (see chapter 13), most of the fleeting phenomenal contents we enjoy in vision are never coded into long-term memory. Only those that are attended and selected for further processing can be later recalled. Therefore, much of the phenomenal visual field leaves no traces behind in the hippocampus. Tracing backward from the hippocampus might lead us toward the contents of reflective consciousness rather than the total contents of consciousness. It may also lead us toward many areas that have nothing to do with consciousness, as the hippocampus is densely connected to a multitude of different areas.

The Anatomy of the Phenomenal Level: Local or Holistic?

The correlates of particular contents of consciousness can be found in widely distributed cortical areas. Activity in many extrastriate visual areas in the occipital and temporal lobes correlates with visual awareness of objects or particular visual features. The parietal lobe appears to be most important for bodily awareness and awareness of space. As far as phenomenal consciousness is concerned, only frontal areas do not seem to be necessary. They are probably involved in higher-order forms of consciousness, such as reflective consciousness, self-awareness, and working memory.

It seems that large-scale interaction between different areas is required for the phenomenal level to come about. Thus, the neural basis of consciousness should not be expected to be anatomically localized in any single area or cortical lobe. Instead, the mechanisms of consciousness consist of networks in the brain that connect the diverse contents of consciousness into one coherent whole. The constitutive mechanisms of consciousness must include *an anatomically widespread complex network.*

The correlates of particular contents of consciousness may be localizable, however. But the system that *realizes* and *unifies* the phenomenal contents should have a more holistic character. The neural correlates of phenomenal space might reveal the mechanisms responsible for global phenomenal unity.

The Network Underlying Phenomenal Space

In hemispatial neglect half of phenomenal space disappears. Hence, the precise localization of the damage causing neglect should reveal where the mechanisms of phenomenal space are localized in the brain. Typically, the lesions causing neglect in different patients overlap in the inferoposterior parietal region (Farah, 2000). However, this traditional view has been questioned, because the region of maximal lesion overlap across neglect patients does not necessarily reflect the areas where the mechanisms are localized. Instead, it may merely reflect the vulnerability of these regions to damage after stroke, for example.

Subtraction of lesion overlap in patients *with and without* spatial neglect yields a different picture. The center of lesion overlap specifically associated with hemispatial neglect is now found not in the parietal lobe, but in the *temporal* lobe (Karnath, Ferber, & Himmelbach, 2001). Moreover, spatial neglect is not only associated with *cortical* injury but is also frequently observed after *subcortical* lesions in the right hemisphere, even in the absence of any cortical damage.

The picture that emerges from the anatomy of neglect suggests that there must be a *complex anatomical network* involved in the construction of phenomenal space. The network includes several cortical and subcortical nodes. Damage to *any* of the major anatomical components of the network disrupts the contralateral space, wiping out one half of the phenomenal world.

According to the latest studies, the network underlying phenomenal space interconnects at least the following anatomical structures: the superior temporal gyrus in the cerebral cortex, the pulvinar in the thalamus, and the putamen in the basal ganglia (Karnath, Himmelbach, & Rorden, 2002). Lesions of thalamic nuclei with widespread cortical projections cause a neglect syndrome also in animals (Steriade, 2001).

The Thalamocortical System and the Conscious State

To be in the conscious state is to have the underlying phenomenal space currently realized in the brain. Only in that case are particular phenomenal experiences enabled. Several theorists have suggested that the state of being conscious is dependent on neural activity in thalamocorticothalamic loops (Newman, 1995; Llinás et al., 1998).

Circumstances that lead to loss of the conscious state might be used to test these theoretical ideas. Epileptic absence seizures, general anesthesia, and NREM sleep are all states in which the phenomenal level is temporarily disabled. All of them involve remarkable changes in thalamocortical function.

Epileptic absence seizures involve a brief transient loss of consciousness. The cause of this loss appears to be disruption of the high-frequency thalamocortical oscillations. Suddenly, large numbers of thalamocortical loops are recruited to a much stronger, low-frequency (about 3 Hz) pattern of oscillatory activity (Kostopoulos, 2001). Thus, high-frequency oscillations in the thalamocortical system appear necessary for supporting the phenomenal level.

A functional brain-imaging experiment on the loss of consciousness during anesthesia also points to the importance of the thalamus (Alkire, Haier, & Fallon, 2000). Two different anesthetic agents were applied independently: halothane and isoflurane. Each caused specific relative reductions of regional cerebral glucose metabolism, primarily in the thalamus. They probably induced the state of unconsciousness by creating a hyperpolarization block of thalamocortical neurons. The researchers concluded that a reduction of thalamocortical output may underlie the loss of consciousness in anesthesia.

During NREM sleep, full-blown world simulation (vivid dreaming) rarely happens. In the deep stages of NREM sleep, the contents of consciousness are either sparse or totally missing. Brain imaging studies have revealed that during NREM sleep, glucose and oxygen utilization in the thalamus is radically lowered. This finding supports the idea that the thalamic level is strongly deactivated in NREM sleep (Hobson et al., 2000).

The data from various sources thus point in the direction that high-frequency oscillatory activity in the thalamocortical networks plays a decisive role in the mechanisms of the conscious state as such.

The thalamus forms complex feedback circuits with the cortex. Two types of thalamocortical networks can be distinguished: diffuse and focused. The anatomical basis of the diffuse networks involves a specific type of thalamic cell called the *matrix neuron* (Jones, 2001). Matrix neurons are widely distributed throughout the thalamus and can be found in every thalamic nucleus. They project to the superficial layers of the cortex. The projections are diffuse and range across several cortical areas. By contrast, another type of thalamic cells called the *core neuron* is found only in certain thalamic nuclei. Core neurons project in a focused manner to the deep layers of only specific cortical areas.

The two types of thalamocortical circuits form oscillatory loops of coherent neural activity between the thalamus and the cortex. Here is one hypothesis worth considering: The diffuse thalamocortical network formed by the matrix neurons might be the anatomical basis of the phenomenal coordinate system. The specific thalamocortical circuits might be the anatomical basis for forming the particular contents of consciousness. The physiological mechanism acting in these circuits is high-frequency synchronous oscillation, binding contents and space together.

The top-down constraints from neuropsychology appear to be consistent with the above hypothesis. Damage to the thalamus, especially the pulvinar nucleus, causes hemispatial neglect (Karnath et al., 2002)— and there is a large population of matrix cells in the pulvinar (Jones, 2001). Thus, the connectivity of the matrix cells might play a central role in the construction of phenomenal space, especially visual space.

Different visual cortical areas appear to have independent access to phenomenal space, so that cortical damage to one area may wipe out a particular phenomenal feature but leave others intact (see chapter 11). All visual cortical areas have their own, independent connections with the thalamus. Conversely, when the phenomenal space itself is damaged, then no visual features have access to the phenomenal level. The independent access of phenomenal features to phenomenal space and the block of all access with the disappearance of phenomenal space could be accounted for by the architecture of thalamocortical connectivity.

The overall picture that emerges from current theories is that the neural constituents of consciousness are not spatially localized in one precise place in the brain. Instead, they probably form a complex system of corticocortical and thalamocortical networks, each contributing some essential features to the phenomenal level of organization.

The Physiological Mechanisms of the Phenomenal Level

Deciphering the anatomical location is only the first part of the task of identifying the neural substrate of consciousness. It is at least as important to determine the nature of the neurophysiological mechanisms that might be involved in the generation of consciousness. A candidate mechanism would have to be capable of accounting for the features of the phenomenal level, and would have to comprise higher levels of organization in the brain.

Synchronicity as a Mechanism of Consciousness

Synchronous neural activity at high frequencies is the leading candidate among the potential neurophysiological mechanisms of consciousness. As we observed in chapter 16, gamma-band oscillatory activity is involved in the conscious perception of unified visual objects both in humans and animals. Synchronization related to visual awareness of objects has been detected by invasive microelectrodes as well as noninvasive scalp electrodes (Singer, 1999; Gray, 1999; Tallon-Baudry & Bertrand, 1999; Revonsuo et al., 1997).

Some theorists (e.g., Engel et al., 1999) propose that gamma-band synchronous activity in the cortex is necessary for consciousness. Others (e.g., Llinás & Paré 1996, Newman & Grace, 1999) regard synchronicity in thalamocortical loops and subcortical circuits as more important for consciousness. The anatomy and physiology of thalamocortical connections seem just right for producing large-scale synchronous patterns. Thalamic cells show inherent oscillatory rhythmicity, and their connections to the cortex support both specific loops and widespread loops of coherent activity.

There are both empirical and theoretical reasons to believe that synchronicity might serve as a mechanism of consciousness. Empirical evidence from a variety of sources points to a connection between consciousness and gamma-band synchronicity (see chapter 4 for evidence regarding dreaming and chapter 16 for evidence regarding binding). Theoretically, synchronicity might be a way to establish higher levels of electrophysiological organization in the brain. As the phenomenal level is a higher level of biological organization, perhaps it could be based on neural synchronicity.

If synchronicity is a constitutive mechanism of consciousness, then synchronous patterns of activation should correspond in some way to the patterns of phenomenal experience. One theory of synchronicity (Roelfsema & Singer, 1998; Roelfsema et al., 1996) in fact postulates holistic patterns of neural synchrony that resemble the percepts we have in visual awareness. Thus, in principle, neural synchrony is capable of supporting higher-level electrophysiological entities that are isomorphic with the contents of visual consciousness.

Singer (2000) proposes that "metarepresentations" are the higher-level neural entities on which consciousness is based. Metarepresentations have a rich combinatorial complexity, the ability to reconfigure themselves rapidly, and the ability to handle contents that are completely unpredictable. Temporary association of neurons into functionally coherent assemblies could be the way to build metarepresentations. The assemblies could be defined by synchronization.

In principle, it seems possible to build higher-level electrophysiological entities resembling the phenomenal objects in consciousness by using synchronicity of large neural assemblies as the mechanism. Thus, synchronicity could be the microlevel mechanism underlying the phenomenal *contents* of consciousness.

The Dynamic Core: A Higher Level of Neural Organization?

The dynamic core hypothesis (G. M. Edelman & Tononi, 2000) describes a holistic neural mechanism that might be the basis of consciousness as a unified whole. The dynamic core is a cluster of neuronal groups that strongly interact among themselves. The cluster as a whole has distinct functional or physiological (rather than anatomical) borders with the rest of the brain.

The idea of a "functional cluster" is interesting, because a "level of organization" is defined as a *cluster of closely interacting parts.* The parts of a level interact more closely and directly with each other than with entities outside that level. Consequently, if a dynamic core really exists in the brain, it would count as a higher level of neurophysiological organization.

Where in the brain is the dynamic core localized? Reentrant connections in the thalamocortical systems are involved, but otherwise it is not localizable:

> A dynamic core is a process rather than a thing or a place, and it is defined in terms of neural interactions rather than in terms of neural connection, location, or activity. . . . it is in general spatially distributed and thus cannot be localized in a single place in the brain. . . . The term "dynamic core" deliberately does not refer to a unique, invariant set of brain areas . . . , and the core may change in composition over time. (G. M. Edelman & Tononi, 2000, p. 146)

The dynamic core hypothesis denies that the local, intrinsic properties of neurons could in some mysterious way have a privileged correlation with consciousness. Thus, the idea is that the level of organization at which the dynamic core resides is higher than the level of single neurons, and the properties of single neurons are not by themselves decisive as to whether the neuron in some sense contributes to the dynamic core.

Interactive Feedback Loops

Lamme and Roelfsema (2000) suggest that the difference between nonconscious visual processes and subjective visual awareness is based on two different sweeps of neural information processing that occur during visual perception. A *fast feedforward sweep* reaches the furthest areas in the visual processing stream within 100 ms. However, then a second, *feedback processing sweep* is initiated through recurrent connections. It travels backward toward the earlier stages in the processing hierarchy. The recurrent sweep is closely connected to visual awareness (figure 19.1).

This implies that the emergence of a stimulus to visual awareness happens with a temporal delay of over 100 ms. This is supported by the well-established fact that a visual

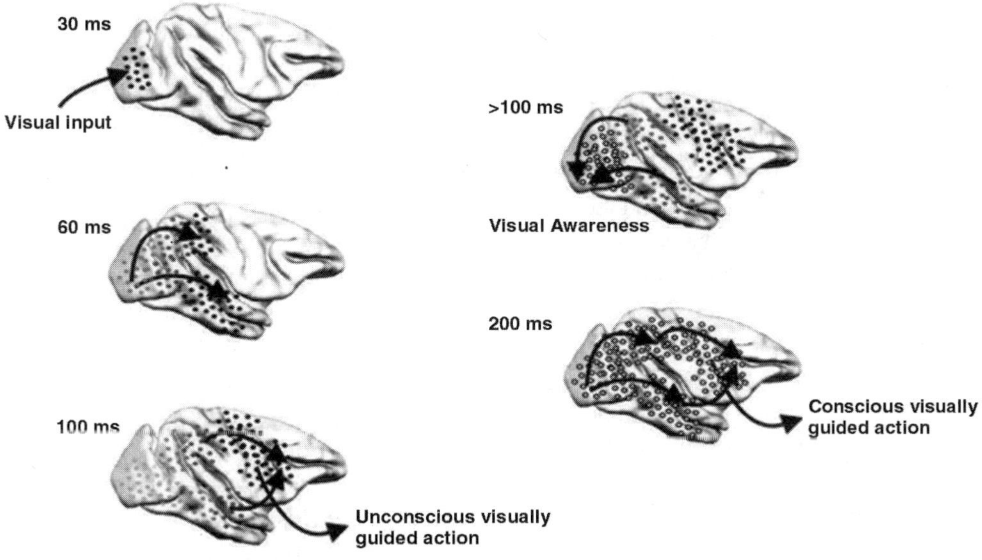

Figure 19.1
Recurrent feedback loops and visual awareness. The first wave of feedforward processing does not involve phenomenal consciousness. At 30 ms from stimulus onset, the visual information enters the brain (the primary visual area V1). From 30 to 100 ms the feedforward wave of processing travels through extrastriate visual areas and from there reaches frontal areas. This rapid, nonconscious processing guides visual action outside of consciousness. After 100 ms from stimulus onset begins the second, backward wave of recurrent processing that feeds the activity in extrastriate visual areas back toward lower-level areas such as V1. This backward wave of processing modulates the contents of phenomenal consciousness. At still longer latencies (after 200 ms) the conscious visual information may be used in visual action guided by phenomenally conscious information (subjective seeing of the stimulus). (Modified from figure 2 in Lamme, V. A. (2000). Neural mechanisms of visual awareness: A linking proposition, *Brain and Mind, 1*, 385–406, with the kind permission of Kluwer Academic Publishers.)

backward mask presented within 100 ms after the target stimulus strongly reduces visibility of the target. The late mask is effective even when presented well after the stimulus because the mask disrupts the recurrent interaction between early and late visual areas, critical for awareness. The mask arrives at the early cortical areas just in time to barricade the formation of the recurrent loop crucial for visual awareness of the previous stimulus.

Also, experiments on the timing of the electrophysiological correlates of visual awareness support the idea that sensory information modulates the phenomenal level only in relatively late time windows, well after 100 ms from stimulus onset. Visual awareness negativity (VAN) is the earliest correlate of phenomenal consciousness in vision. Our research group has identified this response in human event-related brain potentials in several experiments (Koivisto & Revonsuo, 2003; Ojanen, Revonsuo & Sams, 2003; Wilenius-Emet, Revonsuo, & Ojanen, 2004). VAN is the earliest difference wave that remains when the same physical stimuli are shown to the subject under two conditions: one preventing awareness of the stimuli, the other allowing awareness. Hence, VAN reflects the difference between the presence and the absence of visual consciousness of the stimuli. When full-contrast stimuli are shown, VAN typically starts to emerge around 120–150 ms, and it peaks around 200 to 300 ms. VAN thus probably reflects the neural events that take place as the input from the sensory channel modulates the phenomenal level.

Now we are in the position to briefly summarize what happens in the brain when a visual stimulus is presented and, consequently, enters consciousness. The main players in these events are the forward and backward sweeps of cortical activation, and the concomitant activity in thalamocortical circuits. The first, the rapid feedforward sweep, probably only establishes short-lived local centers of synchronous oscillatory activity in cortical areas along the ventral and dorsal visual streams. As such, the islands of synchronicity persist for a few hundred milliseconds but remain at a nonconscious level (Tallon-Baudry, 2003). The backward sweep, recruiting both corticocortical and thalamocortical connections, generates strong global synchronicity between all the active areas across ventral and dorsal areas. The global wave of synchronicity, spreading simultaneously in the cortical areas and in the specific and diffuse thalamocortical loops, functionally connects all of them together. At that point the phenomenal contents may finally enter phenomenal space.

The Master Loop Hypothesis

In the light of the theory and evidence reviewed above, I am putting forward a—admittedly speculative—hypothesis concerning the constitutive mechanisms of consciousness.

The phenomenal level of organization is a rapidly reorganizing loop of bioelectrical activity in the brain. It emerges at the intersection where two types of recurrent electrophysiological loops meet: one modality-independent, fundamental, spatially unified loop and many modality-specific loops that contribute their particular phenomenal content to the phenomenal level. They deliver their specific contributions by activating and modulating the otherwise dormant qualities in phenomenal space. The interaction between the loops induces particular qualities and simultaneously organizes them into complex spatiotemporal patterns.

The loops involve corticocortical as well as thalamocortical connections. At the cortical level, convergence zones where the two kinds of loops (modality-specific and modality-independent) meet are to be found in the inferior parietal lobe and the superior temporal lobe. At the subcortical level, the thalamus is the key structure. Its diffuse, nonspecific projections to the cortex may be involved in the construction of phenomenal space, and its specific connections to the construction of the objects to be embedded in the space.

According to this hypothesis the neural substrate of consciousness consists of large-scale electrophysiological or bioelectrical activity patterns that are enormously complex (probably involving millions of neurons and billions of synapses). Synchronous oscillations or other forms of spatiotemporally coherent neural activity in the large-scale networks are the mechanism by which the conscious state, the subphenomenal space, and its phenomenal contents are realized in the brain. The networks are characterized by an architecture of recurrent connectivity. That special architecture supports closed loops of coherent bioelectrical activity. The loops extend "horizontally" across the cortex (like the feedback sweep in the ventral visual stream) and also "vertically" between the cortex and the thalamus ("specific" and "nonspecific" thalamocortical loops).

Finally, we are now in a position to delineate what *kind* of biological phenomenon we are searching for when trying to discover NCC in the brain. The top-down strategy suggests that the phenomenal level is internally integrated, continuously and rapidly reorganizes itself, has a center-surround structure in an egocentric frame of reference, and an immense combinatorial capacity. The bottom-up strategy suggests that the phenomenal level is based on the coherent and rapidly changing activity of large-scale recurrent neural networks. They are anatomically distributed within the brain but they create physiologically integrated loops of bioelectrical activity.

Difficult though it may be, try to imagine this sort of a spatially distributed master loop: a constantly changing but unified bioelectrical phenomenon somehow realized within the depths of the living brain. Perhaps you will get at least a faint idea of what the biological research program should be searching for. The challenge for neuroscience is to get an empirical grip on the levels of organization that could support exactly *this* type of biological phenomenon. The question we need to face next is, Can this kind of a phenomenon be captured with the currently available methods of neuroscience?

Summary

When neuroscientists look for the phenomenal level in the brain, they ought to have some idea of what such a thing might look like and where it might lurk in the brain. In order to sketch an initial idea about that, both top-down and bottom-up constraints should be used. Top-down constraints take the features of subjective experience as the starting point, and try to descend from them to the features of the constitutive mechanisms. Bottom-up constraints look at neural systems that could realize large-scale coherent states and thus be plausible candidates for mechanisms of consciousness.

The evidence concerning the neural basis of consciousness comes from many different empirical and theoretical sources. When the sources are integrated with each other, a converging picture starts to emerge. As to the neural correlates of visual consciousness, the primary visual area and frontal cortex do not seem to be necessary. Extrastriate cortex and occipitotemporal areas along the ventral visual stream seem necessary for particular visual features and coherent visual objects in consciousness. Parietal areas are necessary for the body image and the self. A network of thalamocorticosubcortical connections seems necessary for phenomenal space and for the state of being conscious. Coherent neural activity at high frequencies in these areas is the prime candidate for the physiological mechanism that might constitute consciousness.

The phenomenal level is not localized in any single cortical lobe, but involves a large distributed network of recurrent neural activities in corticocortical and thalamocortical loops. The speculative master loop hypothesis postulates that one type of these loops is content-specific and modulates the other type of loop which is nonspecific. The latter loop corresponds to unified phenomenal space, the former to the bundles of qualities we experience as the phenomenal contents directly present for us in experiential space. Where the two different types of loop interface in dynamic interaction, there reside the constitutive mechanisms of consciousness.

20 The Methods of Neuroscience in the Search for Consciousness

We now have a preliminary idea of what neuroscience is looking for when it chases the neural mechanisms of consciousness in the brain: the phenomenal level of organization, realized as a master loop of bioelectrical activity in corticocortical and thalamocortical loops.

Experiments seeking the neural correlates of consciousness (NCC) aim at observing neural phenomena that covary with the phenomenal level. An NCC experiment thus attempts to *isolate* the neural effects arising at the phenomenal level from all other effects arising at purely nonconscious levels. Ideally, the physical stimulation in these experiments is held constant. Yet, in the experimental condition the stimulus modulates the phenomenal level, whereas in the control condition it does not interact with the phenomenal level in any way. If visual stimuli are used, the stimulus is *seen subjectively* in the experimental condition, whereas in the control condition it remains entirely outside of visual consciousness.

In an NCC experiment, the crucial difference between the experimental and control conditions in terms of phenomenology is this: in the former, the stimulus information is *present in* phenomenal consciousness, whereas in the latter the same information is *absent from* phenomenal consciousness. Consequently, there *must* be *some* empirically detectable difference between these two conditions in terms of neural activity. The crucial difference reflects neural events directly associated with the phenomenal level.

Another relevant experimental approach is to vary the presence and absence of the conscious *state* as such, rather than specific contents of consciousness. Thus, in the control condition the phenomenal level is present in the brain (normal waking state); in the experimental condition the phenomenal level is absent from the brain (as during general anesthesia or dreamless slow-wave sleep).

The two approaches complete each other: the first tells us what happens when the phenomenal level is modulated by input information; the second tells us what happens when the phenomenal level is temporarily wiped out altogether (or when it reappears).

The question we are concerned with in this chapter[1] is this: Even if the experimental design of the NCC experiments is perfect, what aspects of neural activity can be captured by the currently available research instruments of neuroscience? Some of the most prominent methods will be evaluated in the light of this question: single-cell recordings, functional brain imaging with PET and fMRI, and extracranial neuroelectric (EEG) and neuromagnetic (MEG) measures. We will try to find the answers to the following questions:

1. What are the neural phenomena actually observed or measured by these methods?
2. Do the measurements reflect such levels of organization in the brain where the phenomenal level or its constituent mechanisms are to be found?
3. Are any of these methods serious candidates for passing the dream catcher test?

Single-Cell Recordings with Invasive Microelectrodes

In extracellular single-cell recordings, a microelectrode is inserted into an animal's living brain. It is placed so that it registers the electrical activity of a single cell or a few nearby cells only. The electrode can be used to monitor the firing rate of the neuron during sensory stimulation, thus giving the researchers an idea about what kind of sensory information makes the neuron become active, and what it does not care about.

Single-cell recordings in monkeys have been used to correlate neuronal firing rates with the content of visual awareness during *binocular rivalry.* In binocular rivalry, two different pictures are shown, one to each eye. They cannot be fused to form one coherent percept; thus the pictures start to alternate in visual awareness, so that only one can be subjectively seen at any one time. The physical stimuli stay constant all the time. Thus, this arrangement offers a way to dissociate the phenomenal content of consciousness (which keeps changing) from the physical stimuli (which stays the same).

In the famous study by Sheinberg and Logothetis (1997), the single-cell activity of cortical neurons was recorded in the macaque monkey during binocular rivalry. The researchers first identified some single cells that selectively responded only to a certain visual image, say a face, and others that selectively responded only to another image, say a banana. The monkeys were trained to make specific behavioral responses to each stimulus. When the two stimuli were shown simultaneously under a rivalrous condition, the behavioral responses were taken to reflect the content of the monkeys' subjective visual awareness.

The researchers recorded the responses of single units in the monkeys' temporal cortical areas. The activity of about 90% of the recorded cells in superior temporal sulcus and inferior temporal cortex covaried with and reliably predicted the behavioral response of the animals, and thus signified the content of the animals' visual awareness.

If we read the original paper by Sheinberg and Logothetits carefully, we find that they recorded changes in the firing rate of fifty single cells in an 8×8 mm^2 cortical area. This is a rather narrow sample of all the potentially recordable cells in that area (hundreds of thousands of cells and millions of synapses). As the retinal images of even small objects will activate thousands of cells, the sample of fifty neurons must be only a tiny fraction of the cells activated by or participating in the construction of visual awareness.

Single-cell recordings furthermore involve a general methodological problem in sampling neuronal activity. When the microelectrode is inserted into the brain, its tip should be located so that it picks up the signals from some clearly isolable neurons. However, some types of neurons are more easily found in this procedure than others. Consequently, the recorded cells may form a biased sample, a subpopulation of particularly responsive cells that allowed clear isolation during the recording. What the neurons that are not so easily isolable are doing remains unclear.

Even so, the crucial issue is this: In single cell recordings, is it possible to acquire data that directly reflect the contents of the phenomenal level? According to the master loop hypothesis, the phenomenal level is a higher level of bioelectrical organization, realized as complex patterns of neural synchrony in corticothalamocortical loops. Patterns at the phenomenal level are thus constituted by temporally coded (rather than rate-coded) neural activities in massive networks of cell populations (rather than at the level of single cells). Major portions of them lie below (rather than at) the cortex. As single cell recordings typically reflect rate-coded activities of single cells in the cortex, the data acquired do not directly reflect the large-scale bioelectrical patterns constituting the phenomenal level.

If the temporal coding hypothesis turns out to be true for the brain in general, and crucial for the realization of the phenomenal level in particular, how informative are single-cell studies where firing rates only are recorded? Features of temporal coding (synchronicity of neural signals) appear to be independent of firing rates. Thus, it may be that a measurement revealing firing rates is largely blind to the levels of organization based on synchronicity. For example, Friston and Frackowiak (1997) write that

> In short, one would like to be confident that whatever aspect of neuronal interactions are measured, they relate in some systematic way to a neuronal code. . . . From the perspective of neuroimaging the distinction between temporal coding and rate coding is important because it is conceivable that changes in temporal patterning of impulses can change without any necessary change in the rate of firing. (p. 493)

Also Singer (1999) notes the possibility of such a dissociation:

> However, when synchronization occurs on a fast time scale with correlation peaks narrower than the average interspike intervals, it can be entirely independent of discharge rate . . . internally generated synchrony can only be assessed by direct correlation analysis of simultaneously recorded neurons. (p. 54)

The dissociation between firing rate and synchronicity was demonstrated in a study of binocular rivalry in the cat. An increase was observed in the synchronicity of V1 neurons representing the winning stimulus in binocular rivalry, although *no change in firing rate was detected* (Engel et al., 1999). Consequently, a measurement of single-cell firing rates appears to be blind to the levels of electrophysiological organization where, according to the master loop hypothesis, the phenomenal level might be realized.

Furthermore, it appears that the data pertaining to single-cell firing rates are *not explanatorily adequate* for finding consciousness in the brain. We have no idea how the firing rate of an isolated neuron is supposed to contribute to a subject's phenomenology. Consequently, we have no clue how to reconstruct any aspect of the subject's phenomenology from the firing rate data alone. A direct explanatory connection between the single-cell data and the phenomenal level seems to be missing.

To illustrate this, let us consider what happens when during the binocular rivalry experiment, the monkey becomes aware of the image of a banana. At the same time particular cells in the temporal lobe can be observed to increase their firing rate. Even if this correlation holds time after time, we are none the wiser as to what exactly the firing of a particular cell contributes to the phenomenal level and how it delivers its contribution. If we prevented the cell from firing, would the visual percept in the monkey's phenomenology change in color or form or size or contrast or part-whole organization, or in some entirely different property? Or would it change at all? What is the *mechanism* whereby the firing modulates the subjective visual percept at the phenomenal level? There is no mechanistic model that would connect the single-cell level with the phenomenal level, revealing a direct explanatory interrelation. Nor is it easy to imagine how such a model could be constructed.

Single-cell firing rates that correlate with visual awareness, however, may justify the conclusion that the activity of the cells *somehow* contributes to the construction of consciousness. Certainly, that is a remarkable result in itself, an important first step in the search for consciousness in the brain. Still, the genuine discovery and explanation of the phenomenal level will require much more than that.

The gap between single-cell data and consciousness is a gap between different levels of organization. When firing rates are recorded from single cells, electrophysiological activity is being observed at a *very* low level of neural organization. The data reveal isolated activities of the elementary microlevel parts in the brain. The phenomenal level resides several levels higher up in the hierarchy.

If the master loop hypothesis has any truth to it, then research instruments sensitive to the patterns of oscillatory synchrony in corticocortical and thalamocortical loops are required. It seems plausible that at least thousands, if not millions, of cells will be participating in the construction of the pattern underlying, say, a coherent phenomenal object. Only data that allow the reconstruction of those patterns might ever pass the dream catcher test.

Rat Dreams Discovered in the Brain?

We shall now return to the fascinating experiment about rat dreams, introduced briefly in chapter 17 (Louie and Wilson, 2001). It was publicized in the popular press which reported that the researchers could tell, on the basis of brain measurements from sleeping rats, what the rats were dreaming about. Certainly, the experiment requires a closer analysis. What exactly was measured, and on what basis was the content of the rats' dreams inferred from the measurements?

As *Newsweek* reported (5 February 2001), the researchers could tell precisely what part of the maze the rats dreamed they were in. But one is left wondering how exactly they managed to achieve that miraculous feat. Did the scientists actually *find* the phenomenal level of organization in the rats' brains? Perhaps a reconstruction of their data showed the animals' virtual dream reality, where the rats' viewpoint was embedded within a complex spatiotemporally organized environment resembling the subjective perception of the maze.

The true story turns out to be not all that exciting. The researchers isolated multiple active pyramidal cells (the number ranged between eight and thirteen) in the awake rats' hippocampus while the rats were running in a circular maze in search of a food reward (this is called the RUN condition). When the animal was running in the maze, the recorded ensemble of cells displayed a characteristic pattern of spiking activity. The researchers deemed that pattern "a unique signature of the behavioral experience." The pattern of neural activity was strongly dependent on the animal's position in the maze.

Next, they recorded the activity of the same ensemble during REM sleep. Subsequently, they tried to find matches in the pattern of activity between the RUN and the REM recordings at the time scale of several tens of seconds. Forty-four percent of the REM episodes correlated significantly with RUN episodes. However, the match was not exact in the temporal scale: the REM pattern of activation tended to develop at a *slower* pace than that in the RUN episodes. Also, patterns of theta frequency activity in the hippocampus corresponded between the two states, which suggests that a similar internal state existed in both REM sleep and wakefulness.

These findings are very exciting, but unfortunately they fall short of conclusively showing what the rats dreamed about, or even that they dreamed at all. An alternative explanation suggests that the patterns of activation in the hippocampus reflect some entirely *nonconscious* encoding of information into hippocampal spatial maps. The corresponding activity during REM sleep accordingly reflects *nonconscious memory consolidation processes* rather than dreaming about the place. There is no reason to invoke the phenomenal level of organization to explain the data. No feature of the data can distinguish between the two alternative explanations, one of which is in terms of entirely nonconscious spatial processing, the other in terms of the phenomenal level and subjective experience.

One aspect of the data speaks against the dream hypothesis. The fact that the REM patterns tended to be slower than the RUN patterns means that if the rats were dreaming, their dreams must have unfolded in slow motion or in an altered time frame. While certainly a possibility, it is not supported by what we know about the sense of time in human dreams. In an ingenious experiment, human subjects estimated the passage of

10 seconds first in the awake state. Then they slept in the sleep laboratory. Their task was to become lucid during dreaming, and then estimate the passage of 10 seconds. As they were well-trained lucid dreamers, they were able to give voluntary eye movement signals, objectively detectable in the electro-oculograph, at the beginning and at the end of the 10-second period. Thus, the time estimations performed during wakefulness and lucid dreaming during REM sleep could be directly compared with each other and with objective timing. No significant distortion of the sense of time during REM sleep dreaming was noted in these studies (LaBerge, 1990). In other studies, small electric shocks were given to subjects in REM sleep, after which they were awakened and asked to estimate how long ago they were stimulated (30 seconds or 3 minutes). Almost every time the subjects chose the right answer (Pivik, 1991). At least in humans, dreams appear to unfold at the same pace as waking experience, not in slow motion or in an altered time frame.

The main problem with the rat dream hypothesis is this: The cell activity recordings only allow the tracking of the representational content of neural activity patterns, not the reconstruction of the phenomenal content (if any) associated with them. To say that a subject—even if only a puny rat—is dreaming about *being in a certain place* is to state that there is a specific pattern realized at the phenomenal level in the subject's brain. To establish that a pattern of neural activity during REM reveals a specific dream content in the subject's consciousness requires that not only the representational contents of neural activity but the phenomenal contents of consciousness can be directly reconstructed from the data.

This is *not* to say that experiments such as that of Louie and Wilson (2001) are worthless. On the contrary, they give us good reasons to believe that the rat's brain re-creates an internal state closely resembling the awake state during REM sleep. Certainly, the data are *consistent* with the interpretation that the rats dream about something, and maybe even about running their maze. Unfortunately it cannot exclude the possibility that the activity recorded is entirely nonphenomenal, not accompanied by any experiences at all. Tracking the representational content of the firing rate of even multiple cells does not provide us with an explanation of how the phenomenal level emerges from such activity, or even show conclusively that it emerges at all.

The recording of firing rate patterns from about ten individual neurons is not sufficient to a dream catcher method. It probably does not even come very close to being such a thing. A much larger number of cells would probably have to be recorded, and the recordings should not be restricted to firing rates or to hippocampal neurons. Such an achievement is going to be technically very difficult, and therefore attempts to identify synchronous assemblies are still at the very beginning:

> Thus, if it is the case that the generation of the metarepresentations required for consciousness involves the organization of highly distributed assemblies, we are a long way from the direct iden-

tification of the neuronal correlates of even the simplest forms of consciousness. (Singer, 2000, p. 134)

Extracranial Electrical (EEG) and Magnetic (MEG) Recordings

Electroencephalography and magnetoencephalography are popular methods in cognitive neuroscience, and also in the search for the neural correlates of visual awareness (e.g., Vanni, Revonsuo, Saarinen, & Hari, 1996; Revonsuo et al., 1997; Tallon-Baudry & Bertrand, 1999; Koivisto & Revonsuo, 2003; Wilenius-Emet et al., 2004). But what is the nature of the signals that we pick from the brain with EEG and MEG? What levels of organization in the brain do they reflect?

EEG and MEG detect large-scale electrophysiological phenomena in the brain, and they are capable of doing this with the fine temporal resolution of a millisecond. EEG detects the changes in the electrical fields of the brain as reflected at the scalp; MEG detects the changes in the magnetic fields that accompany electrical phenomena in the brain.

This sounds very promising, for here we are dealing with electrophysiological phenomena at a high temporal resolution. According to the master loop hypothesis, the phenomenal level is a complex and rapidly changing electrophysiological phenomenon at a high level of organization in the brain. Can EEG and MEG thus discover the phenomenal level in the brain?

The electrical potentials and magnetic fields detectable by EEG and MEG outside the skull are believed to be determined by the net current from postsynaptic potentials produced by pyramidal cell apical dendrites. For a typical detectable response to be generated, simultaneous activation of about 10^7 synapses in a cortical area of 1 cm^2, altogether containing about 10^{10} synapses, is sufficient. The neuroelectrical sources are assumed to be dipoles that have a positive and a negative pole in opposite directions from the source. MEG, however, is only sensitive to a subset of such sources: tangentially oriented, superficial neuroelectric sources, mostly located in cortical sulci. Only that kind of neuroelectric source generates a detectable magnetic field outside the head where the recording instrument resides. EEG is most sensitive to radially oriented neuroelectric sources in cortical gyri, but not completely blind to tangential sources either. EEG signals are spatially spread when they are conducted through tissues and skull onto the scalp surface where the sensors are placed. By contrast, MEG signals do not suffer from spatial blurring (Nunez, 1995) (figure 20.1).

Unfortunately, the electrical potentials or magnetic fields recorded outside the skull do not carry any definite information about their point of origin within the brain. Furthermore, it is mathematically impossible to determine the location of the actual electrical sources in the brain with any certainty if we only know the distribution of the electrical or magnetic field as it appears outside the skull. Any given field pattern

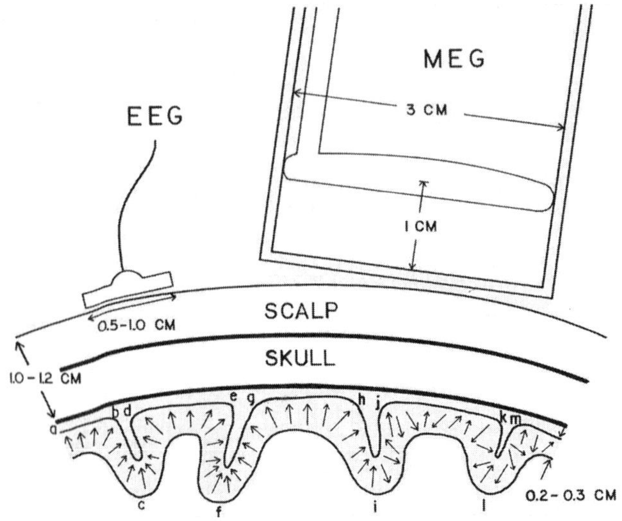

Figure 20.1
EEG and MEG signal sources. The scalp EEG sensor electrode is separated by over 1 cm from the cortical surface. The scalp, the skull, and various membranes stand between the sensor and the brain's electrophysiological phenomena. EEG is most sensitive to correlated dipole layers in gyri, such as in *a–b, d–e,* and *g–h;* it is less sensitive to correlated dipole layers in sulci such as *h–i,* and completely insensitive to opposing dipole layers in sulci such as *b–c–d* and *e–f–g,* and to randomly oriented dipole layers, such as *i–j–k–l–m.* The MEG sensor coil is separated by at least 2 cm from the cortical surface. MEG is most sensitive to correlated dipole layers in sulci, such as *h–i,* and much less sensitive to all other sources. (From Nunez, P. L. (1990) Physical principles and neurophysical mechanisms underlying event related potentials. In J. Rohrboush, R. Johnson, & R. Parasuraman (Eds.), *Event-related potentials of the brain* (pp. 19–36). New York: Oxford University Press. © Oxford University Press, Inc. Used by permission of Oxford University Press.)

outside the skull could have been brought about by an infinite variety of different current source generators. Mathematically, there is no way to go back from the observed pattern outside the skull to the ones inside the brain that actually brought about the neuroelectric phenomena. This drawback is known as the *inverse problem.*

Consequently, the neural generators need to be *modeled.* Typically a single dipolar source is assigned to a certain location in a model of the head. Then the correspondence is calculated between the model and the actual observations of the electrical or magnetic field. When the correspondence becomes good enough (i.e., the assigned sources create a field outside the head closely similar to the one that was actually observed), then the researcher *assumes* that the sources were where the model shows them to be. Thus, the source model is basically an educated guess as to how many dipolar sources there are, where they may be located, and what the time course of their activation is. Any of these assumptions might be wrong. The results of such modeling can, however, be presented in a graphical form by superimposing the assigned sources on a structural MR image of the brain. When looking at such an image we are easily led to believe that we can directly "see" how different parts of the brain activate or "light up" in response to certain types of stimuli.

EEG and MEG detect fast changes in the gross synchronous activity of millions of synapses in selected areas on the cortical surface. If the sources are too small or incoherently oriented or asynchronously activated, they do not generate any signals detectable with EEG or MEG. Of course, neuroscientists are well aware of these limitations:

> Even if the complete electric and magnetic field around the head could be measured precisely, an infinite number of current distributions in the brain could still be constructed that would explain the measured fields. For example, it is always possible that some sources are missed, whatever the measurement set-up . . . even when MEG is complemented with EEG, silent sources are possible. (Näätänen, Ilmoniemi & Alho, 1994, p. 391)

EEG and MEG signals can detect the presence, the temporal duration and the latency of large-scale synchronous events in the electrophysiology of the brain. EEG and MEG studies have revealed that gamma-band synchronization is associated with the perception of coherent objects in visual awareness (Tallon-Baudry & Bertrand, 1999). Still, there is a crucial difference between detecting the mere *presence* of a biological phenomenon and constructing a *model of its mechanistic details.*

For example, we could have some method that detects the presence or activity level of protein synthesis in different types of cells. Such a measurement would reveal one aspect of the internal "activity level" of the cells, or be a biological correlate of protein synthesis. But biologists would like to know more about protein synthesis than what such a correlation could ever convey. Even if we had a precise description of the "activity level" of every single cell of an animal, that would not amount to a description of the mechanistic details of how protein synthesis actually works. For that, we need a multilevel mechanistic model of the transcription and translation of DNA and RNA molecules to sequences of amino acids.

In a similar vein, the current brain-sensing and -imaging methods detect "brain activity" or even "synchronous neural activity" that correlates with conscious perception. Yet, descriptions of the level of activity do not amount to a description of the mechanistic details. How exactly does bioelectrical activity constitute complex spatiotemporal patterns within neural tissue? In what respects do those patterns correspond to the patterns of phenomenal experience? We should expect the multilevel mechanistic models of conscious perception to be at least as detailed and complex as the models that explain how all the thousands of different types of complex proteins are built up from amino acids within the cells of all living organisms.

What do EEG and MEG data reveal about the actual neural phenomena that generated the signals? The source models represent the center of gravity of the electrophysiological activity as a large featureless point on the surface of the cortex, typically superimposed on a structural MR image (e.g., Vanni et al., 1996). It is not possible to reconstruct from the data the actual spatiotemporal patterns of synchronicity within neural tissue that contributed to the detected signal. Therefore, it seems that it will not be possible to reconstruct any features of the phenomenal level of organization either, if that level is indeed based on the detailed patterns of large-scale coherent electrophysiological activity.

EEG and MEG data will not allow the *discovery of* the phenomenal level in the brain, in the strict sense of "discover." Neither of these methods in their present form constitutes a dream catcher. In fact, as half a century of studies on the EEG correlates of REM sleep and dreaming confirm, no aspects of the phenomenal content of dreams—of the organization at the phenomenal level during sleep—have so far been reliably reconstructed or predicted from the EEG signal recorded during dreaming. Only a general correlation between EEG and dreaming has been established. Across the different sleep stages, the more desynchronized the EEG (the more there is high-frequency activity with low amplitude), the greater the recall of dreaming and the more dreamlike the recalled material. But more detailed correlations between dream content and the EEG signal are hard to find. Even when a given EEG pattern is constantly maintained, there may be a large variation in both the incidence and quality of mental activity. Conversely, even when marked differences in EEG patterns exist, there may be only slight differences in dream recall (Pivik, 1991).

While it is unlikely that EEG or MEG would pass the dream catcher test, they are extremely useful in the search for the NCC. First, they can be used to demonstrate that there are detectable electrophysiological differences between the presence and the absence of subjective experience. As EEG and MEG can track electrophysiological events with high temporal resolution, they reveal the time windows in which conscious processing differs from nonconscious processing or when stimulus information enters consciousness (Koivisto, Revonsuo, & Lehtonen, in press). Furthermore, as phenomenal consciousness of a stimulus must precede reflective consciousness of the same stimulus, it may be possible to differentiate the correlates of phenomenal and reflective consciousness from each other. It should also be possible to differentiate the effects of attentional selection from the effects of consciousness as such (Koivisto, Revonsuo, & Salminen, 2005). The signals contain rich information about activity at different frequency bands, so it is possible to test, say, whether gamma-band activity is specifically associated with consciousness. Thus, despite their obvious limitations, many research groups, including my own, have used and will continue to use these methods in NCC research.

Functional Brain Imaging with PET and fMRI

No doubt PET and fMRI are the methods that have produced the most spectacular images of the brain. They show us which brain areas "light up" during binocular rivalry (Tong, Nakayama, Vaughan, & Kanwisher, 1998), visual hallucination (ffytche et al.,

1998), or dreaming (Maquet et al. 1996; Braun et al., 1998). Apparently, the images reveal what happens in the brain when subjective phenomenal experience is realized in consciousness. But what is actually shown in such images? Do we really "see" consciousness there, as a brightly colored area in a computer-generated slice of the brain?

EEG and MEG were found to be relatively gross methods for detecting the patterns of neural activity in the brain, and their ability to accurately localize of the origin of the signals was found to be poor. PET and fMRI are quite another story. They give relatively good spatial resolution: we can find out with reasonable accuracy *where* in the brain the signals that we detected were generated. The bad news is that temporal resolution is disastrously poor: we need to collect signals for a PET image for several seconds or even minutes. In fMRI the images can be generated somewhat faster, but still far too slowly to capture the rapid reorganization of phenomenal content at the millisecond scale.

A comment by Mazziotta (1996) on temporal resolution is relevant here:

> Turning to the speed of measuring biological events relevant to brain activity, an obvious and general rule may be offered. That is, the speed of the measurement must be faster than the speed of the biological event to obtain an accurate measure of it. (p. 397)

In the case of PET and fMRI trying to image consciousness, it appears to be just the opposite: the speed of the biological event (the reorganization of the phenomenal level when a new stimulus enters visual awareness) is typically *much* faster than the speed of the measurement.

However, the worst is yet to come. *Neither of these methods detects signals directly generated by neuroelectric activity.* Neither PET nor fMRI detects electrophysiological or bioelectrical signals. Instead, PET detects gamma rays that originate when a positron is annihilated in the brain. The positron is generated when a radioactive isotope in the tracer compound (say, radioactively labeled water or glucose analogue molecules) in the bloodstream decays. The distribution of the radioactive tracer reflects where blood flow or glucose metabolism increases in the brain, relative to a control condition. This distribution is supposed to give a general idea of "brain activation" in the experimental condition (figure 20.2).

In fMRI, it is the relative amount of oxygenated vs. deoxygenated blood that is being detected, for these two forms display slightly differing magnetic properties. fMRI signals originate in the vasculature where there is venous blood. Its oxygenation level rises during brain activity and thus brings about the fMRI signal. The signal is generated several steps away from actual neural activity. Heightened electrophysiological activity first leads to an increase in the local cerebral metabolism. Then the increase in the local metabolism leads to the increase in regional cerebral blood flow. The vascular supply where this response is realized is regulated at a spatial scale (0.5–1.5 mm in humans) that is several orders of magnitude larger than individual neurons. This fact limits the ultimate spatial resolution achievable with fMRI (Menon & Kim, 1999).

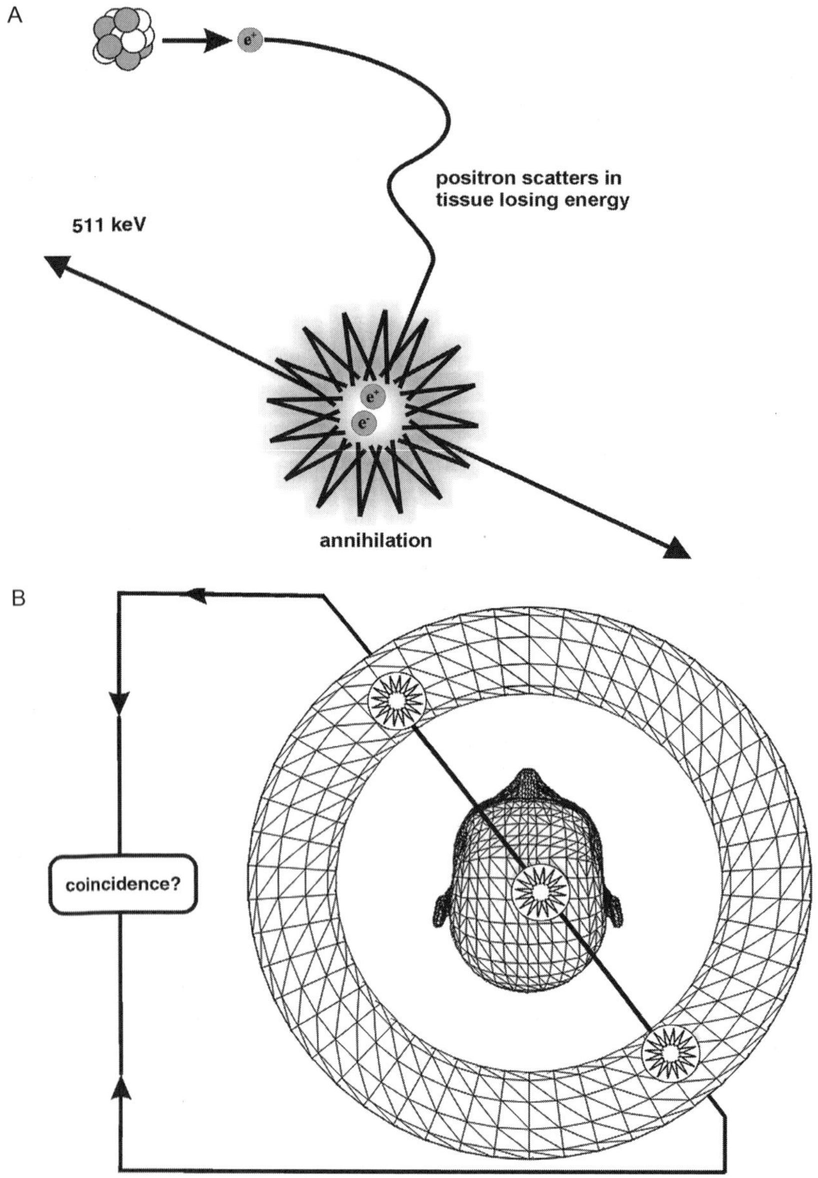

Figure 20.2
Positron emission tomography (PET). (A) A positron is emitted when the radioisotope (in the labeled tracer molecule) decays in the bloodstream or within brain tissue. The positron scatters randomly to the surrounding tissue, losing energy, until it collides with its antiparticle, an electron. Both are instantly annihilated, producing two gamma rays that travel in exactly opposite directions. (B) The PET scanner is a ring of gamma ray detectors. A signal is recorded when two gamma rays are detected simultaneously on exactly opposite sides of the head (coincidence detection). The signal defines a line of response along which the annihilation

PET and fMRI images are not images of neurons or neuroelectrical activity, but of changes in the *circulatory system* in the brain. The exact relationship between neuronal activity and the associated hemodynamic response is indirect and remains incompletely understood (Friston & Frackowiak, 1997; Logothetis & Wandell, 2004). In the temporal dimension, when neural activity increases in a location, there is a delay of several seconds before blood flow increases ("hemodynamic response function") (Turner, Howseman, Rees, & Josephs, 1997). The fMRI signal starts at 2 seconds and reaches its peak at about 13 seconds from stimulus onset (Menon & Kim, 1999).

The fMRI signal seems to be significantly correlated with a particular aspect of neural activity, the same aspect as is measured by local field potentials (LFPs). They reflect the *input* to an area rather than the action potentials generated within that area (its output) (Logothetis & Wandell, 2004). Therefore it might be possible to detect an fMRI signal in an area that has no electrophysiological single-unit activity (i.e., where the neurons are not firing, although they are receiving signals from other neurons).

Mazziotta (1996) characterizes the relationship between electrophysiological events and the signals actually detected by functional imaging in the following way:

> . . . indirect measures of variables, such as cerebral blood flow and volume . . . are assumed to be both delayed and dispersed relative to the electrophysiological event that initiates them. In addition, the coupling between such events may not always be tightly linked either in magnitude or in timing. (p. 397)

The colorful computer-generated images produced by PET and fMRI are not "images of mind" (Posner & Raichle, 1994) or, strictly speaking, even "neuroimages," but rather "images of blood flow" or "blood oxygenation levels" in the brain. Or, in fact, they are statistical color-coded maps of changes in blood flow or oxygenation level. These maps are typically superimposed on structural MRI images, which mostly reflect proton densities of different tissues, and give good spatial resolution and contrast beween different tissues.

If we assume that increased blood flow in an area reflects increased neuronal activity there—a well justified assumption—then we can safely say that PET and fMRI images can be used to localize activated brain areas during different tasks. After all, that is why they are widely used in cognitive neuroscience. But the specific *theoretical* question that interests us in the present discussion is whether these images reveal the levels of biological organization where consciousness is likely to be realized. The answer to this question is negative. First, neuroimaging may be insensitive to temporal codes (neural

happened. A combination of lines of response from several different angles are used to construct cross-sectional images that reflect the concentration of the positron-emitting compound in the tissue. (Modified from Cherry, S. R. & Phelps, M. E. (1996). Imaging brain function with positron emission tomography. In A. W. Toga & J. C. Mazziotta (Eds.), *Brain mapping, the methods* (pp. 191–221). San Diego: Academic Press. © 1996, with permission of Elsevier, Inc.)

synchronization), because the hemodynamic responses are probably largely functions of the rate of firing:

> What then are the implications of this conclusion [that the brain uses temporal codes] to neuroimaging? If our measurements are sensitive only to discharge rate, they are potentially blind to a whole temporal dimension of neuronal discourse. In short, we could be measuring the wrong thing. (Friston & Frackowiak, 1997, p. 494)

Second, nobody believes that consciousness is realized in blood flow or within the circulatory system in the brain. An image of the spatial volumes (voxels) where blood flow increased in a "conscious" as compared to a "nonconscious" condition may give us a clue about the anatomical location of neural populations that increase their firing rate in the "conscious" condition. It is not an image directly depicting those neurons, and even less is it an image depicting the complex electrophysiological patterns that are generated by, say, fast synchronous oscillations in those neurons. It is simply impossible to derive, from those kind of data, the organization of the electrophysiological phenomena assumed to constitute the phenomenal level. Consequently, it is equally impossible to arrive at a multilevel mechanistic model of the phenomenal level by looking at hemodynamic responses only.

Are there any new technological developments around the corner that will solve these problems? There is no doubt that fMRI is rapidly developing, that single-event fMRI is becoming more and more popular, and that the fastest imaging techniques can make a single image in 50 milliseconds. However, it is of little help to be able to make an image very rapidly as long as the event being imaged, the hemodynamic response itself, remains much slower. There may be one way to get around that problem: There is a small early negative hemodynamic response at 500 milliseconds (Ernst & Henning, 1994) that can be detected with fMRI. It could provide us with better temporal and spatial resolution. So far there are few studies that have actually managed to utilize this response (but see Duong, Kim, Ugurbil, and Kim [2000]), and even if it could be utilized in NCC experiments with humans, the images are still directly based on vascular, not electrophysiological, events. The same basic limitation applies also to the fast early hemodynamic response: the presence or organization of patterns of synchronous neural activity cannot be deciphered from images of vascular events.

Brain imaging has further methodological limitations (Revonsuo, 2001a; Van Orden & Paap, 1997; Stufflebeam & Bechtel, 1997), such as the use of relative, not absolute, measures. Typically, one condition is subtracted from the other, and only the difference is reported. The brain maps where areas neatly "light up" in all colors of the rainbow actually show the results of complex statistical comparisons between the experimental and control conditions. The "lighting up" is in most cases just a way to present the statistically significant pixels or voxels in a color-coded scale. When a brain area lights up in the brain map of an imaging experiment, we are not really witnessing a phenomenon of nature as such (as we might by looking into the microscope or telescope). The maps do not show the actual phenomena, but only the probabilities that the tracer molecule density or the MR signal was significantly different in one condition as compared to another one at the coordinates represented by the spatial arrangement of the pixels. What lights up in the PET and fMRI brain maps are the statistical P-values reflecting changes in blood flow or oxygenation levels, not neurons or consciousness.

The interpretation of the relative differences in brain activation is extremely difficult. Brain images only reveal that during the experimental condition, a region is more active than it was in the control condition. This can be interpreted as showing that the activated regions are *somehow* involved in the task, but they show nothing about *how* the task is done or *what* the activated area is doing. Since the PET measurement itself only reveals that a part of the brain is "active" during the performance of the task, the clues as to *what* that part is doing *must come from elsewhere.* To link structure and function, a task analysis or decomposition must be made with the help of an explicit cognitive model of the cognitive functions in question. But in that case the task decomposition will critically depend on the cognitive model one chooses to use, and usually there is no single, universally accepted model available. Consequently, the PET data and the subtractions made are interpreted in the light of the chosen model. However, different decompositions or models of the same cognitive function will yield entirely different interpretations of the same data, or lead to entirely different experimental designs. Thus, PET experiments and data are always subject to multiple interpretations depending on the cognitive models used, because the data in themselves do not reveal what the area is doing (Stufflebeam & Bechtel, 1997).

In their paper "PET: Exploring the Myth and the Method," the philosophers Stufflebeam and Bechtel (1997) conclude:

> Merely finding increased blood flow in areas of the brain during performance of a particular task does not reveal the function of that locus . . . PET only shows that a part of the brain is active during the performance of a particular task. It cannot give any direct indication of exactly what that part is doing. (pp. 99–100)

All these facts point to the conclusion that the underlying neurophysiological levels of organization cannot be reconstructed from signals acquired by using PET or fMRI. Therefore, these methods (at least in their present form) cannot uncover the phenomenal level of organization in the brain.

Prospects for the Discovery of Consciousness

Consciousness, or the phenomenal level of organization, probably resides at higher levels of complex electrophysiological and bioelectrical phenomena in the brain. We have few theories describing how such phenomena might be organized at the levels of millions of interacting cells in widely distributed cell populations. A conjecture of at least some plausibility depicts the phenomenal level as a dynamically changing master loop of coherent recurrent activity at the intersection of multiple thalamocortical and corticocortical processing loops.

Currently no methods exist for directly imaging (or otherwise capturing empirically) the levels of electrophysiological organization in the brain that would allow the reconstruction of the contents of a subject's consciousness.[2] The brain data we have available do not allow outlining a multilevel model of the phenomenal level and its relation to other biological levels of organization in the brain. Thus, for the time being, discovering consciousness in the brain is not feasible.

I have been perhaps overly critical of the methods of cognitive neuroscience. But it should be noted that this critical analysis only applies as far as the *literal discovery* of the phenomenal level of organization in the brain is concerned. I have only tried to figure out whether our current research instruments could be used as dream catchers. Although they cannot, they are wonderful research instruments for many other purposes all the same. My purpose thus is *not* to argue that all the current methods of cognitive neuroscience are totally useless for consciousness research. On the contrary, brain sensing and imaging do reveal many interesting (but indirect) *correlations* between brain activity and consciousness.

For the time being we will have to base our theories and models of the neural basis of consciousness on the correlations between neural activity and subjective experience. My message is, We can make progress with the currently available technology, but we won't reach our final destination with it. My claim can be summarized in the following way:

> The brain-sensing and -imaging methods currently available in cognitive neuroscience are limited in that they cannot take us *all the way* to the actual discovery of the neural *constituents* of consciousness.

This claim should *not* be confused with another, much stronger claim, which I explicitly reject:

> The brain-sensing and -imaging methods currently available in cognitive neuroscience are limited in that, by using them, we cannot make *any* significant progress in the study of the neural *correlates* of consciousness.

Certainly, we *can* make progress in NCC research, but we should also bear in mind that the results of the research do not amount to the literal discovery of consciousness. None of the data we get from the current research instruments can reveal a level of organization in the brain that would somehow correspond to our phenomenology, and we should not even expect them to find any such thing. The correlations we have detected are not sufficient for the construction of a multilevel model of consciousness, because the phenomena that constitute the sources of the signals (e.g., blood oxygenation levels, single-cell firing rates) detected by our best currently available research instruments are rather distant from the phenomenal level. Still, even the currently available signals might contain correlative information revealing when the phenomenal level is "on" and when it is "off" (say the difference between the conscious vs. unconscious state during anesthesia), or when a conspicuous change occurs in its global content (say during binocular rivalry). But this information, though very exciting in itself, is still hopelessly indirect and coarse for the purpose of building a detailed theoretical model.

In the philosophy of science, it has been noted that the development of science depends at least as much on new research instruments as it does on new ideas (Giere, 1988). Many biological phenomena could not have been discovered without the proper equipment and the development of very specific methods. For example, the complex internal structure of the mitochondrion could only be discovered with the electron microscope. Before the appropriate methodology was available the complete explanation of biological respiration and oxidative phosphorylation remained unknown (Bechtel & Richardson, 1992). In cognitive neuroscience, both our theories about the large-scale organization of brain activity and our instruments to observe such phenomena are still quite limited. Even if we forget about consciousness for the moment, there is a lot to be discovered in the brain. New methods and theoretical frameworks will be necessary to make those discoveries. We should not overestimate the state of our current understanding or the capabilities of the currently available research instruments; we are only beginning to open some restricted empirical windows to the living brain.

The difficulty in discovering and explaining consciousness is due to our crude research instruments and lack of established theories in neuroscience rather than to the mystical nature of consciousness. I am *not* implying that discovering consciousness in the brain is impossible in principle. I merely want to point out that even if consciousness turns out to be a real biological phenomenon in the brain, even our best research instruments are not *yet* capable of discovering empirically the relevant biological levels of organization in the brain.

Summary

A survey of the principal methods in the cognitive neuroscience of consciousness was conducted. The biological signals detected by invasive microelectrodes, extracranial electromagnetic measures (EEG, MEG), and functional brain imaging (PET, fMRI) do not allow reconstruction of the phenomenal level in the brain. Thus, none of them in their present form is a viable candidate for dream catcher, a method whose data would directly mirror the contents, organization, and dynamics of the phenomenal level. Present neuroscience should not be expected to discover the phenomenal level. If the research instruments evolve further, the discovery of consciousness may become feasible.

21 The Future Explanation of Consciousness

Ideally, neuroscience should provide us with a complete theoretical model of the mind-brain. It would describe all the levels of organization residing in the brain and explain their interrelations. In the complete multilevel model of the brain, the phenomenal level and its constitutive mechanisms would *have to* be included as well.

Theoretical modeling of all the different levels of organization in the brain requires access to empirical data from each level. If only neuroscience had the methodology that is required to access *every single level of organization in the brain,* then the phenomenal level and its constitutive mechanisms would *necessarily* be discovered as well. At present, we are incapable of making all the required discoveries due to the methodological limitations discussed in the previous chapter. Nonetheless, it should be possible to *imagine* the *general outline* of the required discoveries and explanations. Thought experiments might give us a clue as to how the problem of consciousness could be eventually solved through empirical means.

In this chapter we examine future prospects for the discovery and explanation of consciousness. First, if a merely unintelligible correlation between the neural and the phenomenal will not suffice for an explanation, then what would? Second, when we try to discover a particular phenomenon in the brain, we should have a clear idea of what such a phenomenon is supposed to look like. The neuroscience of consciousness is trying to find the subjective *world-for-me* in the brain, but what exactly does a subjective world *look like* from an objective vantage point? Third, what exactly would be required of a brain-sensing or -imaging method for it to acquire data directly from the phenomenal level in the brain?

The exploration of these issues will gradually lead us toward a vision of a future science of consciousness where the phenomenal level is but one level of biological organization among others in a multilevel model of the mind-brain.

The Explanatory Power of Models

We already know what would *not* count as a genuine explanation of consciousness: unintelligible correlations between phenomenal facts and neural facts. They are the *data* that require explanation, not the explanation. According to biological realism, phenomenal and neural facts refer to different levels of organization in the brain. In the multilevel framework of explanation, the observed correlations between lower- and higher-level phenomena are theoretically explained by multilevel mechanistic models. The theoretical model shows how and why the two types of phenomena are empirically correlated in the first place; it establishes the required intelligible connection between them.

In the multilevel framework, a theoretical explanation thus comes in the form of a detailed model of the explanandum. But what exactly is it that provides a model with genuine explanatory power? It seems that fruitful theoretical models possess two vitally important characteristics. First, a truly explanatory model must be related in an appropriate way to the *reality* being modeled. Second, the model must be properly related to the *human mind.* The explanatory power of the model is based on fulfilling these two relationships simultaneously.

Let us first consider the relationship to reality. In the philosophy of science, a naturalistic approach regards explanation as *a relation between models and reality* (Giere, 1988). Theoretical models in science are abstract entities that describe and explain (aspects of) real phenomena out there in the world. They manage to do this because the models bear a *similarity relationship* to the real entities out there that they are models of. Similarity is always a matter of degree: the strongest form of similarity would be perfect isomorphism between the model and the real phenomenon. That is usually too strong a requirement, not met by any actual models in science (Giere, 1988).

One major goal in scientific model-building thus is to reach as close a similarity relationship as possible with the modeled phenomenon. Ideal scientific models should be constructed with this requirement in mind. The major features and relations of the entities at any particular level of organization should be reproduced or closely mirrored by the model depicting that level. The larger the amount of features and relations taken into account by the model, and the closer the similarity relationship between the model and the reality, the closer the model is to being the perfect model of the phenomenon.

Similarity to reality cannot be the *only* criterion for scientific model-building, though. If it were, one serious problem would arise. It would lead to the absurd conclusion that the perfect model of a phenomenon must be a perfect *duplicate* of the phenomenon itself! That would make modeling easy, but explanation difficult. The perfect model of a biological organism could be constructed by simply cloning the organism. But if one aims to *understand* how a cell works, duplicating the cell and calling it the perfect model would hardly be of any help.

Thus, an explanatory model must fulfill further requirements. Explanation does not just consist of relations between models and reality; it also involves a relationship to human cognitive activity. The explanation of a phenomenon should be accompanied by an *understanding* of how the phenomenon works. For a model to increase human understanding, the model must represent reality in a manner that renders the otherwise inaccessible features of reality directly *accessible* to human consciousness.

A model with genuine explanatory power, when consciously apprehended by the scientist, is experienced as a pattern of phenomenal features in consciousness. The model as a stimulus thus creates its own surrogate object at the phenomenal level. The surrogate in consciousness opens up specific, appropriate semantic windows. Thus, semantic-conceptual knowledge is being attached to the surrogate. For example, knowledge about DNA and its chemical constituents is brought to consciousness when one appreciates a macroscopic model of the double helix molecular structure.

Understanding is conscious mental activity. Explaining and understanding natural phenomena cannot happen without consciousness being involved in the process. Even a perfect model, if totally inaccessible to conscious minds that could use it for understanding the phenomenon, is no explanation. To constitute an explanation, a model must be interpretable by the scientist *as* a model of a certain phenomenon. He must be able to cognitively construe in his conscious mind how the entities, interactions, and causal processes depicted by the model are supposed to work in reality.

Explanatory Models: Mirrors of Reality Accessible to Conscious Understanding

An ideal model thus mirrors reality as closely as possible, but at the same time the model is easily accessible to the human cognitive system. An ideal level of description in science depicts the corresponding level of organization in reality in the following way: The structure, organization, dynamics, and the constitutive and causal relationships of entities at that level are preserved in the model. At the same time, the model can be appreciated and comprehended by human observers. I call this view of mechanistic explanation the *mirror metaphor of explanation.* According to it, models that yield genuine explanations in the biological sciences are, at bottom, *cognitively accessible accurate mirrors of nature.* Like images reflected in a mirror, they convey the structure, organization, and dynamics of the phenomena they reflect. Like mirrors, they render the otherwise hidden corners of the world accessible to us.

Multilevel mechanistic models in the biological sciences fulfil the requirements of the mirror metaphor. Typically, the models employ analogical, visualizable, macroscopic representations of complex microlevel mechanisms. This modeling strategy is evident already at the chemical levels of description. Macromolecules with complicated 3D structures are modeled by macroscopic images or simulations that preserve the 3D configuration. The spatial structure of protein molecules, for example, would be impossible to grasp without such explicit analogical models. The models may be even concrete stick-and-ball constructions. The double helix of the DNA molecule is often presented in that way. In fact, Watson and Crick utilized the stick-and-ball approach as tools of thought when they first discovered the structure of DNA. Nowadays molecular and other complex microstructures are more efficiently depicted by 3D computer simulations that may be visualized from any angle.

Even the structural formulas of chemical substances may be regarded as rough analogical representations of the molecular structure, or as schematic topological and geometrical representations of the molecules (Del Re, 1998). The symbol for benzene, for example, directly reflects the spatial structure of the molecule: six carbon atoms forming a ring, connected to each other by three single bonds and three double bonds.

While it is true that molecules could in principle be fully described by quantum-mechanical equations, and their behavior in principle fully predicted with the help of quantum mechanics, in practice those descriptions are not workable. The problem with them is that they are not accessible to the human cognitive system. It would be immensely demanding to formulate the quantum-level descriptions of chemical events. Even if they could be constructed, it would probably be humanly impossible to comprehend them. Thus, they would not count as explanatory models of the phenomena, because they violate one of the two main requirements of explanation. Although they might be accurate mirrors of nature, the images they reflect are in principle inaccessible to the human cognitive system. The visualizable, analogue models of molecular structure would anyway have to be used by scientists as tools for *really* understanding the mechanistic story behind chemical phenomena.

Therefore, when it comes to the phenomenal level, the ideal explanatory model should also fulfill the two requirements of the mirror metaphor. The multilevel model of consciousness should mirror reality as closely as possible, while retaining easy access to the scientist's conscious mind where it promotes understanding. The model that explains consciousness should, first, show similarity relationships to the real thing with respect to the structural, dynamical, and qualitative aspects of consciousness. Second, it should modulate the contents of the scientist's consciousness in such a manner that a transparent surrogate of the real thing is created in the scientist's own consciousness. The surrogate in consciousness consequently becomes connected to appropriate semantic-conceptual knowledge, and conscious understanding of the phenomenon follows.

Mechanistic explanation, at bottom, implies "seeing how a thing works." Certainly, according to the mirror metaphor of explanation, with the help of an appropriate model the scientist may literally *see* how something works. Consequently, we now know what would be required of a genuine explanation of consciousness, too. The explanatory model depicting the mechanisms of consciousness should allow us to literally *see* how the phenomenal level works in the brain.

Modeling Consciousness: A Hall of Mirrors?

Explaining consciousness might, however, be more tricky than explaining other biological phenomena. When consciousness is involved in understanding other phenomena, transparent surrogates depicting the phenomena can easily be created at the phenomenal level. To take a concrete example, when we visually observe a neuron in brain tissue (with the help of some complex research instruments and tissue preparations), what really happens, subjectively, is that we experience a certain structured pattern of phenomenal features at the phenomenal level in our own brain. The brain attaches a semantic interpretation to that pattern by opening the appropriate semantic windows. As we peer into the microscope and the pattern of phenomenal features clears up, takes color and shape, we suddenly realize that *that* pattern must be a single individual neuron.

We should remember that the pattern we experience is not as such the neuron. Instead, it is a pattern of phenomenal features, a semantic window in our own consciousness. The actual neuron is at the *other* end of the etiological pathway to consciousness; it is the first link in the causal chain that modulates the phenomenal content of consciousness.

Santiago Ramón y Cajal, the father of the neuron doctrine, was among the first persons to ever have had that kind of experience, which he described as follows:

> Against a clear background stood black threadlets, some slender and smooth, some thick and thorny, in a pattern punctuated by small dense spots, stellate or fusiform. All was sharp as a sketch with Chinese ink on transparent Japanese paper. . . . [A]ll was clear and plain as a diagram. A look was enough. Dumbfounded, I could not take my eye from the microscope. (Sherrington, 1935, cited in Gazzaniga et al., 2002, p. 11)

Now, applying this analysis to the empirical exploration of the phenomenal level itself, we get into some sort of a circle (but not a vicious one, I hope). It goes like this: A model of the phenomenal level is a model of a system in the brain that *itself* models or images the world, by constructing organized patterns of phenomenal features and by opening the corresponding semantic windows. A mechanistic model of the phenomenal level is, therefore, *a model of a world-modeling system in the brain.*

To explain consciousness, a theoretical model would be required that creates transparent surrogates in consciousness, only this time depicting consciousness itself! How could consciousness contain a transparent surrogate of itself? The mirror metaphor of explanation, when applied to consciousness, appears to leads us ever deeper into a hall of mirrors.

What Would the Phenomenal Level Look Like?

To find a way out from the hall of mirrors, we should figure out how a world-modeling system could be observed or modeled from the outside, by using "objective" methods and measurements. The incorrect image is to think of the phenomenal level as some sort of a concrete bubble-like space inside the brain, with a homuncular body image in the center, and then try to figure out how such a system of a "homunculus-inside-a-bubble" would look like from the outside.

Why is that image mistaken? Quite simply because the phenomenal level *only has an inside*! There is no way to "see" or "observe" it from the outside as if it were a real soap bubble, which *does* have an inside as well as an outside. It is possible to observe or model the phenomenal level *only from the egocentric perspective from which it is experienced.* The patterns of phenomenal properties are tied to the first-person perspective; no other perspective on the system is conceivable. Forcing any other perspective on the phenomenal level would violate the similarity relationship between the model and the reality.

The traditional "third-person perspective," however, invites the image that the observer is separated from the observed: out there under the lens is the specimen, the object of observation, and in here, at the other end of the microscope, is the scientist, the observer employing the third-person perspective on the phenomenon. The phenomenon, let us say a tissue preparation, is placed before the observer and, when consciously perceived, it gives rise to the appropriate semantic windows in his consciousness.

But when we "observe" or model consciousness itself, the traditional observer/object distinction cannot be applied. Because the phenomenal level has a first-person ontology and an egocentric frame of reference, it would have to look like the subject's own *internal* point of view, not like an outsider's external point of view of a soap-bubble miniature model of the world. There is no phenomenal bubble inside the brain that could be "opened" from the outside like a shell to see into the phenomenal level hidden inside the shell. On the contrary, the data structures that directly reflect the phenomenal level should reconstruct the patterns and organization of phenomenal features from the subject's egocentric point of view.

This conception should be kept in mind when the phenomenal level is empirically sought for in the brain. To be able to tell whether or not some sample of brain data depicts the phenomenal level, *we must know what such a thing would look like.*

What Would Be Required of the Method That Can Capture the Phenomenal Level?

The method that acquires data from the phenomenal level would have to access patterns of coherent electrophysiological activity in corticocortical and thalamocortical loops. To imagine what a future "consciousness-imaging" method might be like is to construct a piece of speculative fiction, but then, the currently available brain-sensing and -imaging methods would have been regarded as science fiction as recently as the 1950s. Thus, it may be that today's science fiction is tomorrow's standard scientific procedure.

Somehow, the method would have to collect signals that originate in the organized patterns of large-scale electrophysiological activity. The signals should preserve fine-grained information about the spatial organization and the temporal dynamics of the patterns. Hence the signals would have to *trace* those patterns and *originate from* them. I have no idea how such patterns could be traced, and I fear that neither does anybody else.

Nonetheless, let us assume for the moment that there will be some way to do it. Perhaps one day it will be possible to develop *electrophysiological tracers* that reveal the organized patterns of bioelectricity realized in reentrant loops. The basic idea could be analogous to PET tracers, but rather than spreading through the bloodstream to oxygen- and glucose-hungry neurons in the brain, the dream catcher tracers would spread selectively along with the patterns of coherent electrical activity. The distribution of the tracer, as well as the signals acquired, would reflect the spatiotemporal organization of the bioelectrical patterns. Separate tracers would be used for different frequency ranges or for different types of coherent activity, so that several independent, organized patterns, realized by distinct activities, could be revealed at the same time.

When we imagine this method, we should remember the basic principle of biological measurement: the speed of the measurement must be faster than the speed of the biological event under observation to obtain an accurate measure of it. Therefore, the temporal resolution of the method would have to be at the very least less than 100 milliseconds. Thus, the dream catcher should be capable of creating a full image of the large-scale coherent electrophysiological patterns, or recording the full range of data, more than ten times per second. The global patterns of organized bioelectrical activity that constitute the phenomenal level change at about the rate of once in 100 to 300 milliseconds. On the other hand, the synchronous oscillations on which the phenomenal level is based at the underlying microlevels are probably within the gamma range (20–80 Hz). To capture the dynamics of the phenomenal level and its underlying micromechanisms, the recording must be capable of distinguishing between different patterns at least at that rate. The temporal resolution of the recording must be at least as high as the rate of reorganization of the phenomenal level.

The spatial resolution of the method would have to be such that the constitutive mechanisms of any two different points or regions in the phenomenal coordinate system can be told apart from each other. It is difficult to say what that comes to in terms of spatial scale in the brain. What is the objective spatial scale in which the subjective just-noticeable differences of spatial location are realized within the phenomenal level? We may speculate that it must be coarser than the spatial scale of single neurons, but certainly much finer than the scale of 1 mm^3. The scale of the bioelectrical events, however, may not be directly comparable to the scale of the structural neural building blocks that support the activity. The only thing we can be sure about is that it does not hurt to have as fine a spatial resolution as possible.

Let us assume that the dream catcher samples data at the rate of 100 Hz, and it can resolve spatial details in that activity that take place in volumes of space at around 0.0001 mm^3. The signals it collects originate at levels where organized electrophysiological patterns are realized in recurrent loops of coherent activity. The dream catcher thus must be capable of scanning the whole 3D volume of the cerebrum simultaneously and it must be able to collect signals from a wide range of different frequencies across the whole brain, especially in corticocortical and thalamocortical loops.

It goes without saying that the complexity of the data collected by the dream catcher is monstrous. How could anybody make any sense of such a data set? Well, the data collected by PET, fMRI, or MEG are also very complex (though they surely pale beside dream catcher data), but when properly processed, the results of the measurements can be presented in ways that are not all that difficult to interpret.

The way to think about the dream catcher project is to see it as a natural outgrowth of the branch of neuroscience now known by the name "brain mapping" (or "cartography of the brain"). Toga and Mazziotta (1996) note that maps are indispensable in several branches of science, for *a map can represent virtually our complete understanding of an object.* Cartography has become a way of organizing scientific data, representing it, and communicating results. The visualization of data and phenomena is an essential element in cartography.

Thus, brain mapping or cartography is just another aspect of the pervasiveness of the multilevel mechanistic approach and the mirror metaphor of explanation in neuroscience. Theories, multilevel models, and explanations of the brain are not clothed in sets of laws, propositions, or sentences, but in visualizations: 3D maps, diagrams, and computer animations representing the complex, multilevel organization of biological phenomena in the brain. It would be awkward to try to present the same information in a propositional form, and if presented in that way, it would most likely become entirely indecipherable, whereas a visualizable multilevel model can make an enormous amount of reality-mirroring data easily accessible to the scientist's cognitive system.

Progress in brain mapping is linked to advances in both of the two relations specified by the mirror metaphor of explanation. The models bear an ever closer relation to the biological reality inside the brain, due to advances in data acquisition from several different spatial and temporal scales and levels in the brain. The models furthermore are better and better accessed by the human cognitive system, due to advances in technical abilities to visualize and animate the images depicting complex neural phenomena in real time—or sometimes even in a slowed-down or otherwise altered time scale—with the help of computer technology.

The development in brain modeling seems to lead to ever more detailed visualization of data (and phenomena) in a meaningful spatial framework in a 3D volume. The goal is to construct realistic visualizable models that have high temporal and spatial resolution, include several different levels of description at the same time, and allow the scientist to move from one level of description downward to the lower-level mechanisms of a phenomenon or upward to its role as a component in higher-level mechanisms or backward in time to see the etiological causal chain that brought the phenomenon about. Currently we can already see combinations of anatomical and functional data in a 3D spatial framework; for example, how an electrical field (measured by high-density EEG) develops on the surface of the cortex (as depicted by a structural 3D-reconstructed MR image).

If brain mapping ultimately strives to create a map that represents virtually our complete understanding of the brain, then that kind of a map will have to include a description of the phenomenal level of organization as well. For such a project to succeed, more developed technology for the processing, visualization, and modeling of the data will be required. The phenomenal level includes an astronomical number of different kinds of phenomenal features and their combinations. The domain in which the data are presented should have a comparable variety of representational complexity. Visualization on a flat, 2D computer display, used for the visualization of the structure of complex macromolecules, will not be sufficient.

How could the representational complexity of data presentation be increased? One way to do it would be to engage not only the visual modality but also other sensory modalities. Thus, a full-scale multimodal virtual reality system may have to be used to "visualize" the phenomenal level of organization, just like a 3D spherical model of the Earth has to be used, rather than a 2D projection, to capture the physical reality of our planet realistically.

The Multilevel Modeling of Consciousness

The appropriate modeling system would produce more than "visualizations" of the data, because sensory modalities other than vision would have to be used as well. Hence, it would be more accurate to talk about "phenomenalizing" the data: translating it into all the different sensory modalities that we can experience. The model of the phenomenal level should show similarity relationships to the real thing with respect to the structural, dynamical, and qualitative aspects of consciousness. I suspect that it is very difficult to construct a model of the phenomenal level that bears the appropriate similarity relationships to phenomenal reality, *unless the phenomenal level itself is used as the output domain where the model is presented.*

The situation in a future Center for Phenomenal Neuroscience might look like this. Let us assume, in accordance with the dream catcher test, that the research group is trying to register the content of the subject's phenomenal level during dreaming. The researchers place the subjects in a whole-head dream catcher scanner for one night. Data are recorded during several REM sleep periods when the subjects are dreaming (i.e., when the phenomenal level of organization is realized in their brains). When a large enough database has been collected, analyses and modeling of the data begin. Instead of looking at EEG curves and 2D topographic current density maps on computer displays (like most present-day EEG researchers do), the phenomenal neuroscientists enter a multimodal simulator to explore and model the data. They start by modeling the lower levels of organization: the firing rates of small neural populations. The events can be presented as auditory, visual, or as multimodality, dynamic patterns, in a 3D anatomical frame of reference. They note that, during REM sleep, several neural populations are firing almost as actively as during the waking state, whereas others are shut down.

The team then proceeds to the modeling of the higher levels of coherent bioelectrical activity at multiple frequency bands, especially in corticocortical and thalamocortical loops. At the level of large-scale activity, involving millions of neurons in the cortex and thalamus, several coherent electrophysiological loops are observed to be in tight interaction with each other in the millisecond time scale. One of the coherent loops seems to be the cornerstone of the higher-level interaction. It enables the cooperation of all the other loops: its existence is necessary for the interaction to occur at all. This master loop of coherent activity is based on a constant oscillatory synchrony at high frequency, creating an overall unified *field* of activity.

The researchers set out to model this activity in more detail. They figure out that its lower-level neural generators are embedded in the thalamocortical matrix neurons. The model that makes the best overall fit for this coherent activity is in terms of a 3D, centered coordinate system.

The other patterns of activity that are in interaction with the master loop seem to be able to modulate its local states. One particularly interesting pattern of activity has a relatively fixed, centralized location in the coordinate system: all the other patterns contributed by the other loops seem to shift their position in the master loop in relation to this central pattern. That complex pattern is best made available for the researchers by transforming it into states of a whole-body data suit, so that its modeling can be conducted in terms of bodily sensations. The other patterns can be best modeled by using visual and auditory patterns in the multimodal simulation.

This multimodality phenomenalization of the data leads to a surprising effect. First, at the lower levels of organization, the researchers observed complex patterns of bioelectrical activity from the outside. But as they modeled the higher levels, they suddenly noticed that they were no longer in the midst of just another complex pattern of neurophysiological data. Instead, they found themselves in the middle of data patterns that started to look more and more like a perceptual *world.* At a higher level of electrophysiological organization, the data invited a particular interpretation. They could be optimally modeled as a single centered 3D coordinate system. It was best displayed for the researchers as a spatial egocentric frame of reference in the multimodal simulation.

Moving still one level up, they encounter what from the lower level seemed like the interaction of many recurrent loops of activity. Several organized patterns are found at this higher level. The spatiotemporal patterns of electrophysiological data are curiously reminisient of coherent objects, people, and a perceptual environment. However, the coherence of the organization of those patterns varies from moment to moment, suggesting that there is always a single central region with maximum coherence, and a more vague periphery where the patterns are less recognizable. Furthermore, there is a pattern of activity that lies in the origin of the coordinate system. When visualized, this data pattern looks like a human body, seen through the eyes of its owner. It contains the visual components of a body image. Another loop contributing to this activity can be transformed to somatosensory stimulation and it nicely coincides, in terms of coordinates of the basic loop, with the tactile components of the body image

Some parts of the data cannot be meaningfully modeled, especially the part that would have been located inside the body image in the coordinate system. The researchers wonder whether that might be because those data would need to be represented in a format not accessible for them to model: patterns of properties *inside* the body image: body sensations, emotions, inner speech, semantic interpretations of percepts, and so on. They see that an even more advanced phenomenalization of the data would have to be developed to capture all aspects of the modeled phenomenon at this level of organization.

After decades of progress in the field of phenomenal neuroscience, the next generation of researchers finally manage to solve the problem of how to present all the data in a form that respects the phenomenon to be modeled. They construct a *dream presenter* system, to display and model the data collected by the dream catcher. In the meantime they have figured out how the multiple loops of activity interact and contribute to the master loop. They have also noted that the relevant neurophysiological organization is very flexible, especially during REM sleep. The flexibility of electrophysiological patterns corresponds to the flexibility of subjective dream content: the body image of the dreamer may be unusual, the virtual objects may rapidly transform their shape, and the semantic windows opened by virtual objects may be quite dissimilar from the corresponding ones during waking, creating strange subjective interpretations of familiar patterns.

In effect, if it would be possible to bring about a REM-like state for a subject and control the construction and modulation of the master loop, then it would also be possible to make the subject experience a wide variety of phenomenal contents: a different kind of body, or any kinds of internal body sensations, or weird interpretations of and beliefs about the perceptual world, and so on. Presenting a data set in the dream presenter system would be equivalent to a controlled dream experience, or to a fully immersive virtual reality simulation where even internal experiences can be simulated. In the dream presenter, you can temporarily become somebody else and see the world not only through the eyes but through the body and the interpretations and memories of another person. And all this without any tampering with the anatomical structure of your brain. Modulating the complex electrophysiological patterns in your brain is sufficient, in a manner similar to what happens in your own dreams every night. After all, in our dreams, we sometimes experience, believe, and falsely remember the strangest things anyone could ever imagine.

Thus, you step into the ultimate dream presenter and want to phenomenalize the data collected from the phenomenal level of a dreaming subject. The dream presenter models the data by putting you into a REM-like state. Consequently, it takes control of the master loop in your own brain. You experience not only the visuospatial world of the dream, but you also interpret it exactly as the subject did; you have a body image identical to the one the original dreamer had, and in your mind the inner mental musings are present in the same way the subject experienced them when dreaming.

The only proper way to model the data recorded from the phenomenal level is to *translate it back to the states of the system that is surely able to present the data:* the phenomenal level. The dream presenter fulfils the requirements of the mirror metaphor of explanation: first, it faithfully mirrors the reality it is supposed to model, and second, it presents the data in a cognitively accessible way.

However, what makes the dream presenter an *explanatory* model of the phenomenal level is *not* simply its capability to *reproduce* in the observer the phenomenal contents of the subject. Make no mistake: sheer reproduction of a phenomenon does not entail explanation of the phenomenon.

In addition to just blindly mirroring reality, an explanatory model should make the structure, organization, temporal dynamics, and the causal and hierarchical relationships of the modeled phenomenon cognitively accessible for the scientists, so that they can see how the phenomenon works. The dream presenter can be used to construct a full-scale, multilevel mechanistic model of the phenomenal level of organization in the brain. Not only can the spatiotemporal patterns of phenomenal features be faithfully modeled but it is possible furthermore to move freely and smoothly between the different levels of organization surrounding the phenomenal level, across the different spatiotemporal scales, and forward and backward in the temporal dimension. These dimensions of the model correspond to the downward-looking (or constitutive), upward-looking (or contextual), and backward-looking (or etiological) explanations in mechanistic models.

Furthermore, it is possible to predict from the model what happens at the phenomenal level in different circumstances. If the lower levels of organization are somehow manipulated, as in altered states of consciousness or due to structural brain injury, it is possible to model the effects of the lower-level changes to the higher-level phenomenal organization. Conversely, if we have a detailed phenomenal description of the experiences of a brain-injured patient, then it will be possible to model the damage to the lower-level mechanisms that brings about exactly those types of changes at the phenomenal level. If an epileptic patient reports a particular experiential aura every time a seizure is about to start, or a patient with Charles Bonnet syndrome hallucinates faces in one part of the visual field, the multilevel mechanistic model should be able to illuminate the etiological and constitutive basis of these peculiar patterns and bundles of phenomenal features.

The dream presenter would be the ultimate multilevel mechanistic model of consciousness. It would reveal the hierarchical relationships between different levels of organization surrounding the phenomenal level, and the temporal evolution of events along the etiological pathway, causally modulating the phenomenal level. The ability to model interlevel and cross-level relationships, and to predict phenomenal consequences from neural facts (and vice versa) provide the dream presenter with genuine explanatory power.

Implications of Modeling Consciousness

Dream technology could not only acquire and display "observations" of a particular person's particular phenomenal states but it could also be used to construct general theoretical models of human phenomenology. Let us call the project of creating a universal model of the states and phenomenal contents of human consciousness the *Human Phenome Project.* Such a project would be feasible only if some sort of dream technology were available.

With the help of the dream catcher and the dream presenter, it would be possible to systematically model the whole range of possible states and contents of the phenomenal level. Thereby we will gain a better insight into what happens at the phenomenal level in, say, neglect, synesthesia, or apperceptive agnosia. Models of unusual phenomenal states could be constructed, and they could be appreciated by anybody through the dream presenter system. Again, the fully explanatory model of such distorted phenomenology will be a *multilevel* model, including models of the lower levels of organization and the etiological pathways to the phenomenal level. Thus, it would be possible to see how the coherent loops interact at the lower levels of organization or what happens at neural processing stages temporally preceding and modulating the phenomenal level. This would lead to an understanding of what goes wrong in the underlying and preceding nonphenomenal mechanisms when abnormal phenomenology results at the phenomenal level.

A proper model of the phenomenal level would provide us with a standardized map of the human phenome: the Human Phenome Project. Like the project of mapping the human genome, or the human brain, the Human Phenome Project would be an attempt to depict the general structure and organization of the phenomenal level in the human brain. Whereas information about the human genome can be printed on paper or displayed on a computer screen, information about the human phenome can be fully understood or communicated only when the output domain is a system of corresponding self-presenting features: another phenomenal level of organization.

One important difference between models of other biological phenomena and those of the phenomenal level is that in the phenomenal level there is a dimension not found in other systems. In a model of the phenomenal level, it is especially challenging to establish the similarity relationship between the model and the reality for that dimension. That is the *qualitative* dimension of phenomenal experience.

The notion of isomorphism does not seem to capture that dimension. A perfect model of some ordinary biological phenomenon could bear the relationship of perfect isomorphism to the real system. All parts of the model would stand in the same configuration to the whole model as all the parts of the real system stand to the whole real system. Thus, isomorphism concerns the structural features of the system and its model. But in the case of the phenomenal level, the structure and organization is built out of qualitative "parts"; therefore the perfect model of the phenomenal realm would not only have to be isomorphic but also "isoqualitative." All the phenomenal qualities in the model should stand in the same relation to each other and the whole model as all the phenomenal qualities in a real consciousness stand to each other and to the entire sphere of consciousness. Again, we end up with the view that the only way to present a scientific model that faithfully captures the reality is to use the phenomenal level itself as the modeling domain.

A traditional question in the philosophy of mind is whether phenomenal properties can be expressed in neurophysiological language. No, if by "neurophysiological language" one means the conceptual system of current neuroscience. But as I have tried to show, those descriptive systems will change, and the "language" of neuroscience will be more and more nonpropositional, involving visualizable models and systematic maps of different levels of organization in the brain. Thus, there will never be a simple identity statement for consciousness (or a set of such statements for different aspects of consciousness), such as, "The experience of blue = 40 Hz activity in XYZ-neurons." The immediately lower levels of description that underlie sensory-perceptual experience cannot be described propositionally. Their systematic description is feasible only in the form of a complex phenomenalized model. States of the phenomenal coordinate system are complex, dynamic electrophysiological patterns whose propositional description would be so long and so complicated that no one would ever be able to write it down. Or even if it could somehow be written down, no one would be able read or understand it. It would be about as impossible in practice as the description of the smallest unit of life, a single living cell, in terms of a chemical formula of the cell. No biologist would say that the ideal explanatory model of a living organism would be in the form of a long chemical formula describing every compound and biochemical process in the organism. In that sense, *a living organism as a unified whole cannot be described in the language of chemical formulas,* because no one could understand such a description. An explanation that no one can understand is hardly a good scientific explanation. Models of living organisms have to depict the higher-level structural components (e.g., organs, tissues, cells, organelles), their hierarchical composition and causal interactions. Chemical formulas come into play at lower levels.

In one sense it will be possible to express phenomenal properties in neurophysiological language if one accepts the fact that the "language" of neuroscience will be at least partly embedded in phenomenal experience: multilevel visualized and phenomenalized models will be used to communicate theoretical ideas. The language of future neuroscience is not going to be the kind of language that analytic philosophy has traditionally been dealing with.

Models of Nonhuman Phenomenology

The requirement of qualitative similarity in models of the phenomenal level places restrictions on how faithful to the original phenomena our models of nonhuman phenomenology can be. However, these restrictions may not be as limiting as many philosophers have anticipated, for the requirement of a *practically useful* (rather than theoretically perfect) model is not absolute isomorphism and isoqualitativism, but only a sufficient degree of structural and qualitative similarity. Thus, it may be possible to construct reasonably good models of, say, bat phenomenology by using the human phenomenal level as the modeling domain. The model would be an approximation just as most scientific models are. If dream technology became available, it would probably be possible to construct reasonably good models of the phenomenal levels of even radically alien species. After all, some of our spontaneous dreams do contain radically altered phenomenology. All that "phenodiversity" is attainable without any structural alterations in the brain. For example, people sometimes report dreams where their body image is radically altered, or where they experience being an animal, or engaging in actions (e.g., flying) not possible during their waking lives.

Furthermore, although there may be some intractable qualitative differences between human and alien experience, yet there probably are many similarities in the spatiotemporal organization of the experiences. The organization can be mirrored by using the human repertoire of qualities to reconstruct a closely similar configuration. The phenomenal level of organization in different mammalian species probably has common evolutionary roots: the function of the system is to construct a meaningful unified simulated space in the brain. The world simulation mirrors the original sources of the stimulation by creating their transparent surrogates at the phenomenal level. The simulation is used for computing and monitoring the current and future trajectories of the organism through its behavioral environment. The phenomenal level in all mammals is thus likely to be similar: a 3D, unified, egocentric spatiotemporal frame of reference where different qualitative dimensions construct simulated objects that open semantic windows and make the surrounding physical world transparent and meaningful.

The differences among species are not in the phenomenal patterns, but rather in the semantic windows opened. We should expect that the world-imaging systems of different species probably regard entirely different things as meaningful. For a bat, flying insects are modeled at the phenomenal level as moving virtual objects that are very desirable as something to be pursued, captured, and eaten. Also, other bats are highly conspicuous virtual objects in the bat's world, as possible mates or rivals. Human beings probably are just vague moving objects that should be avoided if they get too near; otherwise they can be mostly ignored.

The intractability of alien phenomenology has been exaggerated, especially by those philosophers who oppose the idea that consciousness can be naturalistically explained. The common factor behind the phenomenal levels of all conscious creatures is the biological function of consciousness as a navigational system operating in a phenomenal, meaningful virtual space in the brain, attempting to model and simulate the adaptively important external sources of stimulation.

If we had dream technology available, would it be possible to solve empirically questions such as which biological processes are accompanied by experience, or which living (or even nonliving) creatures are conscious subjects and which mere nonconscious objects? This problem will boil down to the empirically tractable question: Does a particular biological creature realize, in at least a minimal form, the phenomenal level of organization? From the human case we would know that the phenomenal level is realized by highly specific neurophysiological phenomena—the coherent master loop interacting with several other loops of neural activity. If a system includes nothing that even remotely resembles the constitutive mechanisms of the human phenomenal level, then there is no phenomenal level and no consciousness there: the system is a mere object or zombie.

If there is doubt about some specific property as to whether or not it is capable of supporting the phenomenal level, its phenomenality could be empirically tested by using the dream presenter technology. The device would simply reproduce that very phenomenon in your own brain and try to incorporate it into the constitutive mechanisms of the phenomenal level. If that could be done somehow and a new kind of experience would result for you, then the phenomenon does realize an aspect of the phenomenal level. But in general the constitutive basis of the phenomenal level will only include such specific neurophysiological phenomena that, once we know more about them, it will be immediately obvious to us which systems are and which ones are not even remote candidates for having any phenomenal level of organization.

The phenomenal level is the only natural phenomenon we are fully acquainted with. Therefore, when the phenomenal level is discovered empirically in the brain, we will *not* discover some exotic, alien physical or computational phenomenon. We will not find some strange entity that we cannot make any sense of. A scientific account of the phenomenal level is not going to be expressed as a complicated propositional description in exotic symbols or impenetrable formalisms, so that somehow only that sort of an impenetrable formula is supposed to capture the seat of subjectivity in the universe. Instead, we will find the very phenomenon that has been with us all the time, from the very beginning: the familiar world of virtual objects spatially organized around a virtual self.

The science-fiction scenario of dream technology I have described should not *itself* be taken as an *explanation* of consciousness. It is just one possible metatheoretical scenario that shows how empirical research *could,* in principle, eventually solve the problem of consciousness. The actual details will have to be discovered empirically and the actual theories and models constructed on that basis. No amount of philosophical speculation or science-fiction story-telling is going to deliver them. But the crucial point of the thought experiment is this: *Objective neural mechanisms and subjective consciousness can be seen as lying along the same gapless continuum in nature.* The continuum will be created by both sides giving in a little. Consciousness will have to be "objectified" as the phenomenal level of organization in the brain. Neuroscience will have to be "subjectified": the phenomenal level is an integral part of the biological brain, and to capture it empirically, the data must be phenomenalized and subjective consciousness itself used as the domain of theoretical modeling. Consciousness and neuroscience meet at the bridge across the troubled waters of the explanatory gap, each coming halfway to meet the other.

The Connection between the Phenomenal and the Nonphenomenal

A critic might object that this dream technology scenario, even if it were otherwise conceivable, does not provide us with any intelligible connection between phenomenal features and neurophysiological properties. I think that such an objection would have to be based on a lingering but mistaken image of the situation; an image that still treats the phenomenal realm as entirely separate from the neural. On the one hand, one envisions a group of neurons engaging in synchronous activity; on the other hand, one imagines some sort of phenomenal glow around the synchronously firing population. There is supposed to be no physical explanation as to why and how the phenomenal glow is attached to exactly *that* sort of activity instead of some other type.

But that kind of an image depicts consciousness not as a separate level of organization, but as an epiphenomenal echo of "real" neurophysiology. We should exchange this image for the correct one, where consciousness is seen as a causally potent level of organization of its own, as part and parcel of "real" neurophysiology, not as something extra attached to, or merely correlating with, some already objectively describable level of organization. Once we see that there is such a higher level of phenomenal organization in the brain, and that it is in principle discoverable empirically, then it becomes much more difficult to maintain that there is no intelligible link with brain states and consciousness. Consciousness has simply turned out to be a brain state at the phenomenal level of organization.

Let me continue to play the critic and suggest that perhaps the wedge of the explanatory gap could be driven between the phenomenal level and the immediately underlying levels of its constitutive mechanisms. The mechanistic model of these levels may make it intelligible *that* there is such a thing as a phenomenal level in the brain, but does it make its experientiality *necessary*? In other words, once the organized patterns corresponding to phenomenology have been found in the brain, it will be difficult to deny that consciousness is just one level of organization in the brain, but perhaps one question will remain: Why is this particular level an *experiential* level; whence comes its experientiality or phenomenality? Could there not be a unified model of the world in the brain with complex organized patterns and what-have-you, but all of that would be nothing experiential, just another nonconscious level of organization in the brain? Or could we not take the phenomenality of the phenomenal level away and just leave all the complex patterns there?

Unfortunately, I do not see how that could be done. If you take away the phenomenal features themselves, the patterns built out of them (the virtual objects, the virtual body, etc.) cease to exist. It is as impossible to take phenomenal features away but leave the patterns as it is to take all the Hs and Os away but leave the wetness of water, or to take all the base pairs away but preserve the double helix structure of DNA. Experientiality is the basic building block of the phenomenal level, and the phenomenal coordinate system is the only place where those building blocks reside. Take either one away, and the phenomenal level ceases to exist.

Still, the critic stubbornly insists, some deep reason seems to be missing for *why* the patterns realized in the phenomenal coordinate system must be *experiential* patterns as opposed to zombie patterns. We know for a fact *that* they are experiential patterns, but do we know *why* they *must* be such? My reply is that the deep reason lies precisely in what the experientiality consists of: phenomenality consists in there being *self-presenting* features at one level of organization in the brain. What it takes to construct a self-presenting property (as opposed to a relational, nonexperiential property) from lower-level properties which themselves are not self-presenting is not a purely philosophical problem but one that must be figured out by future empirical research.

The mystery crystallizes at the very interface between the phenomenal level and its constituent mechanisms. Somehow, it seems to us, we fully understand how nonconscious physical entities, neurons, for example, can interact and create complex nonconscious electrophysiological patterns, but when we move upward to a higher level of organization, we suddenly need to add consciousness to the picture. But how are we supposed to do that? This depiction of the problem presupposes that the idea of nonconscious phenomena out there in physical space is entirely nonmysterious, whereas the only mystery is how consciousness gets added to it. But if we approach the problem from the opposite direction of the first-person perspective, we may say that the only world we are ever acquainted with is the world made of phenomenal experience. After all, we live in one all the time, whether awake or dreaming, have always lived in one, and can never escape its confines. Thus, if we start at the phenomenal level of organization instead—for at least *that* level of organization *must* exist in the world, even if science turns out to be mistaken about all the rest—and try to move toward lower levels of nonconscious organization, we need to somehow *subtract* consciousness from the picture.

Can we really do that? Can we fully grasp the idea of an entirely nonconscious natural world out there? One could argue that we cannot conceive of such a world, because once you take away consciousness, everything just disappears: time, space, objects—at least as we know them through their transparent phenomenal surrogates. An entirely nonconscious world is rather difficult for us to imagine, because the only thing we know about absolute nonconsciousness is that while it reigns, existence itself seems to cease. How could any kind of a world be built out of fully nonconscious properties? Thus, the burden of proof in this matter is divided equally: We do not really understand how anything could exist in a conscious form, but neither do we really understand how anything could exist in an entirely nonconscious form. Since we do not really understand how *anything* can exist, whether conscious or nonconscious, we should not confuse *that* problem—the problem of existence per se—with the problem of the *relation* between the conscious and nonconscious realms. The mere existence of either type of reality is perhaps beyond our grasp, but after that has been granted, the relationship between these two kinds of realities is no longer all that mysterious.

In fact, I am inclined to think that the nature of conscious existence—the phenomenal level of organization—is more intelligible (or even more "real") than, say, the nature of quantum existence. There is no good reason to think that the true and fundamental nature of all reality is hidden at the smallest conceivable spatial and temporal grains. What seem to remain at those levels of description are precise mathematical tools for predicting the behavior of enigmatic quantum phenomena, but what seems to be missing is any clear ontology. What, precisely, is the nature of those phenomena, and in what sense do they even exist? It is as if physical existence itself would cease to be unambiguous or definitive at those ultimate microlevels of physical organization.

But perhaps that is exactly what we should expect if we take seriously the view that physical (and biological) reality is a layered hierarchical structure, and the levels of organization are ontological, not observer-relative constructions that merely echo the "true" levels of some ontologically supreme microphysical reality. Why should we suppose that there is only one "real" level of existence, and that "real" reality is to be found at some infinitesimal spatiotemporal scale that almost escapes measurement and understanding? Why could it not be the other way around? Perhaps entities and events do not become less real when we move toward coarser spatial and temporal scales to higher levels of organization, and more real when we move toward smaller scales and to lower levels of organization. On the contrary, perhaps (metaphorically speaking) some sort of critical ontological mass must be acquired, in terms of spatial and temporal grain and level of complexity, before even unambiguous physical *existence* is possible. Perhaps the higher levels of organization are, in some sense at least, *more* rather than less real than their lower-level microconstituents. Taking advantage of this feature, Mother Nature manages to make something out of almost nothing, more real things out of less real ones.

The phenomenal level for sure is very real, but it might be a mistake to think that its reality could (or should) be somehow better understood from the vantage point of far lower levels of organization. Every phenomenon is best understood at its own level of description and in relation to the immediately surrounding levels. Descending to far-fetched microphysical levels will likely make the phenomenon disappear from view altogether. Even if it could be somehow described at that level, the description would be needlessly complicated and detailed, if intelligible at all. The impracticability of microphysicalism surfaces already in the relationship between quantum mechanics and chemistry.[1] The special sciences (chemistry, biology, psychology) need not envy physics for the fact that only it is supposed to deal with the ultimately "real" in the physical world. In fact microphysics seems to deal with the less and less real, with less and less tangible entities, found at less and less intelligible spatial and temporal microscales. Ontologically tangible entities and structures only arise at the higher levels of organization, life and consciousness being the most fascinating products of the natural ontological progression.

How, then, does a nonconscious phenomenon *produce* or *become* a conscious phenomenon? The problem with this characterization is that we easily imagine some nonconscious entity (a neuron, say) somehow "producing" consciousness. But that image is misguided. Nonconscious phenomena do not mysteriously become conscious phenomena, or unaccountably "emit" them. Rather, at one level of organization there are nonconscious phenomena that, when collectively interrelated, form a higher level of organization where there are conscious phenomena. The nonconscious phenomena do not mysteriously emit consciousness, they collectively constitute it. To ask, "How does a nonconscious phenomenon produce or become a conscious phenomenon?," is like asking, "How does a subatomic particle become an atom?" or "How does a water molecule emit liquidity?" or "How does a DNA molecule become alive?" The questions ascribe a higher-level feature to a lower-level entity, which in none of the cases makes any sense. Furthermore, it makes as little sense to ask, "Why is this experience of color (say, seeing the sun near the horizon as a red-orange circle) exactly like this?" Well, things are what they are: a pattern of phenomenal features is what it is, an electron is what it is, and a DNA molecule is what it is, and not something else. Does it make sense to ask, "Why is an electron an electron?" or " Why is a DNA molecule a DNA molecule?" I do not think these questions make any sense, and therefore require no explanation.

Instead of these misguided questions, we should form an image of a multilevel hierarchical organization in nature, where it is possible to move from one level to another, without any gaps. Yet, at the different levels, quite dissimilar entities and events are found. In the cases where we truly understand the mechanisms behind complex biological phenomena, we move across the levels and see that even a gapless natural continuum can support all sorts of radically different things.

Does the question, "Why is phenomenal yellow constituted by one type of neurophysiological output from the color module in V4, and phenomenal blue by another type?" make any sense? It seems to make a bit more sense than the questions we considered above. The six elementary colors that humans experience *must* be linked to the underlying mechanism in something like the way that the type of chemical element is tied to the underlying number of protons and electrons inside the atom. The phenomenology of elementary colors is a top-down constraint on the constitutive mechanism of chromatic visual awareness. Anyone with access to both levels of organization (the lower-level constitutive mechanism and the higher-level phenomenal color experience) will see the necessity of their connection. But we do not yet have access to a detailed description of the mechanism (say, the electrophysiological outputs of V4 that modulate the phenomenal level).

Somebody without access to color experiences will not understand the connection between the levels, because he does not even understand what the explanandum is. In the philosophical literature the famous fictional neuroscientist Mary who has been raised in a black-and-white environment is a case in point (Jackson, 1986). Mary simply cannot possess the full, perfect description of the human brain (or color vision), because perfect neuroscience of the brain will have to also include a perfect model of the phenomenal level. The theoretical model of the phenomenal level, however, cannot be communicated propositionally or printed in black-and-white figures: it can only be presented and grasped through a full chromatic phenomenalization. Thus, *Mary's own brain is a crucial part of the machinery required for displaying and understanding the perfect neuroscientific model of color vision.* Therefore, she cannot have a perfect knowledge of neuroscience, because she cannot grasp the perfect model of color vision. It cannot be made available to her because her brain lacks the relevant electrophysiological technology through which the perfect model of the six elementary color qualities, for example, could be displayed to her. Mary is doomed to be ignorant of crucial aspects of phenomenal neuroscience. The multilevel models produced by that branch of neuroscience cannot be fully presented to her.

Or if we grant that the perfect models of color vision are accessible to Mary, and that she does possess truly perfect scientific knowledge of color vision, then she will already know what red looks like and will experience no surprise when she is released from her black-and-white environment. In any case, Mary cannot at the same time lack all acquaintance with color qualities and possess the perfect science of color vision, because in future phenomenal neuroscience, the latter will necessarily involve the former.

In closing, the problem of understanding phenomenal consciousness seems to boil down to the problem of mechanistically modeling "self-presentation."[2] Do we have any idea why some levels of biological organization may "feel" or "sense" their own existence, whereas others have no means for sensing any existence at all? I can only offer some speculations about this. Most physical phenomena exist in the dark, hidden even from themselves. They are not present for themselves and nothing is present for them. Somehow, for a physical or biological system to sense its own existence, it must be capable of being present for itself in a special way. It must make an appearance to itself, in order to create its own, self-contained, inner presence: the world-for-me.

The "self-sensing" capability might be the result of the system being connected to itself in a particular way at the lower levels of organization, which would support a special type of global unity at the higher level. Every part of the system should become present to every other part simultaneously, to create their spatial copresence in the same phenomenal world. Thick interconnections from every part to every other part and to the whole should thus be required at the lower levels. This kind of neural architecture might be found in the thalamocortical loops. An integrated bioelectrical phenomenon emerging in this architecture, based on densely interconnected coexisting elements, might thus come to sense its own existence as the electromagnetic oscillations flow rapidly back and forth through the interconnected neuromatrix. The integrated sphere of neuroelectrical flow may thus become present for itself, a *world-for-itself.*

Summary

To explain consciousness, we first need a clear idea of the nature of explanation. In the biological sciences, multilevel models with genuine explanatory powers have two properties: they faithfully mirror reality and they are fully accessible to human cognition. Models that fulfill these requirements induce genuine conscious understanding.

This conception of explanation can be applied to the case of consciousness. We may at least *imagine* what would be methodologically required from neuroscience for it to discover and explain consciousness. The future technology needed to handle this task is called dream technology. It includes the dream catcher: a method that acquires data directly from the phenomenal level. Such a method is necessary for constructing a model of the phenomenal level that faithfully mirrors the real phenomenon. It further includes the dream presenter: a method that conveys the modeled data in a form accessible to human cognition and understanding. With the help of dream technology, a multilevel model of consciousness becomes feasible. The technology would allow us to see the subjective *worlds-for-someone* as natural parts of the hierarchical continuum of biological levels in the brain.

A challenge for dream technology comes from the qualitative aspects of phenomenal consciousness. It seems, however, entirely conceivable that in the multilevel model of consciousness, the higher-level qualities appear in a natural manner that can be fully understood. Another challenge for the explanation of consciousness comes from the fundamental notion of "presence" and "self-presentation." Although biological self-presentation appears to us to be a magical feat, perhaps it is no more magical than biological self-replication, which also once seemed inexplicable to human science. The key to understanding is to be found in the underlying mechanisms. Thus, there may be particular biological mechanisms that render a biological process present-for-itself. When these mechanisms operate, they generate the sense of inner presence. The multilevel model of consciousness will show what those mechanisms are and where they lie in the brain.

VI The Function and Causal Powers of Consciousness

The phenomenal level in the brain is a *real* biological phenomenon. In biological realism, the criterion for "real" is defined in terms of causal powers: *to be real is to have causal powers* (Kim, 1992, p. 135). Conversely, anything that has no causal powers whatsoever cannot be a real biological (or physical) phenomenon, and, therefore, constitutes neither a proper explanandum nor a proper explanans for biological science.

Causally powerless entities are usually called "epiphenomena" and a doctrine that postulates such entities is called "epiphenomenalism." When it comes to consciousness, two different varieties of epiphenomenalism should be clearly differentiated. *Metaphysical epiphenomenalism* regards consciousness as altogether causally powerless. According to metaphysical epiphenomenalism, consciousness exists and is brought about by physiological activities in the brain, but its existence makes absolutely no difference in anything in the physical world. Consciousness is, causally, a dead end: although it is caused by brain processes, it cannot cause any further brain processes or have any causal influence on behavior. If we accept the principle that to be real is to have causal powers, then metaphysically epiphenomenal consciousness does not fulfil the criterion of "real."

Metaphysical epiphenomenalism has to be strictly separated from *biological* epiphenomenalism. A feature is biologically epiphenomenal if it possesses no such causal powers that increased the inclusive fitness of its owners during their evolutionary history. Thus, biological epiphenomena are not totally devoid of causal powers. They are only devoid of causal powers that make a difference in reproductive success. Many physically real features of biological organisms are biologically but not metaphysically epiphenomenal.

The fact that the heart makes a thudding noise (causes an acoustic phenomenon in the surrounding medium) serves as an example of a biologically epiphenomenal feature. A totally silent heart with equal causal powers for pumping blood would have done just as well in our evolutionary history. The thud of the heartbeat is biologically epiphenomenal. The noise as such does not contribute anything to the biologically significant work that the heart is doing: pumping blood. However, it is not metaphysically epiphenomenal. The noise of the heartbeat has physically real causal powers. Among them is the capability to cause conscious auditory experiences in humans. A skilled cardiologist may use that effect in an initial evaluation of a possible heart condition. Still, the noises emitted by the heart made no difference whatsoever to human inclusive fitness during our evolutionary history.

If consciousness is biologically epiphenomenal, then consciousness made no difference in survival and reproduction during evolutionary history. A totally nonconscious brain would have been precisely as good as a conscious one, just as a totally silent heart would have been exactly as good as a noisy one. According to biological epiphenomenalism, consciousness is merely inconsequential phenomenal "noise," a worthless byproduct generated while the brain carries out the necessary neurobiological and behavioral functions that do make a difference. Phenomenal consciousness is a mere byproduct, both useless and harmless for the organism possessing it. Consciousness does not contribute anything to organism-environment interaction and adaptive behavior, just as the noise of the heartbeat does not contribute to the pumping of blood.

But if the phenomenal level turns out to be biologically epiphenomenal, how could we show that it is not *also* metaphysically epiphenomenal? Consciousness, unlike a heartbeat, does not seem to produce any physical or measurable "noise" that can be detected (unless our verbal reports and other expressions of subjective states are taken as such). In the case of consciousness, it might be difficult to draw a clear line between metaphysical and biological epiphenomenalism. Unless we can clearly demonstrate the causal powers of consciousness, we cannot rule out the threat from epiphenomenalism. However, epiphenomenalist views of consciousness are in conflict with our intuitive ideas about our own conscious minds. Consciousness surely seems to make an enormous difference in our behavior. Therefore, it would be in harmony both with our commonsense ideas about consciousness and with biological realism if the causal powers of consciousness could be clearly pointed out and shown to be biologically useful.

Both metaphysical and biological epiphenomenalism predict that if consciousness could be selectively carved off or knocked out, leaving nonconscious aspects of brain function entirely intact, then nothing of any value for the adaptive behavior or for the reproductive success of the organism would be lost. If epiphenomenalism is true, then purely nonconscious forms of information and representation in the human brain should be able to guide organism-environment interactions just the same, keeping the person out of harm's way without any help from consciousness. Carving off consciousness in this way should bring the causal powers of the purely nonconscious levels of organization out into the open. After consciousness has been subtracted from the picture, the causal powers of the brain should be no less than what they were with consciousness.

Dissociations where the phenomenal level is temporarily obliterated but intricate organism-environment interaction still takes place are experiments of nature that should reveal whether the causal powers of the brain are in any way diminished when consciousness is temporarily disabled. The dissociations between consciousness and behavior can be divided into two broad classes. The first concerns cases in which *a particular type of phenomenal content* (say visual consciousness) *is selectively carved off* while leaving the brain with nonconscious information in the same sensory modality to guide behavior. Blindsight and other forms of implicit perception reported in neuropsychology are paradigmatic cases where nonconscious information of exactly this type guides aspects of behavior (see chapter 22). They reveal that there are nonconscious zombie systems in our brains.

The second type of dissociation concerns cases in which the *whole state of being conscious seems to have been selectively carved off,* yet leaving the zombie-like person capable of interacting with his behavioral environment. Fascinating evidence along these lines comes from sleepwalking, epileptic automatisms, and other pathological deficits of consciousness (see chapter 23).

In the above cases, consciousness is carved off while leaving behavior more or less intact. Conversely, during dreaming, behavior and organism-environment interaction are carved off, leaving consciousness practically intact. What might the latter type of dissociation tell us about the function of consciousness? Dreaming is an internally generated world simulation during sleep. If waking consciousness simulates the world in order to guide the organism safely through the physical world in real time, what function could the offline simulation of a world in the dreaming brain serve?

Offline simulations are useful especially when preparing for potential future situations too dangerous to train in the real world. Perhaps the sleeping brain simulates the phenomenal dream world for us for basically the same reason. That is the central idea in the threat simulation theory of dreaming (see chapter 24), a novel approach to the function of dreaming that is directly derived from biological realism and the world-simulation metaphor.

In the multilevel model of consciousness, to specify the causal powers and the functions of consciousness is to move upward from the phenomenal level and to describe the functional role of consciousness in the context of the whole organism. As it turns out, far from being a powerless epiphenomenon, the phenomenal world simulation in the brain plays a crucial role in organism-environment interaction. Without the internal simulated world, the brain could not determine or follow the behavioral pathways that tend to keep us safe and sound in our dangerous expeditions in the external physical world.

22 Zombies in the Brain: Information That Bypasses Consciousness

In this chapter we explore brain-damaged patients who suffer from a curious pattern of deficits. Some specific type of phenomenal content has been selectively carved off from their consciousness. That is, when shown that type of stimulus, their experience of the stimulus is either totally missing or at least some specific feature of the stimulus is missing from consciousness. Yet, the same stimulus features that are missing from consciousness are not altogether absent from the brain. By contrast, those very features are being processed and represented at nonconscious processing levels and their existence can be revealed in indirect behavioral tasks and physiological measurements.

The empirical findings showing these unexpected dissociations between conscious and nonconscious information in the brain had a crucial impact on the development of cross-disciplinary consciousness research. In the neuropsychological literature the empirical evidence rapidly surfaced during the latter part of 1980s, forcing neuropsychologists to suddenly face the problem of consciousness. Somehow they had to make room for two different types of information-processing in the cognitive machinery: conscious ("explicit") and nonconscious ("implicit"). It seemed as though the human information-processing system had two entirely distinct channels for processing the same input information, and that the scientifically and metaphysically problematic label "consciousness" was the critical factor that differentiates between those channels. No wonder that neuropsychologists were flabbergasted by the evidence, not quite knowing how to deal with it. Their bafflement is well reflected in the comment by Young and de Haan (1990), who investigated nonconscious face processing in prosopagnosic patients in the 1980s:

> We claim no special expertise in approaching the philosophical or psychological problems associated with the study of consciousness and awareness. The truth is that we had no more than a general acquaintance with such issues until they were forced upon us by research findings. (p. 30)

Philosophers soon caught up with the neuropsychologists and started to theorize about these counterintuitive dissociations. Their favorite case was blindsight, discussed at length by Dennett (1991), McGinn (1991), Tye (1995), Block (1995), and Siewert

(1998). Thus, the issue of dissociation triggered lively interaction between the empirical and the philosophical communities on the topic of consciousness—the kind of interaction that was to become the trademark of the emerging field of consciousness research.

By now the literature contains several comprehensive and useful reviews of implicit-explicit dissociations (see, e.g., Young, 1994a,b; Farah, 1994; S. Köhler & Moscovitch, 1997; Weiskrantz, 1997; Rossetti & Revonsuo, 2000), so it is not necessary to cover all of these data in the present context. In the following I give a short and selective overview of the main findings. Thereafter we examine the theoretical implications of these findings to the study of consciousness in general.[1]

Blindsight

Blindsight involves the absence of the phenomenal experience of visual stimuli (in parts of the visual field), but preserved behavioral responses and interactions with the very same stimuli that cannot be subjectively seen. Blindsight was originally reported by Ernst Pöppel and his colleagues as early as in 1973, followed in 1974 by Larry Weiskrantz and his group (Poppel, Held, & Frost, 1973; Weiskrantz, Warrington, Sanders, & Marshall, 1974). The initial reports revealed that patients who apparently had blind regions in their visual fields resulting from brain injury of the primary visual cortex (V1) showed the unexpected capacity of "residual vision" or, as Weiskrantz named it, "blindsight." This meant that the patients, despite their evident blindness, were able to direct their eyes to where a stimulus was located in the "blind" field. Later it was found that such patients were also able to point to unseen stimuli and even to make discriminations between various kinds of stimuli. In these experiments, the patients had to be persuaded to guess or to make forced choices between alternatives, because it was difficult to convince them that the task was not irrational. The patients felt that they were just making random guesses and they were thoroughly amazed when told about the accuracy of their responses. Phenomenologically, the patient does not *see* anything—he or she has no visual experiences in the blind part of visual field, but somehow the behavioral responses are influenced by the unseen stimuli. Weiskrantz (1997) summarized the findings as follows:

> But taken together, subjects with V1 damage have been reported who are able, in their blind hemifields, to detect the presence of stimuli, to locate them in space, to discriminate direction of movement, to discriminate the orientation of lines, to be able to judge whether stimuli in the blind hemifield match or mismatch those in the intact hemifield, and to discriminate between different wavelengths of light. (p. 23)

Blindsight proved to be just the forerunner of a whole bunch of phenomena, nowadays grouped together under the label "implicit knowledge" or "implicit perception" in neuropsychological syndromes. Consequently, a considerable variety of memory deficits and recognition or perceptual impairments were shown to manifest a pattern roughly similar to blindsight. The patient subjectively lacks a cognitive capacity (or a type of phenomenal content is permanently absent from consciousness). Still, when presented with tasks requiring that capacity or information, his brain can be shown to exhibit many kinds of discriminative responses to the critical information. The patient, however, is completely unaware of any such information or that it is influencing his responses. Furthermore, the patient cannot utilize the information in spontaneous everyday behavior.

Somewhere within the brain of such a patient nonconscious information representing the input stimulus is being transformed into representations that guide the patient's behavioral responses toward the stimulus. Still, the same information never becomes manifest at the phenomenal level of subjective experience. Implicit knowledge is knowledge that is expressed in performance without the subject's phenomenal awareness of possessing any such knowledge.

Prosopagnosia

Prosopagnosia, or the inability to recognize familiar people from their faces, constitutes another important source of evidence for implicit knowledge (for a review, see Young [1994a]). The prosopagnosic patient cannot recognize his friends, family members, or celebrities from their faces—he might not recognize even his own face in the mirror. Usually prosopagnosic patients do discriminate faces from other objects—they know when they are looking at a face. The patient is even able to describe facial features or judge the age or sex of the person from the face, but nevertheless he remains totally ignorant of the identity of the person: he does not have the slightest idea whose face he is looking at. To recognize a person, the patient must use something other than facial information: voice, clothes, or hair might trigger recognition (Young & de Haan, 1990).

If we use the concepts introduced in the previous chapters, prosopagnosia can be characterized by saying that the patient has an intact Gestalt window of the face in visual awareness, but no semantic window can be opened that would create conscious access to semantic knowledge about the person whose face is seen. In an explicit task the patient is often totally unable to classify faces according to their familiarity: for him, all faces seem equally unfamiliar.

However, a wide variety of physiological and behavioral experiments have revealed that the patient does recognize the familiar faces, albeit unconsciously. For example, the patient's skin conductance may change when a familiar face is seen (Bauer, 1984; Tranel & Damasio, 1985, 1988). Visually scanning familiar faces compared with scanning some unfamiliar ones his eye movement patterns may systematically differ (Rizzo, Hurtig, & Damasio, 1987). Even the event-related brain potentials might react to the category difference between familiar and unfamiliar faces (Renault, Signoret, Debruille, Breton, & Bolger, 1989). At the behavioral level, there is evidence from priming procedures, interference designs, and learning tasks, which show that at some level the patient's brain has received and discerned correctly the critical information concerning the familiarity of the faces. Not all patients, however, show implicit recognition: there are cases where no implicit effects remain and the whole recognition system seems to be destroyed (Newcombe, Young, & de Haan, 1989). In this type of prosopagnosia even the Gestalt windows of perceived faces seem to be entirely disorganized, and therefore both implicit and explicit recognition fail.

Young and de Haan (1990) described their prosopagnosic patient P.H., who was asked to match two photographs at a time on the grounds of whether the pictures were similar or not. His performance was faster when the faces were familiar, although he did not have any idea of their familiarity. In an interference task it was found that the semantic category of the pictures affected P.H.'s performance. He was supposed to classify printed names into two categories: as politicians or as nonpoliticians. His reaction times to these words became longer if the names were paired with conflicting or misleading faces from the opposite category (say George W. Bush's name paired with a picture of Harrison Ford's face) compared with pairings from the same category or no picture at all. So, although P.H. was unable to tell whether a given face was the face of a politician, this very information interfered with his response speed.

Bruyer (1991) summarized the counterintuitive findings on covert face recognition thus:

> . . . we now have empirical data showing that some prosopagnosic subjects manifest simultaneously covert behavioral signs of recognition and overt behavioral signs of nonrecognition. What is (un)recognized can be the face familiarity, semantic properties of the person seen, or its name. *These data suggest that the "conscious subject" does not recognize or identify familiar faces, while her/his "information processing system" does.* (p. 230, italics added)

Unilateral Neglect

The dramatic loss of awareness of one side of space in neglect is somewhat of a mystery, because the primary sensory pathways for processing the neglected information may still be intact, and yet the patient is not aware of the stimulus. Furthermore, functional brain-imaging data suggest that the occipitotemporal areas in the ventral stream, normally correlating with visual awareness of objects, are still activated by the neglected stimuli (for a review, see Driver & Vuillemier [2001]). Thus, the mystery is, How can the patient remain unaware of stimuli which elicit neural activation in all of the cortical visual areas normally correlating with visual awareness?

The neglected stimulus is being processed at several levels, but the results of the processing do not enter or modulate the phenomenal level. If the stimulus can be grouped together with a perceived stimulus in the intact field to form one coherent perceptual unit according to Gestalt principles, then the stimulus is much less likely to be neglected.

This proves that, at a nonconscious level, basic spatial grouping according to Gestalt laws is applied also to the extinguished stimuli. Different types of experiments have further shown that even the color, shape, identity, or semantic category of an extinguished stimulus may implicitly influence the behavior of the patient (for a review, see Driver & Vuillemier [2001]).

For example, neglect patients can amazingly often judge whether or not two pictures shown are identical or different even though they might claim that there was actually only *one* picture (Volpe, Ledoux, & Gazzaniga, 1979; Karnath & Hartje, 1987). In another kind of experiment, a patient was shown two pictures of a house (Marshall & Halligan, 1988). One was just a plain, ordinary house; the other was identical, apart from bright red flames coming out of the left side of the house. The patient insisted that the pictures were identical, but when asked which one she would like to live in, she consistently preferred the one without flames, although she did not know why and considered the whole question silly. Berti and Rizzolatti (1992) and McGlinchey-Berroth, Milberg, Verfaellie, Alexander, & Kilduff (1993) have shown that semantic priming effects to the processing of pictures can be obtained in neglect patients when a picture or a word is presented to the neglected half-field and consequently remains subjectively unperceived. Thus, information can be extracted from the stimulus at a cross-domain conceptual-semantic level in the absence of phenomenal experience.

Implicit Object-Oriented Action

The most famous of the patients showing implicit action, D.F., had severe visual form agnosia (apperceptive agnosia) and was thus profoundly unable to recognize, verbally describe, or nonverbally illustrate the size, shape, and orientation of visual objects, due to brain damage caused by carbon monoxide poisoning. Nevertheless, she showed amazingly accurate guidance of hand and finger movements directed at the very same objects. When asked to indicate the size of blocks in front of her by showing the width by means of her index finger and thumb, her estimates had nothing to do with the real size of the objects. However, when simply asked to pick up those objects, her index finger and thumb were adjusted to pick up the object with an accuracy comparable to normal subjects (Goodale & Milner, 1992). The evidence supports an interpretation according to which the dorsal stream from V1 to posterior parietal cortex provides visual information to the online control of many kinds of actions. The ventral stream from V1 to inferotemporal cortex provides visual information to enable recognition and, most importantly, conscious visual perception.

On the basis of a number of experiments on similar phenomena in other patients and normal subjects, Rossetti (1998) concluded that sensory processing results in two distinct representations of space: one devoted to conscious identification ("semantic representation") and the other to action ("pragmatic representation"). In specific circumstances, an object-oriented action can be performed at an implicit level, guided by the pragmatic representation in isolation. In the normal case, however, the two representation systems are in tight interaction with each other. The pragmatic representation is created faster than the semantic one, and therefore it can be used even in isolation when an immediate goal-directed movement aimed straight at the stimulus is required.

Other Types of Implicit Knowledge

There are many other forms of implicit knowledge found in different kinds of neuropsychological patients. For example, a phenomenon analogous to blindsight has been reported in the touch modality by Paillard, Michel, & Stelmach (1983): the patient could not consciously experience any tactile sensation when her skin was touched, but she could point to the location accurately with her hand. The researchers called the phenomenon *blindtouch* (see also Rossetti, Rode, & Boisson [1995]). Implicit semantic processing of language in aphasic patients with severe language comprehension difficulties has been demonstrated both behaviorally (Revonsuo, 1995c) and neurophysiologically (Revonsuo & Laine, 1996). These studies show that semantic networks can be activated implicitly in the absence of conscious understanding of stimulus meaning.

Dissociations and Multilevel Mechanistic Explanation

The approach of cognitive neuropsychology (Ellis & Young, 1988) to understanding the human information-processing system is in accordance with the mechanistic explanatory strategy. The basic idea in cognitive neuropsychology is to map the possible *patterns of dissociations* between different cognitive functions in order to figure out which of them can be realized independently. A function that is independent of another one can become damaged while the other function remains intact, and, conversely, the function can remain intact while the other one is compromised. For example, face recognition and written word recognition are independent of each other if it can be shown that there is at least one patient with severely deficient face recognition but entirely intact written word recognition, and another patient with the reverse pattern. Such a situation would constitute a double dissociation between recognizing visually presented faces and words.

Independent cognitive functions that reveal themselves in double dissociations constitute the functional components of the cognitive system, and each component probably also has a specific dedicated neural basis in the brain. Thus, cognitive neuropsychology applies the principles of decomposition and localization of functions. The dissociation between conscious and nonconscious information processing has been interpreted within this explanatory context in cognitive neuropsychology. Several theoretical models have been put forward that attempt to specify the relations between the conscious and the nonconscious components in the human cognitive system. S. Köhler and

Moscovitch (1997) divide these models into three categories: disconnection models, distinct knowledge models, and degraded representation or threshold models.

In disconnection models (e.g., see Schacter, McAndrews & Moscovitch, 1988), nonconscious domain-specific modules normally produce output that feeds into one common conscious awareness system (CAS). If the nonconscious modules become disconnected from the CAS but otherwise remain intact, they can no longer feed information to consciousness. However, they have other output connections through which the same information may be implicitly processed. Thus, disconnection models see implicit information as information that is supposed to be fed into the conscious component of the system but, due to the disruption of the connections, never reaches its proper destination. Therefore, the information never takes a phenomenal form. Instead, it is routed forward in its nonconscious form along pathways that totally bypass consciousness, and thereby the implicit effects come to be expressed in behavior. In this model, *implicit information is produced by modules that are "earlier" than consciousness in a linear, serial processing chain,* but normally in tight interaction with it. Implicit information remains nonconscious because it originates from stages in the processing chain earlier than consciousness. The information is normally supposed to be transformed into conscious information once it enters (or modulates the states of) the one and only unified CAS, but the normal route has been blocked (figure 22.1).

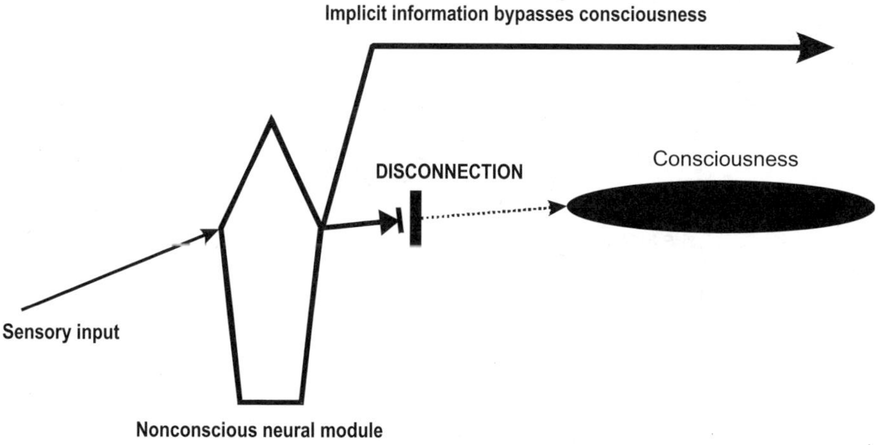

Figure 22.1
Disconnection models. According to this type of model, implicit information remains nonconscious because it resides at an *earlier stage* in the processing chain. The earlier stage is realized by a module that is entirely nonconscious, that is, it has no phenomenal level of organization. The module resides at a stage preceding consciousness in the immediate etiological pathway. The information handled by the module is supposed to be transformed into conscious information once it enters (or modulates the states of) the single, centralized system specialized for consciousness. If the module becomes disconnected from consciousness, its outputs can only modulate other nonconscious systems in the brain. This nonconscious, implicit information consequently reveals itself in various measurable behavioral and neurophysiological responses, but the subject cannot experience or introspectively report it.

In distinct knowledge models the idea is that implicit information resides in processing systems that were never supposed to feed their information into consciousness in the first place: they are thoroughly nonconscious by their very nature. Such processing systems operate *in parallel* with the one(s) subserving explicit knowledge or consciousness, but are usually hidden from view, only exposed in exceptional cases where the conscious processing system is malfunctioning. In such situations, the nonconscious parallel systems go on functioning as ever, transforming specific forms of input into specific forms of output, thus modulating observable behavior nonconsciously (figure 22.2).

Degraded representation models assume that the very same system that generates conscious states also produces nonconscious states, if the system is *inadequately activated* or *partially damaged.* The closely related *activation strength hypothesis of consciousness* holds that the degree of perceptual awareness is encoded neurally as the strength or the "quality" of the underlying neural representation (Kanwisher, 2001). Only nonconscious information transformations occur if the representations that the system produces are degraded or if the activation that the system receives is insufficient. In any case, conscious and nonconscious information (of the same stimulus) does not reside in two different systems, but the difference constitutes two different *states* or *levels of activation* of the very same system. There is no separate system for consciousness—consciousness is a feature of a number of specialized, distributed modules when they are sufficiently activated (this model resembles the "microconsciousness" hypothesis of Semir Zeki, discussed in chapter 19) (figure 22.3).

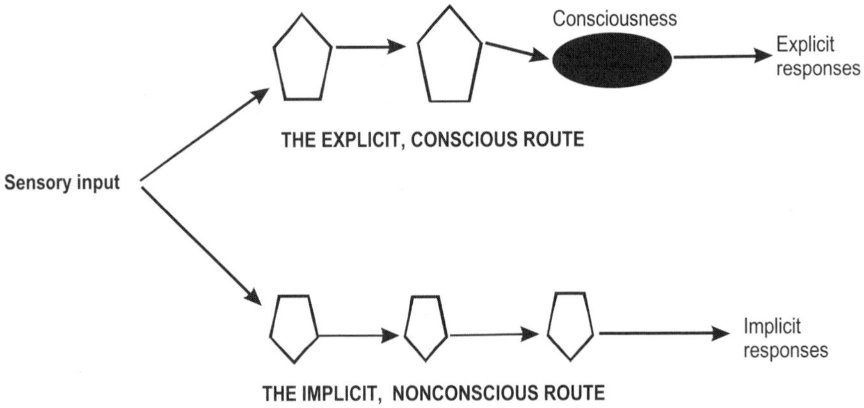

Figure 22.2
Distinct knowledge models. The idea in these models is that explicit and implicit information reside in *separate processing systems* to begin with. The information in the implicit, nonconscious route was never supposed to be fed into consciousness. The modules along the implicit route are thoroughly nonconscious input-output transformers by their very nature. They realize no phenomenal level of organization. Their existence, however, may be manifested only after the explicit processing route is damaged, uncovering the implicit route that continues to function normally.

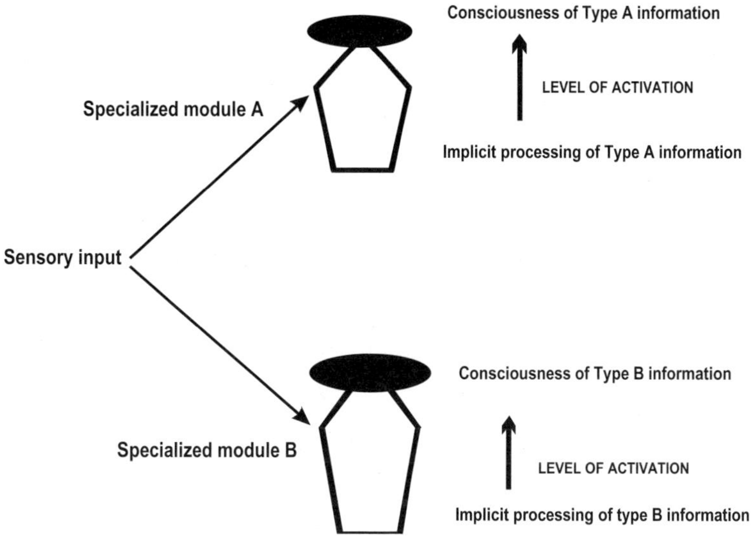

Figure 22.3
Degraded representation models. Conscious and nonconscious information (of the same stimulus) does not reside in two different systems, but the difference consists in two different *states* of the very same system. This view leads to the idea that specialized modules have the capacity to realize the phenomenal level of organization entirely within themselves, independent of other systems. Thus, the full activation of one module produces phenomenal colors, the full activation of another produces phenomenal motion, and so on. Insufficient or deficient activation only produces implicit processing of the same type of information. One problem with this view is that it depicts the phenomenal level as essentially a disunified phenomenon, as having multiple partial realizations throughout the brain (cf. Zeki's "microconsciousness" theory). Such a view is difficult to reconcile with the actual phenomenal unity of consciousness.

S. Köhler and Moscovitch (1997) conclude that the distinct knowledge model can explain most of the available data on implicit visual processing, whereas the two other models seem more restricted. The most convincing evidence for the distinct knowledge model comes from implicit processing in blindsight and visual form agnosia. Implicit object-oriented action in visual form agnosia is typically explained by referring to two distinct visual pathways, the ventral and the dorsal. In several cases of implicit processing findings support this interpretation. Bridgeman (2000) argues that there is overwhelming evidence for the existence of two branches of visual processing: one "cognitive" branch supporting conscious perception, the other a "sensorimotor" branch supporting visually guided behavior. Pisella and Rossetti (2000) show that there are two distinct ways of encoding spatial information for action: one system using "perceptual" or "semantic" representations at the explicit or conscious level, one sensorimotor system using short-lived "pragmatic" motor representations at the implicit or nonconscious level.

Thus, there are completely nonconscious systems in the brain that take in sensory input, process and transform it in complex ways, and deliver representations that modulate external reactions or behavior in various ways. Sometimes they have been called "zombie systems," or even "the zombie within the brain," because they are capable of processing sensory input and synthesizing complex behavioral patterns from it in the total absence of phenomenal consciousness. These nonconscious zombie systems *bypass consciousness entirely,* although they may be in interaction with it or influenced by it to some extent.

The Nature of the Nonconscious Zombie Systems

The nonconscious zombie systems tell us what and where consciousness definitely is *not.* Once we know where those systems are located and how they function, we can rule them out as potential candidates for the constitutive mechanisms of consciousness. The neuroanatomical and physiological bases of the zombie systems reveal what kind of neural architecture may guide behavior in the total absence of consciousness. An understanding of the biology and the behavior of the nonconscious information processing systems in the brain can then be contrasted with the positive account of the mechanisms of consciousness. If consciousness is *not* realized in *these* neural systems and *not* carrying out *these sorts* of input-output transformations, then the phenomenal level is to be found elsewhere in the brain and its functions are complementary to the ones that can be carried out by the zombie systems alone.

There is, however, no compelling reason to believe that *all* the different types of implicit information can be best explained by a similar model by referring to two entirely separate systems as the distinct knowledge model does. Covert recognition of faces in prosopagnosia is a case in point. Young and Ellis (2000) argue that, although the implicit effects related to autonomic activation (e.g., those affecting skin conductance responses) are probably realized by neural systems distinct from the ones supporting overt recognition of faces, the behavioral implicit effects, such as associative priming, can be best explained by a degraded representation model. The basic idea of such a model is that, due to dysfunctional connections, the component modules containing the representations of face and person identity do not receive sufficient excitation from earlier stages of processing. Thus the activation received is not enough to reach above the critical threshold of producing overt recognition, but it is enough to support the implicit behavioral effects.

The differing interpretations of implicit, nonconscious information suggest that such information exists in the brain in several different forms. In all likelihood no *single* model can account for all of them. In some cases it seems clear that nonconscious information is routed in the brain along neural pathways completely distinct from those of conscious information. The two serve different functions; one is neither a preliminary nor a degraded form of the other. However, in other cases it seems more reasonable to think that the implicit information resides within the very same processing route as the corresponding conscious information. Along this route there are stages of completely nonconscious processing which in the normal case modulate the conscious stage at the phenomenal level, but in a disrupted system all the effects remain nonconscious, either because of disconnection between processing modules or degradation of certain processing stages (or some combination of these malfunctions).

Thus, on the basis of the dissociation evidence, it is probably fruitless to try to figure out what is *the* nature of the nonconscious systems, and *the* relation of the nonconscious systems to consciousness. Those questions presuppose that at some fundamental level all the different zombie systems are intrinsically similar to each other (or at least that all of them bear a similar relation to the phenomenal level). But that presupposition is baseless. On the contrary, it seems more likely that the nonconscious systems have *no unitary nature.* Why should they? After all, they are defined through a negation: what unites them is the *absence* of consciousness rather than some positive feature that would be shared by all of them. Therefore, it is not reasonable to expect these systems to have any common basic nature. Probably the different models of explicit-implicit dissociations reviewed above are correct about different types of dissociation. If that is the case, then it does not make sense to try to figure out which is the universally correct model, and which ones are incorrect. Nonconscious input-output transformations are probably realized in all of these ways. It just remains to be seen which model is true of which type of implicit processing.

The dissociations seem to tell us quite a lot about the nature of *nonconscious* information in the brain, and the *separation* of the nonconscious effects from the conscious ones in the brain. Perhaps the more intriguing question is , however, what we can learn about consciousness *itself,* and of the *interaction* between the nonconscious and the conscious. Defining the possible interaction between the components of a system is a crucial step in the development of mechanistic explanations.

How far apart from each other are the conscious and the nonconscious in the light of the dissociation data? The answer to this question depends on the specific type of nonconscious information we are considering. If the nonconscious information resides in a processing system that is entirely separate from conscious forms of information, we are talking about two entirely separate processing systems. But if the nonconscious information is simply a preliminary stage or a weakly activated form of conscious information inside the very same processing system where conscious information resides, then the nonconscious information may be separated from the phenomenal level by only a hairsbreath.

How do the entirely nonconscious zombie systems interact and cooperate with consciousness? First, we should note that these systems do indeed *cooperate* with consciousness instead of *competing* with it. The zombie systems do not have any goals of their own, independent of those determined at the level of conscious intention. In fact, these systems appear to be *slave* systems that ensure that whatever the goals determined at the level of consciousness are, these fast zombies will go for them without asking any questions. This slavelike obedience makes them even more deserving of the name "zombie." Without the conscious selection of goals, the automatic system for visually guided actions would not be able to take any behavioral initiative on its own. And vice versa, without the automatic systems, consciousness would not be able to guide all the details required in programming goal-directed behavior successfully and carrying it out rapidly.

Second, it seems that information can flow from the phenomenal level to the nonconscious zombie systems, but not the other way round (Bridgeman, 2000). In some cases of visually guided actions, when a delayed response to the stimulus is required, the nonconscious system cannot store the relevant representations, but must rely on those delivered by the conscious system. This also shows clearly that the nonconscious system is a servant of the consciously selected goals. Interestingly, the information available through the phenomenal level is not as accurate for the purposes of motor programming as the normal direct online input of this zombie system is, for the representations filtered through the phenomenal level include distortions and illusions that the nonconscious system is not otherwise inclined to generate.

The interaction appears to happen at a stage of processing where detailed motor programs are rapidly activated. That stage is not a part of the phenomenal level: we are not conscious of the motor programs needed to execute a certain action. We do not activate the motor programs at the level of consciousness, because then we would need to know exactly which muscle groups should be used, in which order they should be used, how much muscle power is needed, and so on. Hence this is a nonconscious stage that can be modulated both by the phenomenal level and by the nonconscious zombie systems. Usually that happens in smooth cooperation, but sometimes dissociations occur so that the resulting motor programs are guided only by nonconscious information or by conscious information. The contribution of both streams of information thus converges at the nonconscious stage of motor programming. There the information from the phenomenal level flows and mixes with the stream of nonconscious representations flowing from the nonconscious zombie systems.

The Nature of Consciousness in the Light of the Dissociations

Perhaps one of the most intriguing questions is whether the dissociation evidence challenges the idea that the phenomenal level constitutes one single globally unified system. In any case most cognitive neuropsychologists are not willing to postulate a single system of consciousness to describe and explain the dissociations. Young (1994b) thinks that on the basis of neuropsychological evidence, consciousness is not likely to be a single homogeneous entity. Nevertheless, he considers it an appealing hypothesis that the contents of consciousness correspond to the information that is made available to executive mechanisms, which seems to imply that at least the *outputs* of conscious processing do share common features. Farah (1994) does not accept the model which postulates one single system of consciousness: "There is currently no evidence for a dedicated conscious awareness system, distinct from the systems that perform specific perceptual or cognitive functions" (p. 72).

I believe that the conflict between the global phenomenal unity of consciousness and the dissociation data is more apparent than real. The evidence for the single unified system comes from a different level of organization than the evidence against it. When consciousness is considered as it appears in subjective experience at the phenomenal level, it constitutes one unified system. If, however, the lower-level mechanisms below (or preceding) the phenomenal level are considered, then the picture is quite different. A multitude of widely distributed anatomical areas that participate in perceptual functions seem to be involved in the realization of consciousness: the conscious percept of a face is constructed by activity in one place; the conscious percept of color in another place, and so on. But it should be noted that *this disunified picture concerns the lower-level mechanisms of consciousness rather than consciousness itself.* The unity of phenomenal consciousness does not imply unity of the lower-level constituent mechanisms or unity of the preceding etiological mechanisms. Therefore, there may be both unity and disunity involved, but at different levels of organization in the micro-macro hierarchy, or at different temporal stages in the etiological mechanisms feeding information to consciousness.

The most compelling evidence to support the idea of a single phenomenal coordinate system comes from the dissociations in neglect and extinction. The ventral occipitotemporal stream usually thought to support visual awareness can be entirely preserved, and stimuli seem to be processed in it, yet the corresponding virtual objects do not appear at the phenomenal level of organization. What is the crucial ingredient, then, that is still missing? Driver and Vuilleumier (2001) suggest that the inferior parietal lobe areas impaired in most neglect patients may serve as an interface between the dorsal and ventral streams, allowing the spatial properties contributed by the dorsal stream to be connected to the visual properties provided by the ventral stream. They correctly note that spatial location is not a phenomenal property on a par with other phenomenal properties (such as color, motion, form), but seems to be somehow special, because losing *that* property will lead to the loss of all the other properties as well. The instantiation of other phenomenal properties is necessarily dependent on the instantiation of the location of those properties:

> . . . perhaps the most intriguing aspect of the human neglect syndrome is that the patient does *not* lose awareness solely for the *location* of neglected stimuli, but for their other properties also, and indeed even for the very existence of the neglected information. . . . It thus appears that when the appropriate representation of stimulus location is lost or degraded, as in neglect after parietal damage, then awareness of other stimulus properties . . . is also lost, *as if our internal representations of external space . . . provided the basic medium for perceptual experience.* (Driver & Vuilleumier, 2001, p. 74)

Converging empirical evidence supports this view. Experiments on the neural correlates of visual awareness lead Kanwisher (2001) to the view that

> . . . [N]eural activity in specific regions within the ventral pathway is apparently correlated with the content of perceptual awareness, whereas neural activity in the dorsal pathway may be correlated instead with the occurrence of perceptual awareness in a completely content-independent fashion. (p.108)

Kanwisher's "content-independent" representation resembles phenomenal space in the respect that to create a spatiotemporally structured representation in consciousness, the domain-specific systems must interact with the domain-general systems. Empirical evidence from multiple sources thus seems to converge on the idea of a unified spatial framework underlying all phenomenal experience.

The Causal Powers of Implicit Information

Implicit information in the brain appears to be not very helpful to the organism. The patients possessing implicit forms of information cannot guide their behavior along the adaptive trajectories in the physical environment that they would be able to choose if the same information were available at the phenomenal level. Consider the following comments by Weiskrantz (1992):

> Certainly the neuropsychological patients who suffer from any of the syndromes . . . are deeply disabled: amnesic patients cannot survive on priming or conditioning alone, nor can prosopagnosic patients overcome their acute embarrasment in not recognizing their children, even though they may be able to process "implicitly" their semantic status, nor can the blindsight subject avoid bumping into lamp-posts, even if they can guess their presence or absence in a forced-choice situation, nor can they compare their "covert" detection with past visual experience. All of these subjects lack the ability to think about or to image the objects that they can respond to in another mode, or to inter-relate them in space and in time; and this deficiency can be crippling. (p. 8)

In the light of this testimony, implicit information seems to have little if any survival value for the organism. The person is just as helpless in interacting with the environment with or without the implicit information in the brain. The overall behavioral trajectory taken is not guided by the nonconscious information in any meaningful way, although some minor effects can be observed. Therefore it is fair to conclude that nonconscious zombie systems do *not* provide the person with information that would match the causal powers of conscious information. The causal contribution of the phenomenal level of organization appears to be unique.

Lahav (1993) provides an illuminating analysis of implicit (or nonconscious) and explicit (or consciously experienced) information, arguing that their effects on behavior are profoundly different. Implicit information can only affect narrow and isolated islands of fixed behavioral responses. Nonconscious information is not integrated with other information in the system, and is limited to exerting specific, isolated, or rigid effects on behavior. Lahav (1993) characterizes "automatic behavior" as behavior that is governed by relatively simple input-output relationships; nonconscious information can only give rise to automatic behavior.

Hence the behavioral trajectories determined and guided by nonconscious information are limited to certain types of situations or behaviors. The information can guide the trajectory of the patient's hand toward the direction of the physical stimulus, and can even make successful contact with the object by picking it up. But such actions are isolated from the organism's overall goals. No spontaneous goal image—a meaningful virtual object—corresponding to the object to be picked up is present at the phenomenal level. Thus, the objects accurately but nonconsciously pointed at or reached toward cannot serve as actual goals that satisfy the needs of the organism. The object cannot create the transparent surrogate at the phenomenal level: the corresponding virtual object and the semantic window for the brain. Only those phenomenal entities would simultaneously reveal both the location and the value of the object for the organism.

What are the special properties of the phenomenal level in guiding the behavior of the organism? First, explicit knowledge, or information that modulates patterns of phenomenal features at the phenomenal level, has the causal power to evoke a *wide range of behaviors,* not just a single, fixed input-output pattern (Lahav, 1993). Depending on the internal state of the organism, a glass of water can evoke a powerful goal image and set an immediate trajectory where all the available behavioral means are utilized to get in contact with that object. But if the individual is not thirsty, the object may be just recognized but treated indifferently.

Second, the different sources of explicit information are *integrated* with each other (Lahav, 1993). When in search of sources of water or nutrition, the organism is sensitive to any cues that might reveal the location of such goals. The distant purling of the stream is integrated with the visual cues of where vegetation is fresh and green. Multimodal information is integrated at the phenomenal level because all sensory modalities modulate the states of the single phenomenal world-simulation system. Therefore, phenomenal features modulated by multiple sensory channels can constitute one unified virtual object present in a single location in the phenomenal world simulation. Consequently, that virtual object can serve as a goal image, setting a behavioral trajectory for the system to follow. By contrast, implicit information is not integrated with any other types of information that guide the organism's behavior. If implicit information guides behavior at all, it does so in isolation (sometimes even running counter to conscious information).

Third, the response to explicit information is *not obligatory* but can be *deliberately selected* from a huge repertoire of behavioral responses (Lahav, 1993). There can be a variety of goal images currently at the phenomenal level, invoked by different types of explicit information, but the system is not blindly forced to take a particular goal and thrown into that trajectory by some totally irresistible forces. At least in organisms that are capable of reflective consciousness, various goal images can be considered in working memory before one of them is accepted as the next goal worthwhile. The relative importance of different goals can be changed by bringing all sorts of information, both internal and external, into consideration. By contrast, implicit information guides behavior automatically when certain conditions are met; we cannot control it or choose its paths—we are not even aware of its existence.

Lahav (1993) concludes that conscious experience expresses information that is available for an entire spectrum of global, integrated, and flexible, nonautomatic behaviors. He thinks this is evidence to the effect that consciousness is *a central junction of information* in the brain.

The story so far looks like this. Conscious information has causal powers in the control of behavior radically different from nonconscious information. Of course, consciousness does not realize or control all the details of motor action; they are taken care of by automatic systems that have no phenomenal level of organization. The special contribution from the phenomenal level is to *select behavioral goals,* relying on the information present at the phenomenal level (semantic windows) and to *determine and monitor the trajectory that leads to the selected goal.*

Summary

We explored the causal powers of conscious and nonconscious information by analyzing dissociations where the representation of a stimulus in consciousness is selectively carved off, leaving only the nonconscious processing of the stimulus to guide behavior. The dissociations reveal that some processing systems in the brain are true zombie systems. They are intrinsically nonconscious input-output transformers: no states or representations or stages of processing are ever conscious in those systems. In other words, *there is no phenomenal level of organization in such systems.*

Still, there is at least one system that realizes the higher phenomenal level of organization. In close interaction with the phenomenal level there are several processing stages and below-threshold representations that are intrinsically nonconscious, only preparing information for inclusion into consciousness at later stages, or only receiving information from the conscious stage and nonconsciously transforming it into the activation of motor programs.

However, once a piece of information does enter the level of consciousness, it seems to acquire causal powers that are qualitatively distinct from the powers of nonconscious information in the brain. Thus, it is not possible to carve off phenomenal content while leaving the causal powers of the brain intact. Phenomenal content is not epiphenomenal but causally potent in the brain. In the overall multilevel model of consciousness, the dissociation and interaction data lay open the functional role that consciousness plays in the brain, as a crucial part of the multilevel mechanisms involved in guiding organism-environment interaction. With the help of these data, it is possible to add important pieces to the upward-looking contextual explanation of consciousness.

23 Zombies and Automatic Behavior

In the clinical literature several phenomena can be found that involve curious zombie-like dissociations between consciousness and the control of behavior. For example, sleepwalking (somnambulism), nocturnal wandering, and automatic behaviors during epileptic seizures seem to involve a nonconscious person engaging in incredibly complex behaviors. These disorders seem even more puzzling than the implicit information found in neuropsychological patients, such as blindsight. In blindsight and similar dissociations of consciousness, only specific phenomenal contents are lost, but the patients surely remain in their normal conscious state while they are displaying the surprisingly accurate behaviors guided by nonconscious information. In this chapter, by contrast, we examine global and goal-directed behaviors that seem to be going on in the absence of the whole *state* of being conscious. The conscious state of these patients seems to have been selectively carved off, yet the person (or at least his body) continues to go about in the world, as if consciousness would be unnecessary for behavioral interactions with the world.

These experiments of nature thus test the plausibility of epiphenomenalism as an empirical hypothesis. If even a single convincing case could be found where the loss of the state of being conscious—temporary loss of the whole phenomenal level—does not notably impair the causal powers of the remaining nonconscious brain mechanisms in guiding organism-environment interactions, then we would be compelled to conclude that the causal powers of phenomenal consciousness are only meager or perhaps nonexistent. In that case, consciousness might be regarded as at least biologically epiphenomenal (without any biologically significant causal powers), or perhaps even metaphysically epiphenomenal (without any causal powers at all).

But before we are entitled to draw any such conclusions, the evidence must be carefully examined. A true zombie should fulfill the following requirements:

1. There is solid evidence of total loss of the phenomenal level (loss of the state of being conscious). There is no phenomenal world simulation present in the brain while the observed behaviors are carried out.

2. The nonconscious brain's causal powers in guiding complex, meaningful behaviors are comparable to the conscious brain's powers. There should be no significant difference between the behavioral pathways computed at the phenomenal level of organization (in the conscious state) and those realized without any contribution from the phenomenal level (in the nonconscious state).

In this chapter, we examine the evidence from sleepwalking, epileptic automatisms, and other enigmatic zombie-like behaviors.[1]

What Counts as Evidence for the Loss of Consciousness?

Are zombie-like individuals truly nonconscious when they manifest complex behaviors? Or are they only in a nonreflective or otherwise confused state of consciousness during the experience, or totally amnesic about the experience afterward? The assumption in the medical and forensic science literature about sleepwalking and nocturnal wandering appears to be that if a person is asleep, he is not conscious, and if there is no consciousness, then acts done by the person cannot be criminal, for he does not know what he is doing (Beran, 1992; Mahowald, Bundlie, Hurwitz, & Schenk, 1990).

However, it seems the term "conscious," as understood in that literature, refers approximately to "aware of one's surroundings and of what one is doing." According to the terminology introduced in this book (see chapter 2), if one loses awareness of the surrounding world and the powers of reflective consciousness, this counts as an altered state of consciousness rather than "loss" of consciousness. True loss of the state of being conscious involves having no phenomenal consciousness whatsoever, not even an altered form of it. The decisive question thus is whether the zombie-like persons still have phenomenal experience of some kind, even if it represents the real world only vaguely, partially, or in a distorted manner.

We have no means of checking, independently of the subjective retrospective reports given by the patients, whether or not the zombie-like person was truly nonconscious during the automatic behavior. An alternative hypothesis would be that the patient experienced an altered state that rendered him aphasic during the episode, and amnesic for it afterward.

If the subject reports that he has no recollection of an episode during which he manifested zombie-like behavior, should we believe him? Not necessarily, for it is perfectly possible to be completely amnesic about a past episode during which one was fully conscious. Lack of any recollection of the episode is a necessary but not sufficient criterion for showing that phenomenal consciousness was absent during the episode. The problem is, how do we tell apart cases of pure amnesia from cases of true loss of consciousness?

This is feasible, at least in the case of epileptic seizures. Some patients can clearly remember what happened just before the onset of the attack, how the seizure began suddenly with an epileptic aura, how they subsequently sank into an abyss of nothingness, a complete blackout, from which they remember nothing. The next thing they remember is waking up from the blackout, not knowing how much time has passed or what has happened. If the person *remembers that he or she lost consciousness* before the memory gap and *regained consciousness* after it, and, furthermore, describes the time of the memory gap as a *complete blackout,* then we should assume that he or she was to all intents and purposes nonconscious and that the state of nonconsciousness was the cause of the amnesia. But of course there still is no *absolute* guarantee that this was the case.

In epileptology, seizures have been identified that seem to imply no loss of consciousness, although they cause total amnesia for the episode. These are called "pure amnestic seizures" (see Palmini, Gloor, and Jones-Gotman [1992], where the following cases are described in detail). The patients may notice a memory gap afterward, but they have no memory of a period of nonconsciousness or of losing their consciousness. For example, one woman was on EEG-video monitoring when seizure activity started in the EEG. She was reading a magazine at the time. She stopped reading. A few seconds later the phone beside her bed rang. She sat up, took the receiver, and had a short, entirely normal conversation with her cousin. The next morning she did not remember having received a phone call. When she saw the video taken of the event, she was incredulous. She only remembered reading the magazine, but drew a total blank about the telephone conversation.

Another patient had a seizure when she was transcribing from stenography into a word processor. She suddenly realized that she had a blank in her memory and did not remember having written the copy she saw on the computer monitor. She then read back what she had written and it was all correct, with the exception of a single typing error. The length of the material she had transcribed without memory was a couple of paragraphs. In another episode she came out of a store and realized that she had a blank in her memory. She inferred that she must have written a check because she had jotted down the amount in her checkbook. She returned to the shop to verify that she had written a check and found that she had done so correctly.

In such pure amnesic attacks there is no reason to believe that the patient lost phenomenal consciousness during the seizure. Rather, these attacks resemble transient global amnesia (TGA), a not uncommon memory disorder in the elderly, where for some minutes or hours, the patient is densely amnesic. The difference between TGA and pure amnesic seizures is that the epileptic patients do not realize during the seizure that there is anything wrong with them; they only realize it afterward when they notice the memory gap. That can be explained by the fact that the seizures are very brief compared to TGA episodes. Thus, they are probably too short for the patients to realize that anything is wrong. Behavior during pure amnesic attacks can be entirely normal, but that is not so surprising as the patient has not lost consciousness. What is absent is the memory encoding of the experiences, not the experiences themselves. Absence of memory encoding does not constitute zombiehood.

Thus, we have to be careful not to confuse loss of memory with loss of consciousness. However, we also have to be careful not to exclude by definition the possibility of true zombiehood. If we automatically infer that a patient *must* have been conscious because her behavior was normal, and automatically attribute the inability to report her experiences during the episode to a memory loss with preserved consciousness, then we exclude zombiehood by definition. Therefore, we are not allowed to infer automatically that normal behavior indicates preservation of consciousness. In some cases we have independent reasons to believe that either consciousness or memory (or both) are absent even though the patient manifests complex behaviors. If there was an actual loss of consciousness, then the subject should remember how she lost and regained her senses. If there is just memory loss, she should report having noticed an inexplicable memory gap, but there should be no memory of gradually losing consciousness or regaining it.

Degrees of Zombiehood

We can carry out many highly complicated tasks without paying any attention to the task, being only very dimly aware of our surroundings as our attention is turned elsewhere. Therefore, an apparently nonconscious person carrying out a routine task that can be done normally with minimal consciousness is no evidence of true zombiehood, but only evidence of the activation of highly overlearned action schemata. We regard automatic behaviors that are routine and can be normally carried out without focal awareness as evidence of weak zombiehood. Although weak zombiehood is not quite true zombiehood, it is a remarkable achievement nevertheless: it implies that a nonconscious person can interact with the environment in fairly complex ways, such as successfully moving from one location to another or accurately picking up objects from the surroundings.

What would be evidence of true or strong zombiehood? First, of course, there must be solid reasons to believe that the person was nonconscious during the episode of apparent zombiehood. His retrospective report should therefore describe that he remembers losing consciousness—how phenomenal contents disappeared and a blackout, a total phenomenal void, commenced. And he should further report that the first thing he remembers after that is how phenomenal contents reappeared. As far as he can tell, he was devoid of phenomenal experience in the meantime. It would be better still if this subjective report could be verified by observations of his behavior and EEG during the onset of the attack. Second, there must be evidence of successful organism-environment interaction during the time of the blackout. The zombie should initiate and carry out tasks that are nonroutine or otherwise normally require high awareness of surroundings and meaningful evaluation of the objects one is in interaction with.

Examples of such tasks would be finding one's way or reaching a nonroutine goal in unfamiliar geographical surroundings; responding appropriately to an unexpected dangerous or desirable object; looking up an unfamiliar phone number and making a phone call; writing a letter that makes sense; or drawing a picture that accurately represents something in the environment. These tasks are open-ended, require the evaluation of surrounding objects, and decisions and choices based on such an evaluation. The content of the task and the meaningfulness of the surrounding objects need to be appreciated. If such tasks can be carried out by persons who otherwise, to all intents and purposes, appear nonconscious and afterward report with high confidence the total absence of experience, then we have evidence of strong zombiehood.

Consequently, I evaluate automatic behavior as providing evidence of (1) no zombiehood if the person is at least dimly conscious during the behavior or in an altered state of consciousness, or if the behaviour is completely reflexlike during nonconsciousness; (2) weak zombiehood if the person is truly nonconscious but can only carry out more or less routine action programs; or (3) strong zombiehood if the person is truly nonconscious but can carry out nonroutine tasks involving new decisions and the processing of the meaning of the task and the surrounding objects. This type of zombie can move in the world along trajectories that are indistinguishable from those realized by conscious humans. Strong zombiehood, if it exists, means that there are (temporary) zombies around us, who can perform almost any task even in the absence of consciousness. They would provide strong empirical evidence of epiphenomenalism.

Sleep-Related Dissociations of Consciousness and Behavior

There are several diagnostic categories referring to complex motor attacks occurring during sleep: night terrors, sleepwalking (somnambulism), nocturnal paroxysmal dystonia, nocturnal wandering, nocturnal seizures, and REM sleep behavior disorder (RBD). All of them, apart from RBD, tend to arise during NREM sleep, and it is unclear whether they are manifestations of basically similar or qualitatively different types of phenomena occurring in the sleeping brain. Descriptions of these automatisms are given below.

NREM-Related Nocturnal Wandering: Case Descriptions

Study 1 Reported by Schenck and Mahowald (1995).

Subject A 43-year-old man who showed frequent and violent nocturnal behaviors 1 to 3 hours after sleep onset.

Documented complex behaviors He often engaged in strenuous activity that he could not duplicate in the daytime (e.g., lifting a large mattress over his head or pushing a heavy dresser across the room) and running out of the house. Once he left the house in pajamas by running through a screen door, entered his automobile, and drove 5 miles to his parents' home where he awakened them by pounding on their door. He frequently injured himself while colliding with doorways and furniture, and from falling down the staircase.

Contents of consciousness during automatic behavior The subject was often but not always amnesic about the attacks afterward. During the attack it was impossible to communicate with the patient or break the spell. His eyes were wide-open, but he did not actually see the environment as it was; instead of seeing his wife, he often perceived a dreamed object or a person with extremely threatening content. For example, the episode of somnambulistic automobile driving was initiated by the belief, formed during dreaming, that someone was in the house and about to attack him. While driving he was only aware that he was driving to his parents' home to escape an intruder at his own home.

Zombie rating No zombiehood. This person is not completely nonconscious during the behavioral attacks; instead, he is in an altered state of consciousness, involving distorted perceptions of his surroundings and delusions of threats. Thus, the phenomenal world simulation in the brain is strongly involved in determining the behavioral trajectory of this man, but the system is only partially modulated by current sensory information. The behavioral trajectory is computed at the phenomenal level by taking into account virtual objects whose counterparts do not exist in the sensory environment. Conversely, some external physical objects are ignored by the trajectories because their counterparts do not exist at the phenomenal level as virtual objects.

Study 2 Reported by Kushida, Clerk, Kirsch, Hotson, and Guilleminault (1995).

Subject A 51-year-old man who would abruptly arise in the night and have violent outbursts for 3 to 4 hours.

Documented complex behaviors He smashed dishes, threw anything within reach, crawled on his hands and knees throughout the house, chased the cats, removed his clothes, walked out of the house partially clothed, and attempted to drive the automobile.

Contents of consciousness during automatic behavior The subject's eyes were open, but glazed and he seemed to be completely removed from the environment. Although he often injured himself during these episodes, he could not recall the cause of his injuries upon awakening in the morning. Immediately after an episode of nocturnal wandering, the patient was confused and disoriented, not able to state his name, not oriented to time or place, and unable to repeat phrases or follow simple commands.

Zombie rating Weak zombiehood. There is no evidence of consciousness during the behaviors, although a gravely altered state of consciousness, coupled with dense amnesia, cannot be ruled out. The behaviors he manifests are complex, involving interactions with the environment and its objects. However, the behaviors are manifestly bizarre and indicate that the meaningfulness of the surrounding objects cannot be appreciated. It seems as if the behavioral trajectories are not controlled by the semantic windows of phenomenal objects. Instead, primitive aggressive and defensive behavioral programs seem to be activated. It is conceivable that some such programs might be released with little involvement from the part of the phenomenal level.

Study 3 Reported by Maselli, Rosenberg, and Spire (1988).

Subjects Twelve patients with nocturnal wandering.

Documented complex behaviors Attacks that were stereotyped for a given patient and consisted of complex automatisms ranging from crawling movements to running through hallways. One patient would drag his wife around the bedroom by her hair; another would kneel at her bed and appear to be praying.

Contents of consciousness during automatic behavior Four patients reported stereotyped frightening images that consisted of moving objects, animals, or persons but no dreamlike plot or narrative. Patients were only dimly aware of their behavior, and seemed surprised when the attacks were described by outside observers.

Zombie rating Weak or no zombiehood. Some patients were in an altered state of consciousness; some may have been completely nonconscious. For those who were in an altered state of consciousness, the behavioral pathways were computed by taking into account frightening virtual objects that had no physical counterparts. For those who were nonconscious during the episodes, the trajectories were controlled by the release of primitive motor programs that led to highly routine, bizarre, or maladaptive behaviors.

Study 4 Reported by Guilleminault, Moscovitch, and Leger (1995).

Subjects Forty-one patients with nocturnal wandering.

Documented complex behaviors Subjects could make series of gestures that were very decisive or threatening (e.g., fist movements, kicking, assumption of a defensive posture). One subject threw his wife on the floor, ran to his two children, took them into his arms, and ran out of the house.

Contents of consciousness during automatic behavior Subjects were unresponsive, appeared distant and unaware of their surroundings. They sometimes ran into furniture and objects, due to what witnesses felt was a lack of awareness of objects that were in their way. The subjects had incomplete memory of the episodes, but often had vague recollections of nightmarish imagery that was always terrifying and always involved some type of perceived threat to the subject or a loved one. Subjects appeared to attempt an escape from a danger that they alone perceived, but their movements were not appropriate for the real situation and surroundings. Onlookers were often ignored or pushed aside. The subject who ran out of the house with his children said afterward that he had believed the house was on fire.

Zombie rating Weak or no zombiehood. As in the previous reports, some patients probably were in an altered state of consciousness and their phenomenal world simulation system presented the behavioral environment in a form not corresponding to physical surroundings. Some of the patients may have been completely nonconscious, but their behaviors were too routine or bizarre to constitute more than weak zombiehood.

Study 5 Reported by Plazzi, Tinuper, Montagna, Provini, and Lugaresi (1995).

Subjects Four patients with epileptic nocturnal wanderings.

Documented complex behaviors Patient 1 got up, walked around, opened the door, stepped into the garden, and then went back to bed. In the sleep laboratory, he jumped out of bed, tried to open the door, and started to jump on and around the bed. When questioned immediately after the episode, he could not report any dream. Patient 2 sat on the bed, got up and left the bed, moving around the room with a motionless facial expression and speaking unintelligibly. Afterward he was aware that something had happened during the night. Patient 3 would suddenly sit up in bed, scream and jump out of bed, walk around the bedroom, unresponsive to calls and with an expressionless face. Afterward, he could not remember what had happened. Patient 4 also got out of bed, put his clothes on, screamed, and went back to sleep. He could not remember the episodes the morning after. In the sleep laboratory he pulled the electrodes from his scalp, and tried to get off the bed. Although alert immediately after the episode, he could remember nothing.

Contents of consciousness during automatic behavior Nonexistent or nonreportable due to amnesia.

Zombie rating Weak zombiehood. All of the patients seemed to be quite nonconscious during the episodes, but the behaviors they manifested are not particularly reasonable or demanding. The behavioral trajectories realized by the patients in the nonconscious state seem to be relatively harmless (and useless), routine motor programs released during sleep.

NREM-Sleep Automatisms: Conclusion

The cases described above represent a mixture of sleepwalking, sleep terrors, nocturnal seizures, and related disorders. Remarkably complex behaviors are realized by these patients during NREM sleep, but as far as it is possible to tell, some of the patients are not entirely nonconscious during the behavior. In many cases some sort of frightening imagery or perceived threat is experienced and sometimes its content is later recalled. This hallucinatory content of consciousness obviously motivates and causes the observed, often violent, behaviors. The behavioral trajectories realized are frequently quite rational and adequate in the light of the perceived threat: the patients attempt to save themselves and their loved ones from, say, threatening intruders or a fire. For example, when aged 10 years, one patient had risen from sleep, rushed into the sitting room where his parents were still sitting, and thrown the butter dish out of the window, believing it to be a bomb (Oswald & Evans, 1985). It appears that the patients first misperceive the real surroundings (there is a mismatch between the external stimulus environment and the internal simulated world), then strong goal images based on the misperception are evoked, and a behavioral trajectory is immediately realized in which the hallucinatory images are treated as if they were real. (This pattern of forceful threat-avoidance behaviors elicited during sleep seems to be closely related to the function of dreaming, to be discussed in chapter 24).

The patients have their eyes open and there is at least some registration of the environment, since in many cases (if not always) furniture is bypassed and stairs are negotiated safely. However, even if there is a degree of conscious experience involved in this registration, the patients do not perceive the environment properly nor can proper judgment be exercised (Mahowald, 1993). There is little evidence that the patients manifesting extremely complex automatic behaviors could be regarded as completely nonconscious zombies. On the contrary, most of the patients seem to be in an altered and confused state of consciousness, a mixture of wakefulness and NREM sleep (Mahowald & Schenck, 1992; Mahowald, Woods & Schenck, 1998). In this state, one's subjective consciousness is focused on one internally generated, usually terrifying image or belief. Appropriate threat avoidance behavior is often realized automatically, violently, and efficiently in the absence of reflective thought, without an awareness of one's altered state, one's actions, or their actual consequences.

Some cases of moderately complex behavior coupled with dense amnesia for the events may, however, indicate nearly complete absence of subjective experience during the episode. Even if in those cases the patients can be regarded as totally nonconscious zombies, their behavior is far from the flexible and integrated types of behavior guided by a consciously apprehended model of the world. Sleep-related automatisms without any remembered mental content tend to consist of routine actions or stereotyped violent behaviors that are not particularly adaptive for the individual. The patients may even be seriously injured by their own actions when bumping into obstacles they are not aware of. This kind of behavior may well be the most that can be managed without the contribution of a consciously experienced simulation of the world. There is no evidence of rational, adaptive, and flexible behavior taking place in the complete absence of consciousness (strong zombiehood). But these cases do fulfill the criterion of weak zombiehood.

REM Sleep Behavior Disorder

REM sleep is normally a state of total paralysis of the voluntary muscles, save for the ones used for breathing and eye movements. Hence, for complex behavior to be manifested during REM sleep, the neural mechanisms responsible for maintaining muscular atonia have to be defective. REM sleep behavior disorder (RBD) refers to a condition in which muscular atonia is removed during REM sleep and complex, often violent behaviors are manifested. Some illustrative cases are described below (figure 23.1).

Consider the case of a 73-year-old man. On occasion, he unintentionally struck his wife. Once he jumped off the end of the bed and awoke on the floor with a bloody lip, head, and knee. During another episode, he leaped from his bed, fell, and struck the right side of his face on a corner of a chest, causing him to wake up immediately. This accident resulted in a subdural hemorrhage. In the sleep laboratory during REM sleep, the patient suddenly exhibited explosive running movements, followed by an arousal. The patient's actions clearly corresponded to what he was dreaming about at the time of the observed behaviors. He sustained the subdural hemorrhage when he dreamed of working on a loading dock and saw a man running. Someone yelled "Stop him!," and the patient had tried to do just that when he jumped out of his bed with the unfortunate consequences (Dyken, Lin-Dyken, Seaba, & Yamada, 1995).

Another patient with RBD, on one occasion, "held his wife's head in a headlock and, while moving his legs as if running, shouted: 'I'm gonna make that touchdown!' He then attempted to throw her head down toward the foot of the bed. When woken up, he recalled a dream in which he was running for a touchdown, and he spiked the football in the end zone" (Boeve, Silber, Fernan, et al. 1998, p. 364). If the RBD patients were woken up during an episode of abnormal sleep behavior, none of them recalled that they had executed violent movements, although all recalled violent dreams at the time of wakening: being pursued by an enemy; trying to protect family members from unknown intruders; fighting off unidentified assailants (Comella, Nardine, Diederich, & Stebbins, 1998).

One patient's EEG, EMG, and ECG were polysomnographically recorded during an attack of violent behavior. The muscle tone was increased and the arms and legs showed bursts of intense twitching, accompanied by observable behavior. After a spontaneous

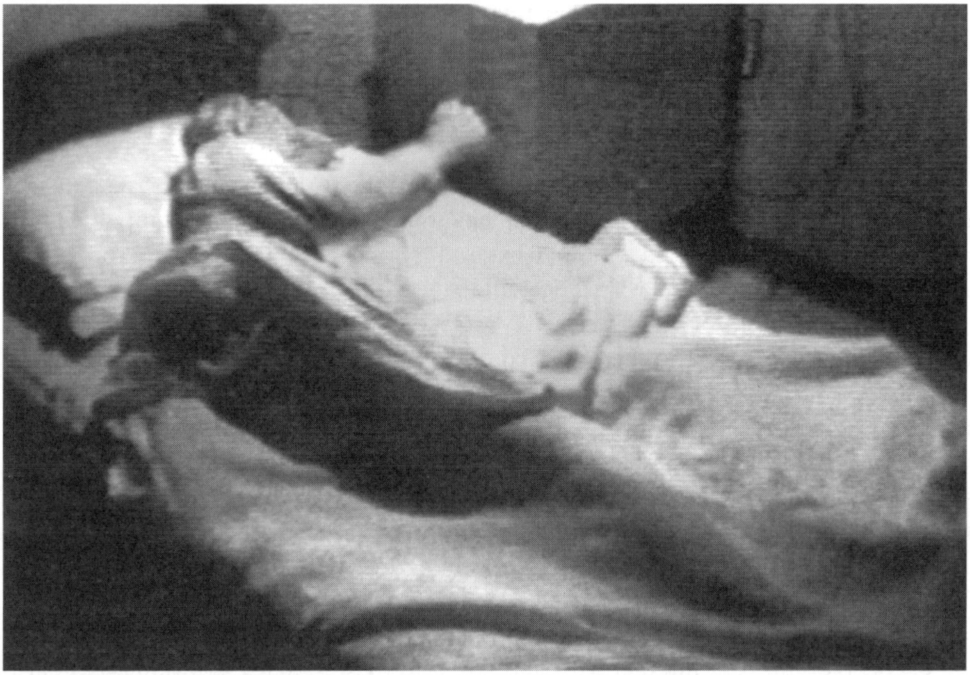

Figure 23.1
Photograph from sleep laboratory video footage of a man with REM sleep behavior disorder. The patient is throwing a punch at a dreamed enemy during a REM sleep dream. RBD patients have vivid, action-filled nightmares that lead to overt, isomorphic enactment of the dreamed movements. (From Schenck, C. H. (1993). REM sleep behavior disorder. In M. A. Carskodon (Ed.), *Encyclopedia of sleep and dreaming* (pp. 409–505). © 1983. Macmillan Reference USA. Reprinted by permission of The Gale Group.)

awakening, the man reported a dream in which he was running and trying to escape skeletons that were awaiting him (Schenck, 1993).

I have personally experienced a couple of times what happens if the muscle inhibition of REM sleep partially gives in during dreaming. On three different occasions, I observed a violent dreamed action at the phenomenal level leading to a corresponding forceful movement of the physical limb. On the first occasion, I dreamed that I was lying on the ground and somebody was coming toward me riding a bicycle. I saw the bicycle wheel rapidly approaching my face, at which point I made a forceful defensive motion, straightening my arm in front of me, in order to fend off the wheel and protect my face. I woke up when my hand hit hard against the bedroom wall. On another occasion I dreamed that I was in a corridor in a big unfamiliar building. From behind one corner, a huge gorilla suddenly appeared and started attacking me. I tried to lift one knee in order to strike the gorilla on the chest and protect my own body. I woke up when my knee hit the bedroom wall with considerable vigor. On the third occasion I dreamed that I was trying to defend (what in the dream was) my house against a violent intruder. I caught the intruder on the staircase going down in front of me. I jumped and attempted to kick the intruder in the head. I did hit the intruder's head (with the dreamed leg), but at the same time my real leg kicked the bedroom furniture, resulting in my waking up (with a couple of aching toes).

The *isomorphism* between dreamed and real movements and trajectories is remarkable. The trajectory of a virtual limb at the phenomenal level will be accompanied by a similar trajectory of the physical limb in external physical space if only the motor commands issued at the cortical level can get all the way through to the muscles.

In conclusion, in RBD there is typically a close correspondence between the virtual action within the dream and the observed real action, which thus is simply the acting out of the dreamed behaviors. During dream enactment the dreamer is far from a nonconscious zombie. On the contrary, the dreamer is right in the center of a vivid subjective dream world, and perfectly unaware of the real surroundings of his physical body. The complex behaviors observed in RBD are guided by the phenomenal contents of consciousness. The subject is, however, totally immersed in the dream world—the phenomenal contents of the simulated world in no manner represent the actual world surrounding the person. The dreamed actions of the dream self and the real actions of the dreamer's physical body will be motivated by events at the phenomenal level. They reflect attempts to interact with and adapt to the simulated world in the dreaming brain.

As there is a radical mismatch between the real physical environment and the world simulation at the phenomenal level, the physical actions realized by the dreamer's physical body prove to be highly maladaptive in the real world, often resulting in injuries to the patients and their bedfellows. As Schenck (1993) notes, in RBD an ironic situation commonly occurs, that in his dream world a husband is desperately fighting to defend his wife from some impending threat while in the real world he is actually beating her up in bed. The trajectories determined at the phenomenal level during dreaming are not particularly useful in the real world. The dream-enacting person will most likely collide violently with real physical objects.

Despite their practical uselessness, dream trajectories (or *dreamwalking,* as Allan Hobson has named RBD) are theoretically significant. *RBD shows that the organism's overall behavioral trajectories are determined by the phenomenal contents of consciousness.* That is to say that the trajectories taken by our physical bodies moving in the physical world are determined by the nature, location, and spatiotemporal relations of the semantic windows in the egocentric phenomenal coordinate system of phenomenal consciousness. If the phenomenal contents of consciousness are formed without being properly modulated by sensory input (as in RBD), then the person will be sent on a fool's errand, a possibly disastrous behavioral trajectory, guided by a misrepresentational internal simulation.

It is clear that RBD provides absolutely no evidence of zombiehood. However, it shows that when guided by dream consciousness, the dreamer behaves in ways that would be adaptive and reasonable in the context of the dream world present in consciousness, although they are not so in the context of the real world where the dreamer's physical body is located.

Automatic Behavior during Epileptic Seizures

Dissociations between consciousness and behavior during epileptic seizures have been described in some detail in the clinical literature. Yet, it is by no means clear what exactly the patients can do and whether they actually are completely nonconscious during the episode. A well-known formulation of this dissociation was given by Penfield (1975). He noted that when epileptic discharge confines itself to one functional mechanism, it will selectively paralyze that mechanism. Consequently, if the mechanisms indispensable for consciousness are involved, then they can be selectively put out of action, which, according to Penfield, converts the individual into a "mindless automaton." Penfield located these areas critical for consciousness in the subcortical gray matter in the higher brain stem (thalamus and basal ganglia); inactivation of these areas produces unconsciousness. Epileptic discharges initiated locally in the temporal or prefrontal cortex may spread to this subcortical network and produce an attack of automatism:

> In an attack of automatism the patient becomes suddenly unconscious, but, since other mechanisms in the brain continue to function, he changes into an automaton. He may wander about, confused and aimless. Or he may continue to carry out whatever purpose his mind was in the act of handing on to his automatic sensory-motor mechanism when the highest brain mechanism went out of action. Or he follows a stereotyped, habitual pattern of behavior. In every case, however, the automaton can make few, if any, decisions for which there has been no precedent. He makes no record of a stream of consciousness. Thus, he will have complete amnesia for the period of epileptic discharge. (Penfield, 1975, p. 39)

Penfield mentioned a patient who could automatically continue playing the piano during a seizure, another who walked home from work, and yet another who drove the car home, although occasionally through red traffic lights. Automatisms are realized by a sensorimotor mechanism which is normally in interaction with, but can become disconnected from, consciousness. The behavior of the automaton reveals, as Penfield observed, what the brain without consciousness can still do:

> The human automaton, which replaces the man when the highest brain mechanism is inactivated, is a thing without the capacity to make completely new decisions. . . . The automaton is incapable of thrilling to the beauty of a sunset or of experiencing contentment, happiness, love, compassion. These, like all awarenesses, are functions of the mind. The automaton is a thing that makes use of the reflexes and the skills, inborn and acquired, that are housed in the computer. . . . This automatic coordinator that is ever active within each of us, seems to be the most amazing of all biological computers. (Penfield, 1975, p. 47)

Thus, Penfield's automaton surely deserves to be described as some sort of zombie, evidently the kind we would classify as representing weak zombiehood.

Very little theoretical attention has been paid to the dissociations in epilepsy between consciousness and behavior. Yet, it is clearly a significant phenomenon for consciousness research. In order to find out more about epileptic automatisms, I have established collaboration with the neurological rehabilitation clinic in Stockholm (Stiftelse Stora Sköndal). There the neuropsychologist Mirja Johanson has collected detailed reports of behavior during seizures from epileptic patients and their family members. The patients were furthermore interviewed about their memories of experiences during seizures, in order to find out whether there was any evidence of subjective experience during the state commonly believed to involve a loss of consciousness. Let us meet some of the most interesting patients (see also Johanson, Revonsuo, Chaplin, & Wedlund [2003]).

Case Reports

Case 1 D.D. is a 38-year-old woman suffering from complex partial epilepsy for over 10 years, with an epileptic focus in the left temporal lobe. Once she had a seizure while on her way to lunch with her colleagues. She recalls nothing of what happened during the seizure. When she regained consciousness she found herself back in the office with a portion of chicken salad (which she does not like) for lunch. Her colleagues said that she got out of the car and walked into a nearby restaurant where she never goes. The restaurant personnel said that she had not said anything, but had just pointed to the salad, bought it, smiled, but avoided eye contact.

In this case we have an example of complex behavior certainly without reflective consciousness and possibly guided only by nonconscious or peripherally conscious information. The goal chosen prior to the seizure (to buy lunch) had been preprogrammed and was therefore carried out automatically though erroneously—the patient bought something she would not have liked to eat and would not have bought in her normal state of mind. This is one of the most complex automatisms so far, involving object recognition (restaurant, food), choice (chicken salad), gestural communication, and complex interaction with objects and persons when paying for the salad. Even if granted that the patient was totally nonconscious during the seizure, the whole behavioural episode constitutes a fairly well overlearned script of "buying lunch." Thus, it would still be regarded only as evidence, even if quite remarkable, of weak zombiehood. The error in choosing something one does not like reveals that the meaning of the surrounding objects was not fully available during the episode. Furthermore, in this case it is quite likely also that memory problems contributed to the patient's not having any idea of what happened during the seizure, for she showed deficient memory performance in neuropsychological testing.

Case 2 J.T. is a 48-year-old woman with complex partial epilepsy and a left temporal focus. She reported a seizure that began with the feeling that she was on the point of vanishing into thin air. She did not remember anything of what happened during the next hour. Her family members reported that she fell sideways onto the sofa, her body first tensed and then relaxed. After about 10 minutes she got up. She turned some lights off. Then she took some children's toys and placed them next to the kitchen sink. Now and then she mumbled incomprehensibly. She was able to walk without bumping into objects. She finally undressed and put her nightgown on, although with some difficulty. The whole time her mouth was distorted and she had a blank stare in her eyes. She went to bed and regained consciousness after some time, but a strong sense of unreality remained long afterward.

In this case we have genuine automatisms (turning off lights, picking up things, undressing and dressing), some of which at least were unreasonable, in the complete or near-complete absence of conscious experience. The automatisms are again quite closely reminiscent of the behaviors manifested by ordinary sleepwalkers. Placing toys next to the kitchen sink reveals that the toys were not recognized but handled as if they were dishes. Therefore, this is another case of weak zombiehood: complex but rather aimless interaction with the environment, nonconscious registration of the surroundings, but no evidence of having access to the full meaning of the objects and one's interactions with them.

Case 3 L.C. is a 26-year-old woman with complex partial epilepsy. During a recent seizure she was cooking. She wanted to buy a red onion, went to the shop, but came back with a yellow onion. She placed it on the floor. She hallucinated hearing the neighbors speaking, and then she realized that she was having a seizure. She called a friend and then lost consciousness. She woke up in bed, and was delighted to see her friend at the bedside. Then she looked at her own hands and saw that they were badly burnt; she was shocked and started to feel the pain. She thought that she must have put her hands on the hot stove while she was nonconscious during the seizure, but she has no recollection of this.

This seizure is very interesting, for it strongly suggests that even an extremely painful stimulus was not consciously registered during the seizure; the patient most likely had been deeply nonconscious—but also behaving in a most unreasonable manner—to have burned her hands that badly. Again, weak zombiehood.

Automatic Behaviors from a Neuropsychological Perspective

There are some neuropsychological findings which may illuminate the mechanisms behind automatic behaviors. Lhermitte, Pillon, and Serdaru (1986) described two types of behaviors that arise in connection with frontal lobe damage. *Utilization behavior* refers to the tendency of perceived objects to trigger corresponding motor programs in which the objects are involved, although no request to use the objects is made. Thus, a comb placed on a table induces combing of one's hair; a glass of water, drinking; a newspaper, reading; and so on. *Imitation behavior* refers to the repetition of whatever behaviors are observed to be done by the examiner (or other people). Such patients seem to be very much dependent on environmental cues, but in the absence of external cues they often show apathy. Lhermitte (1986) called this the environmental dependency syndrome, in which the autonomy of the patient seems to be compromised.

The explanation for such bizarre behavior is that frontal lobe mechanisms normally excerting control over action schemata have become defective, which leads to the automatic activation of action programs, executed without any reflection. This account is consistent with the theory of Stuss, Shallice, Alexander, and Picton (1995) according to which frontal attentional mechanisms control the monitoring, energizing, inhibiting, and competition between rival schemata. Schemata or routine input-output transformations can become automatically activated by sensory input or other schemata, but frontally based attentional mechanisms and reflective consciousness can modulate this activation and thereby implement a degree of choice.

In utilization and imitation behavior the patients are phenomenally conscious, but have impaired reflective consciousness. The crucial question is, Could the automatic activation of action schemata occur also in the absence of phenomenal consciousness, in a nonconscious state? In the absence of the conscious state, the action scripts might still be activated by the same triggers as normally, but since there is no inhibition or monitoring of the activity, the action programs would be released without reflection and perhaps in a state of a very low level of awareness of surroundings. Therefore, nonconscious epileptic patients may carry out complex tasks that are somehow inappropriate. Action scripts are released in the absence of phenomenal experience or reflective control, making the patients do things they would not do if they were able to control their actions and monitor their behavior. Sleepwalkers often do the same sort of things. The mechanisms for releasing the behaviors are probably similar in both cases, although the reason why consciousness is suppressed may be different in these two groups.

Weak zombiehood is probably based on the automatic activation of action programs that can be guided by nonconscious registration of the overall spatial layout of the surroundings, leading to the observed interactions with the environment. An object in the environment is registered at some nonconscious or peripherally conscious level, and it automatically achieves the status of a goal image toward which some routine behavioral trajectory is computed and realized. If the phenomenal world-simulation system is involved at all in guiding these behaviors, it can be regarded as only partially functional, for it seems to not take into account all the information that is normally taken into account when computing and realizing the next behavioral trajectory.

In fact, anyone can experience how nonconscious or peripherally conscious information sometimes automatically guides behavioral trajectories. Just open a box of candies beside you when you watch television, and your hand will automatically perform beautifully accurate and efficient behavioral trajectories between the box of candy and your mouth, at least until the growing feeling of nausea enters the phenomenal level and (hopefully) prevents your hand from continuing on this disastrous path. Often the only way to stop this uncontrollable activity is to either eat them all up, or to move the box to a position out of the reach of your hands.

Summary

My purpose in this chapter was to examine the possibility of real zombies or strong zombiehood existing among us: pathological disorders of consciousness that abolish subjective experience altogether but preserve the causal powers of the brain in guiding complex and entirely normal-looking behavior. In other words, I was searching for empirical evidence of nonconscious systems in the brain that can determine behavioral trajectories for the organism that are indistingushable from those determined by the phenomenal world-simulation system.

Many of the cases regarded as paradigm examples of unconscious behavior turned out not to be what they appear on the surface. Instead, the phenomenal level seems to be present in most cases, although in a distorted or diminished form, an altered state of consciousness. Still, even in those cases the contents of the phenomenal level determine the behavioral pathways taken by the so-called unconscious patients.

Only in a few cases do we have good reason to believe subjective consciousness to have been completely lost. As far as it is possible to tell, this may sometimes happen during sleepwalking or epileptic seizures; at least the patients report experiencing loss and regain of consciousness, but all memory for the events in between is completely lost, even when the patient is interviewed immediately after the episode. Behavior during such episodes is often surprisingly complex, but at the same time clearly abnormal. The nonconscious registration of the environment seems to be restricted in the way that the meaning of the surrounding objects is not available for guiding behavior. A motor program or even a complex event script can be carried out, but in a mechanical way. The meaningfulness of objects, surroundings, and one's own actions seems to be lost with the loss of the simulated world at the phenomenal level. Stimuli cannot evoke meaningful semantic windows for the nonconscious brain, and the trajectories of the nonconsciously guided physical body hardly realize actions that could be regarded as meaningful. The zombie behavior, even when seemingly meaningful for a moment, is not being monitored, and erroneous or aimless courses of action result easily, but are never corrected. Therefore, the behavioral trajectories along which our weak zombies travel often turn out to be either meaningless or even harmful and dangerous for the individual.

In conclusion, no convincing evidence was found of any pathological dissociation where the conscious state (the phenomenal level as a whole) would be completely absent without any significant loss of causal powers, so that complex, adaptive, nonroutine behavior would be possible in the same way it is during normal waking consciousness. This supports the conclusion that consciousness possesses causal powers in the initiation or guidance of behavior unlike those of any purely nonconscious processing systems in the brain. Phenomenal consciousness forms a *meaningful* simulation of the world in the brain, and the brain attempts to guide the organism's interaction with and behavioral adaptation to the world as presented in the content of consciousness at the phenomenal level. When this meaningful world simulation is present in the brain, the person's behavioral trajectories are computed on the basis of it, even if the simulation does not correspond to the person's real physical surroundings (as in RBD). When the meaningful world simulation is absent from the brain, only simple, routine, or meaningless behavioral trajectories can be supported by the nonconscious brain.

24 The Biological Function of Dreaming

Biological realism and the world-simulation metaphor constitute the hard core of the biological research program. Thus they are also expected to lead to new ideas and to guide future research on consciousness in fruitful directions. Consequently, in this final chapter, these ways of thinking about consciousness will lead us toward a novel theory about the biological function of dreaming. This theory is a fresh application and extension of the biological approach to consciousness. Furthermore, it connects biological realism and the world-simulation metaphor with other novel areas in biology of the mind, in particular evolutionary psychology—by suggesting that the function of dreaming is an evolutionary adaptation—and affective neuroscience (Panksepp, 1998)—by stressing the role of emotionally charged dream experiences, especially fear. Another application of the biological research program, not discussed in this book, has already been put forward: a multilevel approach to the description and explanation of hypnosis as an altered state of consciousness (see Kallio & Revonsuo [2003, 2005]).[1]

Waking consciousness is an internal simulation of the external physical environment currently surrounding the organism. This world simulation is modulated in real time by sensory input and thereby provides the brain with telepresence in the organism's behavioral environment. In the brain's transparent surrogate world the spatial distribution of nearby objects is presented in the egocentric coordinate system of phenomenal space. Furthermore, the meaning and the value of each object for the organism is presented in the simulation by connecting the surface Gestalt of the object to long-term memory and affective valence, thus opening a semantic window for each object. Thereby is created the egocentric world of meaningful objects in which we live our conscious lives.

The simulated world of consciousness functions as a navigational system for the brain that otherwise is confined to the darkness inside the skull, isolated from any direct contact with the organism's behavioral environment. On the whole, the brain's primary task is to find safe trajectories across the organism's behavioral space and to guide the organism along those trajectories to goals that promote survival and reproductive success. In mammals at least, the sphere of phenomenal consciousness contributes to this task by creating an integrated model of the probable distal sources of current sensory stimulation. The brain sets and monitors the overall behavioral trajectories by relying on this internal egocentric source model. Consciousness forms the world simulation in which the simulated organism (the "self") navigates among meaningful semantic windows toward important goals while at the same time trying to avoid needless dangers. As the evidence about nonconscious forms of behavior establishes (see the previous chapters), if the brain's phenomenal world simulation is temporarily wiped out (or if it grossly misrepresents the environment), the brain loses most of its ability to guide the organism along safe and meaningful pathways in behavioral space. Therefore, there is no doubt that waking consciousness fulfils a crucial function in organism-environment interaction.

Dreaming is, by the definition introduced in chapter 2, an internal world simulation that emerges during sleep. Why should the dreaming brain generate a highly organized form of phenomenal consciousness? Shouldn't we rather expect to spend our nights in total subjective silence and darkness, in the absence of any form of phenomenal consciousness? At most, we might expect some meaningless, chaotic phenomenology to arise by chance in the sleeping brain every now and then (resembling simple forms of sleep mentation), but an organized, temporally progressing world simulation could hardly arise as a side effect of random cortical stimulation. Furthermore, as we are not engaged in organism-environment interaction during sleep, nor can the brain guide us through behavioral space while we sleep, it seems entirely pointless to engage the internal navigational system of the brain under those circumstances.

Thus, the function of dreaming appears to be a mystery. Biological realism suggests, however, that in order to discover the biological function of dreaming, we should follow the strategy used elsewhere in the biological sciences. Two important points emerge from that approach: First, the *form* of a phenomenon suggests its *function.* Second, the notion of "biological function" has a strict definition that should be followed. These guidelines lead to the conclusion that dreaming does have a well-defined and clearly manifested biological function after all.[2]

What Is a Biological Function?

When we inquire about the "function" of dreaming, we should be clear about what we mean by "function" or "functional." The appropriate sense of "function" in this context is that of a biological, adaptive function. According to Tooby and Cosmides (1992, 1995; see also Cosmides & Tooby [1995]) the biological standard is the only standard of functionality that is relevant to analyzing why brain and cognition are organized in one fashion rather than another. A cognitive system is functional in the evolutionary sense if and only if it promotes the organism's inclusive fitness. That is, the biologically functional system must solve problems that will increase the probability that the organism possessing the system will produce offspring, or that the organism's kin will produce offspring. Evolutionary biology gives the concept of "function" a very specific content: *the function of a system solely refers to how it systematically caused its own propagation in ancestral environments* (Tooby & Cosmides, 1995). If dreaming has an adaptive function, then dreaming must have solved some adaptive problems whose solution tended to enhance survival and promote reproduction in the human ancestral environment, thus causing the persistence of the brain's dream-production mechanisms and their spread in the population.

We should not confuse the biological or natural functions of dreaming with the functions *we* have *invented* for them (Flanagan, 1995). There is an important distinction between what *we* do with dreams once we recall them (e.g., dream interpretation), and *what the dream can do itself* (Breger, 1967; Blagrove, 1996). Natural functions are biologically adaptive functions in the sense defined above, whereas invented functions are derivative psychological or cultural functions. We can put our recalled dreams to a variety of personal or cultural uses, but no matter how enlightening and meaningful such uses may be, they are invented by us, not by natural selection. It is doubtful that any truly natural function of dreaming could be based on the conscious recollection or verbal reporting of dream content, for the natural functions of dreaming, if any, must have been effective in such ancestral conditions and species in which self-reflective dream recollection or reporting was not likely to occur—thus, the natural functions of dreaming cannot have been dependent on them.

Now we are in the position to state our question more specifically. The question we are presently interested in is whether dreaming serves any *natural* functions: *Does the realization of the subjective phenomenal level of organization during sleep—the experience of dreaming or world simulation during sleep—solve any adaptive problems?* That is, did phenomenal dreaming in any way enhance the prospects of the reproduction of humans and their ancestors during evolutionary history? Did dreaming increase the inclusive fitness of the ancestral human?

The primary evolutionary context for considering the possible adaptive function of dream consciousness is the prehistoric Pleistocene environment in which humans (and their bipedal hominid ancestors) lived as hunter-gatherers for hundreds of thousands of years. If dream consciousness is biologically functional, it should have had adaptive value at least in that original environment, under the conditions in which human ancestral populations lived. Whatever the adaptive role of dream consciousness might have been in that long-gone original context, there is no guarantee that the average dreaming brain today, facing a completely different environment than the one in which it evolved, should fulfill any functions that we recognize as adaptive in the present environment.

When put into the proper evolutionary-biological context in this manner, the question, Does world simulation during sleep have a function?, becomes, Did the activation of a simulated world in the ancestral human brain during sleep in some way enhance the probability of reproductive success of ancestral humans in the behavioral environment that they inhabited?

My answer is in the affirmative: the offline simulation of the world we call "dreaming" is specialized in the simulation of particular types of events in the ancestral environment that regularly and severely threatened the reproductive success of humans and their ancestors for millions of years. The world simulation during sleep became specialized in these types of events in order to enhance the probability that subsequent real events of the same type would be negotiated efficiently and successfully.

Traces of the Biological Function of Dreaming

A general rule may be offered when trying to figure out the biological function of a phenomenon: the form of the phenomenon usually suggests its function. When it comes to the biological function of dreaming, we should systematically explore the form and the content of dreams as they appear in large samples of dream reports from different populations. If we pay careful attention to the most conspicuous statistical properties of dreams, perhaps we will spot an underlying thread that leads us to the original function of dreaming.

What kind of traces should we be looking for in the statistical properties of dreams? The traces should be related to a function that can be reasonably well fulfilled by pure mental simulation during sleep. Just as flight simulators are used to train pilots to face emergency situations that would be too risky in reality, perhaps the world simulation during sleep is also specialized in dealing with and preparing for situations too risky to train for in reality. Furthermore, we should expect the dream simulations that fulfill a biological function to have been originally related to events in the ancestral environment that regularly and severely threatened the reproductive success of our ancestors. On the basis of these ideas, we can now formulate an evolutionary hypothesis on the function of dreaming.

The hypothesis I am putting forward states that dreaming (or world simulation during sleep) was originally a biological defense mechanism for simulating threat perception and rehearsing threat avoidance responses and behaviors in the safe virtual environment of the dream world.

If the above hypothesis is on the right track, then we should find clear traces of this function in the statistical properties of dreams, even in the present human population. I will now briefly review the evidence that reveals abundant traces of the threat-simulation function of dreaming.

Traces of the Threat Simulation Function in Normal Dreams

If dreams are specialized in simulating threatening events, then we ought to find that dream content is biased toward including various negative elements (reflecting threats) rather than positive elements. Several prominent features of dream content suggest that this bias indeed exists.

Emotions in Dreams In the classic study of C. S. Hall and Van de Castle (1966) 500 home dream reports from female and 500 from male college students, age 18 to 25, were content-analyzed. About 80% of the over 700 emotions explicitly mentioned in the dream reports were negative, and only 20% positive. The figures remain similar if the dreamer's own emotions only are considered. About half of the negative emotions experienced by the dreamer were classified as "apprehension"; the other half consisted of "sadness," "anger," and "confusion."

In the first normative laboratory study, F. Snyder (1970) collected 635 REM dream reports from students and found that over two thirds of the emotions mentioned in the reports were negative, fear being the most common and anger the next most common. Strauch and Meier (1996) reported a sleep laboratory study in which they not only collected REM dream reported from forty-four subjects but also asked them how they had felt during the dream. The emotions described in response to this question were analyzed. Specific emotions were mentioned in connection with every other dream. Negative emotions appeared twice as often as positive ones, with anger, fear, and stress being the most frequent types of negative emotions. In contrast to specific emotions, general mood states were found to be more often positively than negatively toned.

When emotions are explicitly mentioned in dream reports, they are much more likely to be negative than positive,[3] and they are likely to be appropriate to the dreamed situation (Foulkes, Sullivan, Kerr, & Brown, 1988). These findings are well consistent with the hypothesis that dream content is biased toward simulating threatening events.

Misfortunes in Dreams "Misfortune" names a class of dream event in which a bad outcome happens to a character independent of anything the character has done (C. S. Hall & Van de Castle, 1966). Misfortunes include, for example, mishaps, dangers, and threats. The opposite is called "good fortune." In the C. S. Hall and Van de Castle (1966) normative study, there were altogether 411 cases of misfortune in 1000 dream reports, and only 58 cases of good fortune. Thus, misfortunes in dreams are seven times more frequent than good fortunes. Furthermore, about 70% of the misfortunes happen to the dream self, and accidents, loss of possessions, injuries and illnesses, obstacles, and threats from the environment make up almost 90% of these misfortunes, whereas death and falling are rare types of misfortune (C. S. Hall & Van de Castle, 1966; Domhoff, 1996). Misfortunes therefore typically reflect situations in which the physical well-being or the resources and goals of the dream self are threatened.

Aggression in Dreams Aggression is the most frequent type of social interaction found in dreams, the other classes in the C. S. Hall and Van de Castle (1966) scale being friendliness and sexual interactions. About 45% of the dreams in the normative sample included at least one aggressive interaction. Dreamers are involved in about 80% of the aggressions in their dreams, and when they are involved, they are more often the victim than the aggressor (C. S. Hall & Van de Castle, 1966; Domhoff, 1996).

Summary Negative emotions, misfortunes, and aggression are prominent in the ordinary dreams of the normal population. In most studies they are found to be far more prominent than the corresponding positive dream elements. These findings indicate that various unpleasant and threatening elements are overrepresented or biased in dream content, which supports the view that dreams are specialized in simulating threatening events.

Traces of the Ancestral Environment in Dream Content

"Enemies" in our Dreams Domhoff (1996) defines "enemies" as those dream characters with which the proportion of aggressive encounters of all aggressive plus friendly encounters is over 60%. This calculation on the C. S. Hall and Van de Castle (1966) normative sample reveals that animals and male strangers are the enemies in men's as well as women's dreams. (men vs. animals, 82%; women vs. animals, 77%; men vs. male strangers, 72%; women vs. male strangers, 63%). Encounters with female strangers are not at all so aggressive, but predominantly friendly (men vs. female strangers, 40%; women vs. female strangers, 43%) (Domhoff, 1996). According to C. S. Hall and Domhoff (1963), unknown males are responsible for the high proportion of victimization and physical aggression involving male characters.

C. S. Hall (1955) content-analyzed 106 dreams of being attacked and found that the attacks predominantly represented situations in which the dreamer's life or physical well-being was at stake. The attacker was usually human or a group of humans (70%) but not infrequently an animal (21%). When the sex of the human attacker was identified it was virtually always male. The dreamer usually reacted to the attack by running, escaping, or hiding (unless she woke up). C. S. Hall and Domhoff (1963, 1964) analyzed aggressive and friendly interactions in over 3000 dream reports. They found that interaction was aggressive with 48% of the animal characters in men's dreams and with 29% of the animals in women's dreams.

Van de Castle (1983) compared college students' dreams (over 1000 dream reports altogether) in which humans are the dominating dream characters with those in which animals predominate. He found that dreams with animal figures typically take place in an outdoor setting, have a great deal of activity that is often of a violent nature, and that the dreamer typically experiences fear. If an animal figure initiates an interaction with the dream self, the nature of the interaction is aggression 96% of the time and friendliness only in 4%. Van de Castle writes that "almost without exception, if the animal figure initiates any response to the dreamer, it is some form of threat or hostility" (p. 170).

Why are animals and male strangers our enemies in dreams? Ancestral humans lived in environments in which many animals (e.g., large carnivores, poisonous animals, parasite-carrying animals) presented an ever-present mortal threat to humans. Therefore, behavioral strategies to avoid contact with such animals and to escape or hide if attacked by them obviously were of high survival value. Some deep-rooted human fears and phobias of snakes, spiders, rats, and open spaces are indications that ancient threat-avoidance programs remain with us (I. M. Marks & Nesse, 1994). Dreaming simulates and rehearses these ancestral threat-avoidance programs in order to maintain their efficiency, because the cost of a single failure to respond appropriately when the danger is real may be fatal, while the cost of repeated threat simulations during sleep are rather low.

Our present-day encounters with unfamiliar males in waking life are not predominantly aggressive. In the ancestral human environment, however, intergroup aggression and violent competition over access to valuable resources and territory is likely to have been a common occurrence. Since intergroup warfare and violence was and still is almost exclusively practiced by males (Wrangham & Peterson ,1996; see also Campbell, 1999), encountering male strangers is likely to have been a potentially threatening situation in the ancestral environment, comparable to the threats presented by dangerous animals. Although an overwhelming majority of our current waking-life encounters with animals and male strangers are not particularly aggressive or threatening, dream content still reflects the ancestral conditions in which such encounters were potentially life-threatening. Dreams are biased toward simulating threats that were common in our ancestral environment.

Children's Dreams If dreams are naturally biased toward simulating ancestral threats, then we should expect that the traces of these biases are strongest early in life, when the brain has not yet had the chance to adjust the biases to better fit the child's actual environment. This seems to be the case when it comes to the appearance of animals and aggressions in children's dreams. One of the most prominent differences between child and adult dreams is the much larger number of animal characters in children's dreams. C. S. Hall and Domhoff (1963, 1964) analyzed about 500 dream reports from children aged 2 to 12 years; C. S. Hall later increased the sample to 600 dreams and Domhoff (1996) reported the results from this larger sample. Animal characters make up about 25 to 30% of all characters in the dreams of children 2 to 6 years of age, and about 15% in those 7 to 12 years of age, whereas the normative finding for adult dreams is about 5% (Domhoff, 1996).

Van de Castle (1983) also reported studies on children's dreams. The 741 dream reports (one from each child) were written down by schoolteachers or directly reported by the pupils themselves. The general trend toward a decrease in the frequency of animal dreams as a function of age is clearly manifested. Two-year averages in the percentage of animal dreams for children 4 to 16 years old were 39.4% for 4- to 6-year-olds,

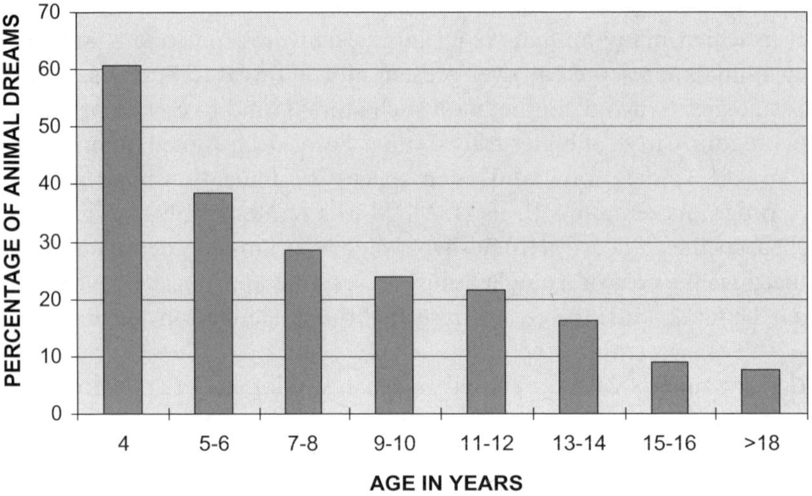

Figure 24.1
Percentage of animal dreams in relationship to age. The figures are based on data reported by Van de Castle (1970).

and 35.5%, 33.6%, 29.8%, 21.9%, and 13.7% for the next consecutive 2-year age groups. In an earlier study on a smaller sample of dreams, Van de Castle (1970) reported closely similar figures (figure 24.1).

In their dreams children surprisingly often encountered such animals that they never or only relatively seldom could encounter in the waking world. Wild or frightening animals (e.g., snakes, bears, monsters, lions, spiders, gorillas, tigers, wolves, and insects) made up nearly 40% of all animal characters in children's dreams in this study, but less than 20% in college students' dreams. Dogs, horses, and cats accounted for 28% of animals in children's dreams but for 38% in college students' dreams (Van de Castle, 1983). Thus, the proportion of domestic animals increases and that of wild animals decreases with age.

Due to the methods of collecting the dream reports, the studies mentioned above may have included a somewhat biased sample of dreams. However, in the laboratory study of Foulkes (1982) animals were also the major characters in the dream reports of children ages 3 to 5 and 5 to 7 years, appearing in 30 to 45% of the reports. Also, the decrease in the number of animal characters with increasing age was confirmed. Strauch (1996) reported results from both home and laboratory REM dreams in Swiss children aged 9 to 11 years. Both types of dreams involved more animals than did young adults' dreams, again confirming the decrease in dream animals with increasing age. Home dreams contained animals about twice as often as laboratory dreams, which was explained by dream report length: home dreams were longer and included more characters. Girls' dreams contained more animals than boys' dreams. In the REM dreams, 102 animals were found. In girls' dreams, tame animals and pets prevailed (63%) over wild native or exotic animals (37%), whereas in boys' dreams, wild animals were much more common than tame ones (61% vs. 39%). Taken together, on average one out of two animals encountered in the child's dream world is an untamed wild animal. For boys around 10 years of age this is the most common type of dream animal.

C. S. Hall and Domhoff (1963) showed that children also have a higher rate of aggression in their dreams than adults. The greatest amount of aggression occurs in the dreams of children aged 2 to 12 years. According to Domhoff (1996), much of this larger amount of aggression is with animals and the child is usually the victim of an attack by the animal. In Strauch's data (1996) of combined REM and home dreams, about 30% of all the animals appearing in 10-year-old children's dreams were in the role of aggressors, compared to 10% in adults' dreams.

J. B. Levine (1991) studied the representation of conflicts in the dreams of seventy-seven children who were about 10 years of age and came from three different cultures: Bedouin, Israeli, and Irish. Conflictual dreams accounted for about two thirds of the reports and were reported about twice as often as nonconflictual dreams in all three cultures. The Bedouin children, who were living in a traditional seminomadic tribe, had dreams that were realistic and concerned with threats to physical survival, usually from the natural world.

Children's dreams thus show strong biases toward simulating a world that contains animals (especially wild animals), aggression, conflicts, animal aggressors, and victimization to a greater degree than their own waking world or the dream world of adults does. These biases decrease with age if the child's real environment is largely devoid of them. It seems unlikely that young children would have had more frequent real waking experiences of such things than teenagers or adults; therefore, it is difficult to explain these biases by referring to the waking lives of the children. These biases seem to be another sign of the fact that the dream production system is well prepared to simulate threatening events consistent with and prevailing in the human ancestral environment. The biases decrease with age, as the child's waking world proves to be quite different from what was anticipated by the dream production mechanisms.

Typical Dreams

Typical dreams (or dream themes) are those that occur in the same general form across large numbers of people over and over again. They thus reflect the kinds of dreams that are rooted deepest in our dream production mechanisms (and in our memory for dreams). Typical dreams are usually studied by presenting a questionnaire with a list of dream themes to large numbers of subjects. The question presented to the subjects is, "Have you ever dreamed of . . . ?" They then check all the alternatives in the list that apply to their own dream life.

As many as 67 to 86% of Canadian undergraduate students in different samples remember dreaming about being chased or pursued, and this is the leading remembered theme in their dreams (Germain, Nielsen, Zadra, & Montplaisir, 2000). In one study, the Typical Dreams Questionnaire, listing fifty-five themes, was administered to almost 1200 first-year university students in three different cities in Canada. The results revealed that "being chased or pursued (but not physically injured)" was again the leading theme. Eighty-two percent of participants reported dreaming about it; 22% reported this being the earliest dream theme they could remember having in their childhood. It was also the theme most frequently given in answer to the additional question: "Which theme occurred *most often* in your life?" All in all, out of fifty-five alternative dream themes, this paradigmatic threat-simulation theme ranked first in prevalence, self-reported earliest emergence, and self-reported frequency. Other threat-simulation themes also ranked high in typicality. Among some of the most prevalent dream themes were also the following:

- Being physically attacked (beaten, stabbed, raped)
- Being frozen with fright
- Being killed
- Falling
- Being on the verge of falling
- Arriving too late
- Trying again and again to do something
- Failing an examination

A web-based survey of 500 participants from all over the world yielded similar results (Garfield, 2001). The three most often reported themes were being chased or attacked (80%), falling or drowning (64%), being lost or trapped (58%).

Recurrent Dreams

Robbins and Houshi (1983) asked 123 university students whether they had ever had recurrent dreams, and if yes, they were asked to describe them. Sixty percent reported that they had had recurrent dreams, many beginning in childhood. A content analysis revealed that only one type of recurrent dream occurred with any frequency: an anxiety dream in which the dreamer was being threatened or pursued. The threatening agents were wild animals, monsters, burglars, or natural forces such as storms, fires, or floods. The dreamer was watching, hiding, or running away. The authors regarded these descriptions as reasonably close to nightmares (Robbins & Houshi, 1983, p. 263).

A. Zadra and Donderi (2000) reviewed the content of recurrent dreams (see also A. L. Zadra, 1996). Threat simulation appears to be prominent in them. First, being chased is the most common theme in the recurrent dreams of both children and adults. Negative affect was far more common than positive affect (about 80% vs. 10%), fear or apprehension was the most frequently reported emotion (occuring in 79% of childhood recurrent dreams) and misfortune was far more frequent than good fortune (42% vs. 4%). All of this is in accordance with the view that the most typical recurrent dreams are powerful threat simulations.

Bad Dreams and Nightmares

A *nightmare* may be defined as "a very disturbing dream that awakens the dreamer." A *bad dream* is "a very disturbing dream that does not awaken the dreamer" (A. Zadra & Donderi, 2000). Estimates of nightmare frequency in the normal population vary, depending on the definitions of what counts as a nightmare and the methods used to quantify their frequency. A. Zadra and Donderi (2000) compared different methods and arrived at the conclusion that in retrospective self-reports, people underestimate the numbers of nightmares and bad dreams that they have had. By contrast, dream logs give the highest and probably the most accurate estimations of their typical occurrence. The researchers thus ended up with the following estimations: normal subjects experience about ten nightmares and about thirty bad dreams per year, that is, about forty "very disturbing dreams" per year. That is close to one (0.77) "very disturbing dream" per week in the normal population.

There is large interindividual variation in nightmare frequency. About 5% of the population is estimated to suffer from chronic, recurring nightmares that occur at least once per week. Also, most children, especially during ages 3 to 6 years, frequently experience bad dreams and nightmares.

Children often dream about being chased or attacked by monsters, animals, or "bad guys." Brenda Mallon (2002) has documented dramatic examples of threat simulation in children's dreams and nightmares (see figures 24.2, 24.3, and 24.4.). Monsters, wild beasts, evil kidnappers, and other enemies chase and torment the children in the dream world: "As you can see from the illustrations, these are not beings we would choose to meet if we had the choice" (Mallon, 2002, p. 21).

The themes in the dreams of lifelong nightmare sufferers are remarkably similar to the themes of recurrent dreams, and the most frequent theme is, again, that of being chased or attacked (Domhoff, 1996; Hartmann, 1984). Such dreams usually begin in childhood and involve being chased by a monster or a wild animal. In adulthood, the chaser was more likely to be a large unfamiliar man, a group of frightening people, or a gang. These dreams can be frequent, seem very vivid and real, but still do not usually reflect any actual events that ever happened to the dreamer (Hartmann, 1998).

Recurrent dreams and lifelong nightmares not directly connected with any real-life events appear to be powerful simulations of rather primitive threats. The origin of these simulations cannot be traced back to the real life of the dreamer. Where do these

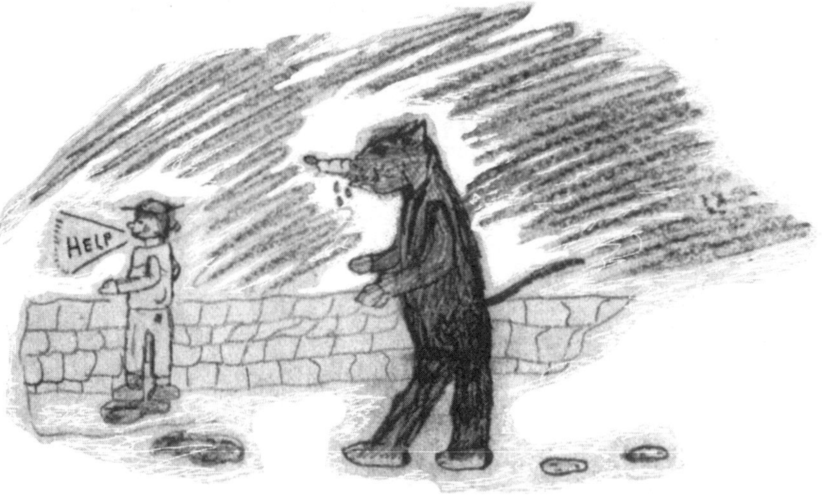

Figure 24.2
Children's dreams as revealed by their own drawings I: Boy being chased by bear. (From Mallon [2002]. *Dream time with children.* London: Jessica Kingsley. Reprinted by permission of the publisher.)

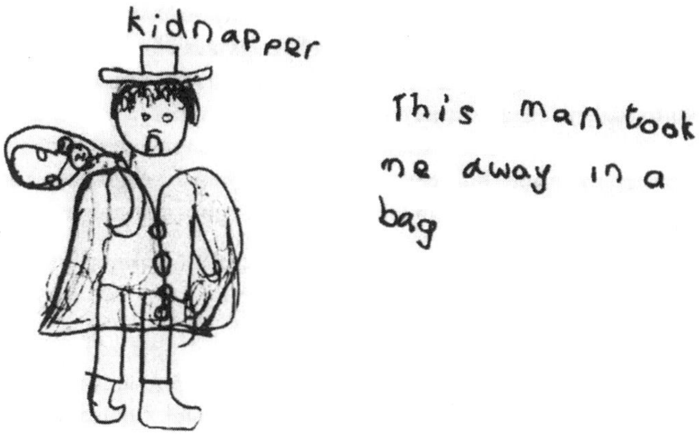

Figure 24.3
Children's dreams as revealed by their own drawings II: Kidnapper. (From Mallon [2002]. *Dream time with children.* London: Jessica Kingsley. Reprinted by permission of the publisher.)

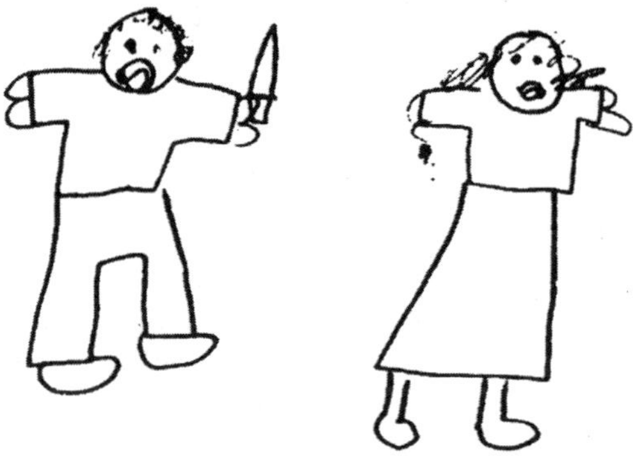

Figure 24.4
Children's dreams as revealed by their own drawings III: Girl chased by knifeman. (Mallon [2002]. *Dream time with children.* London: Jessica Kingsley. Reprinted by permission of the publisher.)

recurrent themes come from? In the light of the human ancestral environment, it makes great sense to simulate violent encounters with animals, strangers, and natural forces, and how to escape from such situations. Therefore, these simulations are incorporated as default values in the threat-simulation system, and they can be activated in almost anybody, at least occasionally. They may be called ancestral "threat scripts": internal models representing the paradigmatic dangers to human reproductive success in the ancestral world.

In conclusion, bad dreams and nightmares are the ultimate forms of threat-simulation dreams. Nightmarish elements frequently occur also in recurrent dreams, children's dreams, typical and universal dreams, as well as in just about anyone's normal dream life every now and then. These elements establish *a continuum of threat-related content* in dreams. Threat-related content seems to be particularly salient in dream production; it is overrepresented in our dream lives (compared to similar situations occurring in our real lives), and thus points toward the original biological function of dreaming.

However, even more decisive evidence for the threat-simulation function emerges when we consider the *impact of real-life experiences on dream content.* Also, in this regard threat-related experiences seem to be unique. They are incorporated into dream simulations with such efficiency and retained there with such persistency that no other types of real experience come even close. Even a single relatively brief exposure to a life-threatening situation may lead to persistent posttraumatic nightmares about the event.

The Effect of Traumatic Experience on Dream Content

Real experiences of actual dangers or life-threatening events are very likely to be incorporated into dreams (Hartmann, 1984, 1996; Barrett, 1996). This is most clearly manifested in cases of posttraumatic nightmares. These are reported by people who have undergone, say, wartime battles, natural catastrophies, terrible accidents, or assault, rape, or torture. The frequency of posttraumatic nightmares depends, among other things, on the degree of threat perceived to be targeted at self and significant others. It appears that the greater the sense of threat created by the experience, the more likely it is that nightmares will follow (Nader, 1996). For example, 100% of twenty-three children who were kidnapped and buried in a truck trailer; 83% of six children who underwent a life-threatening medical operation; 80% of ten children witnessing their mothers being raped; 63% of children exposed to sniper fire on their schoolyard; and 40% of children whose suburb was exposed to radioactivity after a major nuclear power plant accident reported nightmares related to the respective incidents (for a review, see Nader, 1996). Ninety-six percent of 316 Vietnam combat veterans described a combat nightmare in an interview (Wilmer, 1996).

These are very impressive figures, especially in view of the fact that laboratory research has failed to find *any* strong determinants of dream content. Presleep stimuli, such as films depicting violence, are only marginally, if at all, incorporated into dreams. The conclusions of Vogel (1993) in a review of stimulus incorporation in dreams are revealing:

> . . . dream content is remarkably independent of external psychological and physical stimuli both before and during sleep and equally independent of currently measurable physiological processes during sleep. Therefore, the sources of dream content, that is, its themes and its specific elements, remain a mystery. (p. 298)

Laboratory research has failed to find the actual determinants of dream content, probably because it is practically and ethically impossible to expose experimental subjects to situations that evoke a deep enough sense of a threat. The stimuli that are typically used in laboratory research on stimulus incorporation, such as films, never induce anything like a genuine sense of a real threat to one's own life. Therefore they do not function as ecologically valid cues for the dream production mechanisms. We must turn to the cruel experiments inadvertently designed by wars, crime, and nature. The sense of severe personal threat is probably the most powerful factor we know of in the modulation of the content of dreams. The experience of a severe trauma can induce nightmares in almost anyone; the majority of people, especially children, involved in traumatic events do report nightmares; and traumatic nightmares can occur in several stages of sleep (Hartmann, 1984).

Once the dream production system encounters the memory of an event combined with a deep sense of threat, how does it handle it? There seems to be a more or less universal pattern involved in the ways in which posttraumatic dreams are constructed (Hartmann, 1984, 1998). In the first stage, immediately after the traumatic event, the frequency of trauma-related dreams and nightmares increases and the event is being replicated a few times in the dream world, in a form often closely similar to the original experience. The first stage normally lasts a few days or weeks, but in severe posttraumatic disorder it may persist for years. In a longitudinal study of children who were exposed to a sniper attack on the school playground, 42% continued to have bad dreams 14 months after the incident (Nader, Pynoos, Fairbanks, & Frederick, 1990). In another study of a bushfire disaster, 18% of the children continued to have posttraumatic nightmares when studied 26 months after the event (McFarlane, 1987).

Gradually, the nightmares change into increasingly modified versions of the event. At this stage, the original experience is associated with and connected to other similar contents in memory. The resulting dreams may be small variations of the original threat, the original threat mixed with previously experienced ones, and with classic nightmare themes such as being chased or escaping powerful natural forces. Eventually, perhaps after a few weeks or months, the content of dreams returns to approximately normal. Even long after the original trauma, events that are reminiscent of it or unrelated events that also induce a deep sense of threat may trigger the recurrence of the trauma-related nightmares. In posttraumatic stress disorder, this normal development of the dream sequence does not occur, but instead, replications and different variations of the original trauma recur over and over again, even for years (Hartmann, 1984, 1996; Stoddard, Chedekel, & Shakun, 1996).

Threat-Simulation Responses in the Modern World

The September 11 attacks induced threat-simulation dreams across the United States. In the aftermath, people reported dreams about bombs being dropped on their hometowns, seeing planes crash, or being aboard a falling plane with Middle Eastern terrorists (Bulkeley, 2003). In most of these dreams, the people under attack try to escape, fight back, or try to save their family from the ensuing disaster. These dreams were reported even by people who were thousands of miles away from the East Coast and only heard about the attacks through the mass media.

The Gulf War and the Scud missile attacks on Israel constituted a severe threat for the Israeli people. A dream study by Peretz Lavie (1996) demonstrates that the threat activated the threat-simulation system and produced appropriate simulations. In the fifth week of the war almost half of the dreams reported by students at the Technion Faculty of Medicine in Haifa dealt directly or indirectly with the war. The contents of the dreams focused on the greatest personal threat posed by the war, which were the missile attacks of Iraq—Saddam Hussein had threatened to use chemical weapons. Thus, the most important personal defense against such attacks was the gas mask, which became standard equipment for everybody. One of the greatest fears was being caught in a missile attack without the gas mask. According to Lavie (1996) the gas mask became the most common subject of dreams during the Gulf War. Apparently, the dream production system of Israeli students studied by Lavie was presenting threat simulations of situations where survival depended on a fast and appropriate response to a missile attack. One student reported the following dream:

> I dreamed that I was taking a shower when I heard the air raid warning. I ran out of the shower dripping wet, but I could not decide whether I should first dry myself or put on my gas mask. (p. 73)

Lavie himself had the following dream:

> I was on a bus with my gas mask on the floor beside me. When I got off, I realized that I had left my mask behind on the bus, and just as I started to run after it, the air raid warning siren suddenly sounded. (p. 73)

Ordinary as well as posttraumatic nightmares are especially frequent in children (Hartmann, 1984). Nader (1996, pp. 16–17) mentions the following types of trauma-induced threat simulations in children's dreams. Kuwaiti and Croatian children exposed to war dreamed of being personally endangered by someone trying to kill them with a knife, a gun, or bare hands, and of being captured or tortured. Children from Los Angeles who had witnessed their mothers being raped dreamed of the rapist returning, of being threatened, of being severely physically harmed, of directly confronting the assailant, or of taking revenge. A girl who was chased and groped by an unfamiliar man had recurrent dreams in which people or animals chased her. Children who were in a cafeteria when a tornado knocked the wall down with serious consequences dreamed of the wall falling again, of houses being destroyed by a tornado, of branches falling, of being hit by glass, and of trying to find bandages for dead people. After a hurricane, both parents and children dreamed of being threatened by winds or tornadoes coming directly at them.

A child kidnapped in 1976 still suffered from nightmares about 10 years later, repeating aspects of the ordeal in a realistic fashion. Here is one example of such a posttraumatic nightmare that the then 23-year-old man experienced in 1985:

> I had a dream about the kidnapping just a couple of weeks ago. It wasn't the same situation—you know—as on the bus. But it was a bunch of people. We were in a house and this guy had us. And I took a couple of kids and I put them out of this window when the kidnapper wasn't looking. And then when I seen him walk around the corner I took off running. Now, the only thing I can remember—the kidnapper guy was chasing me. And he almost catched me. And I got away. And I got somebody to help me. And we were taking him to the police. We drove around a while and we ended up at that guy's house again. The guy who was supposed to be helping me—like, he really was helping *him* [the kidnapper]. And the dream was pretty, um, it was really real. (Terr, 1990, p. 207)

In a study of 11- to 13-year-old Arab and Jewish children's dreams (Bilu, 1989), all the dreams representing the "other side" were extracted and analyzed. In these 212 dreams, aggression appeared in about 90% of the interactions, while friendliness was virtually nonexistent (4%). Jewish children dreamed about Arab terrorist attacks and camouflaged detonating explosives in public places. In these dreams, the dreamer was usually the recipient of an unprovoked assault initiated by an adult adversary who was typically defeated in the end. Arab children living in a refugee camp dreamed about brutal physical aggression which resulted in death on either side in 25% of the dreams. The dreamers were typically harrassed, expelled, arrested, beaten, injured, or killed. Bilu (1989) comments that the conflict between Arabs and Jews seems to have an even stronger presence in these children's dreams than it does in reality (i.e., it is *overrepresented* in dreams): ". . . the intensity and pervasiveness of the conflict as reflected in the dreams cannot be taken for granted even by those well-acquainted with the situation" (pp. 385–386).

Dreams after trauma reflect the dream production system working at full capacity, producing a regular pattern that proceeds from near-identical replications to increasingly modified variations to gradual fading and possible recurrence. My hypothesis sees posttraumatic nightmares as the ultimate form of the threat-simulation function.

Real Threats as Cues That Activate the Threat-Simulation System

The view that emerges can be summarized as follows: Experiences of real threats are *ecologically valid cues* for the threat-simulation system. Encountering real threats powerfully activates the threat-simulation system. As a consequence, the threat content of dreams becomes more and more dominating, the dreams become more realistic, and the threats as well as the threat avoidance behaviors simulated draw directly from the threats experienced in the real world.

In a study on Palestinian children living under traumatic conditions it was found that the more the children were exposed to trauma, the more negatively emotional and the less bizarre their dreams were. The children exposed to trauma also had better dream recall than other children (Punamäki, 1997). These findings indicate that the dream-production system creates especially vivid and realistic simulations of the threatening events encountered in the real world.

Real threats might even trigger the ontogenetic development of dreaming. Foulkes (1999) argues that adult-like "true" dreaming appears relatively late in childhood, between 7 and 9 years of age. Foulkes's data are, however, based on children who have not been exposed to a particularly threatening environment. By contrast, clinical case reports suggest that the earliest nightmares may be experienced as early as the second year of life (Hartmann, 1998). Some traumatized preschool children report fully developed nightmares, unlike those typical of age (Nader, 1996). Thus, traumatic experiences may actually trigger or significantly boost the development of the dream-production system. Conversely, lack of real life-threatening events might hold it back, or at least preserve the dream-production system in a resting state, although it would already be capable of generating threat simulations if only exposed to the ecologically valid cues.

Selection Pressures and Ancestral Threats

Next, we need to consider whether the human ancestral environment was the kind of place that contained the relevant ecologically valid cues for constantly activating the threat-simulation system, and whether there was likely to be a selectional advantage from improved threat avoidance skills so that repeated threat simulations were likely to lead to increased reproductive success.

We need to show, first, that there was a high selection pressure in the ancestral environment. How long did people live under those conditions? Which proportion of the population survived to reach reproductive age? Meindl (1992) presented estimates of mortality based on three different hunter-gatherer cemetery sites in Africa and North America where hundreds of skeletons have been unearthed. The oldest of the communities dates back to circa 10,000 years ago. Mean life expectancy in each of the three populations is estimated to have been between 20 and 22 years. Thus, as far as we know, mean life expectancy for ancestral humans was remarkably low compared with that of modern times. According to one estimate (Meindl, 1992), of those who reached 5 years of age in ancestral hunter-gatherer populations, about 25% died before entering the reproductive period and about 70% died before completing it. Thus, mortality rates were high, and only the select few ever got the chance to reproduce successfully.

Second, we need to show that the real threats in the ancestral environment were the kind of events the threat-simulation system is good at simulating. What were the most likely threats to survival in the ancestral environment? How severe were they? Among the primary causes of death in hunter-gatherer populations were probably exposure to predation by large carnivores, exposure to the elements, infectious disease, poor conditions and risky activities during hunting and gathering, and aggression or violent encounters, especially in defense of personal resources or group territory (Landers, 1992; Meindl, 1992).

These estimates render it quite obvious that the life of an average ancestral human was constantly at stake in the original environment. The death or serious injury of close relatives and local group members must have been a common event. Confrontation with extremely dangerous or even life-threatening situations is likely to have been part of everyday life rather than a rare exception. In order to reproduce successfully under those conditions, an individual must have been quite skilled at perceiving and recognizing various threatening situations (e.g., predators, aggressive strangers, poisonous animals, natural forces, social rejection by own group members), at avoiding unnecessary dangers, and when a threatening situation could not be avoided, he must have been able to cope with it by using efficient cognitive and behavioral strategies that promote survival.

In view of the harsh conditions in which our ancestors lived, it is likely that every individual, throughout his life, was continuously exposed to what by modern standards would be considered extremely threatening (and "traumatizing") situations. Therefore, the threat-simulation systems of ancestral humans must have been, first, developing in an environment with abundant threat-related input, and second, repeatedly reactivated by the ecologically valid cues from threatening real-life situations. In this kind of environment, the dreaming brain should be expected to produce a continuous flow of threat-simulation dreams.

Threat Simulation in the Dreams of Contemporary Hunter-Gatherers

If, as we have argued, the dreaming brain is a phylogenetically ancient threat-simulation system with default values reflecting ancestral rather than modern conditions, then we should expect to see this mechanism naturally activated in individuals who live in conditions closely resembling the ancestral ones. We should predict high levels of survival themes, threat simulation, and animal characters in the dreams of such individuals.

Gregor (1981) reported a content analysis of 385 dreams collected among the Mehinaku Indians in Central Brazil whose life had remained essentially traditional at the time of the study. The Mehinaku are an exceptionally fruitful group of informants for a study on dreams, for they have the habit of carefully recalling and often recounting their dreams in the morning. Gregor found that the dreams of the Mehinaku contain significantly more physical aggression, especially involving animals, than dreams from the American normative sample. In his paper, Gregor (1981) provides short summaries of the Mehinaku dream reports. Here are some examples of typical threats in the Mehinaku men's dreams:

- A woman attempted to have sex with him; the jealous husband assaulted him.
- Desired and approached girl, struck by his jealous wife.
- Attacked by a jaguar.
- Stung by wasps while in woods.
- Stung by ant.
- Chased by snake, he turns and kills it.
- Daughter almost drowned, rescued her.
- Stung by bees.
- Had sexual relations with girlfriend, wife saw them and became angry.
- Rescued drowning brother.
- Attacked by a herd of wild pigs.
- Shot at threatening jaguar but missed.
- Killed a threatening snake.

When the 276 dream summaries from the Mehinaku men were content-analyzed (see Revonsuo, 2000b, n. 13), about 60% of them were found to simulate events potentially threatening the dreamer's future reproductive success.

Dream samples from contemporary hunter-gatherer groups are probably as close to ancestral dreams as it is possible for us to get, which is not to say that they should be identical. In any case these studies show that threat simulation is very frequent in the dreams of such individuals, and that the dream-production system tends to generate fairly realistic threat simulations when the world it simulates is not very dissimilar from the ancestral human environment.

Dream Production and Threat Simulation

Dream production is an automatic, hard-wired, regularly activated feature of human brain function. The sources of dreams are selected from long-term memory by reactivating and recombining memory traces that are the most salient for the dream production system. *Salience* is a function of at least two factors: the degree of threat-related or negative emotional charge and the recency of the encoding or reactivation (or other priming) of the memory traces. Therefore, *the most salient memory traces* for dream production consist of the ones encoding *the most threatening events most recently encountered* (or whose memory traces have been otherwise most recently reactivated). The salience of a set of memory traces gradually declines by time or may be overcome by that of other traces: memory traces compete for access to dream production through their salience.

Simulations including elements of the selected threatening memories are then reconstructed by the dream-production mechanisms. In this process the dream-production mechanism tends to use dream settings and stereotyped scripts that are compatible with threats similar to ancestral ones (composing events that involve attacks, fights, pursuits, escapes, intrusions, loss of valuable resources, and events during which the dream self or close kin are endangered). Typical threat simulation dreams, such as nightmares and recurrent dreams, are thus composed of a variable mixture of salient episodic memory traces and suitable threat-simulation scripts. This mechanism is biologically functional (it solved adaptive problems for our ancestors) because in the original environment the dream production system regularly generated simulations of such real events that directly or indirectly threatened the reproductive success of ancestral humans.

Simulating these events rehearses performance at two stages: *threat recognition* and *threat avoidance.* The simulation of threat recognition is supposed to proceed in the following way. Salient emotionally charged memory traces are first selected for dream production. A visuospatial simulation is constructed in the brain activating the visual cortex, especially the occipitotemporal ventral visual stream. When potentially threatening content is presented in the world simulation, the amygdala is activated to evaluate the potential threat. Threat-recognition simulation primes this amygdalocortical network to perform the emotional evaluation of the content of visual awareness as rapidly as possible, in a wide variety of situations in which there is a visual object or event present that is potentially dangerous. The second stage, threat avoidance, consists of the rapid selection of a behavioral response program appropriate to the dangerous situation in question (e.g., fleeing, hiding, defending, attacking, seeking help from others) and the immediate realization of this response. Threat-avoidance simulation primes the connections between specific perceptual-emotional content and specific behavioral responses, and rehearses the efficient, forceful, highly motivated release of these behavioral responses through the activation of cortical motor programs. The efficient, rapid functioning of these threat-recognition and -avoidance networks decreases the latency and increases the sensitivity and efficiency of responding to similar real threats during waking. Therefore threat simulation during dreaming increases the probability of coping successfully with comparable real threats, leading to increased reproductive success.

Why Do We Dream about "Current Concerns"?

The capability for ancestral threat simulation is the essence of the biologically adaptive function of dreaming. However, the threat simulation mechanisms automatically select *any* available memory traces with highest relative salience and use them as a basis for simulation, regardless of the specific content selected; the mechanisms have no "insight" into what they are doing and whether it is biologically functional or not. When the individual's waking environment does not include any threat cues, the sources of dreams are quite varied and may be difficult to trace; almost any recently encoded or reactivated memory traces may be selected for dream production. Therefore, the present hypothesis is not in the least similar to Freud's (empirically untestable) thesis that *all* dreams are at bottom wish fulfillments. According to the threat-simulation theory, not all dreams are, nor should they be, threat simulations. The functionally crucial feature of dreaming is its *capability* for regular and efficient threat simulation in environments where the appropriate threat cues are constantly imminent.

The threat-simulation mechanisms operating in present-day humans who are living in safe environments rarely find salient memory traces corresponding to ancestral or mortal threats. Even the most salient traces typically represent only relatively mild threats. In the absence of truly dangerous threats, the threat-simulation system selects any recently encoded or reactivated emotionally charged memories that happen to have higher salience relative to other traces. The selected traces in such cases are typically about the "current concerns" of the dreamer. The simulation of the current concerns of modern humans probably has little, if any, biological adaptive value. The threat-recognition and -avoidance programs, and especially the selection pressures and increases in reproductive success associated with current concerns, are hardly comparable to those associated with ancestral threats in the ancestral environment.

Are there any ways to *separate* the predictions derived from the threat-simulation theory from current concerns theories or from the *continuity hypothesis* that states that dreams simply *mirror* waking life events? Unlike the continuity hypothesis, the threat-simulation theory predicts that threat simulations are sometimes completely *dissociated* from the waking life of the dreamer. Recurrent dreams and nightmares are often like this. Few people are regularly chased by animals, monsters, aliens, or strangers (or even worried about such far-fetched scenarios). Yet, they may frequently dream about such events. The current concerns and continuity hypothesis theories cannot explain these kinds of dreams. The threat-simulation hypothesis can explain both why we tend to dream about the minor real threats in our lives or our everyday current concerns (e.g., occupational or marital troubles)—they are mild emotionally charged threats that are more salient for dream production than emotionally completely neutral contents—and why we also dream about severe and rather primitive threats ("ancient concerns")—they reflect the threat-simulation scripts embedded in the dream production system as default settings, defining the types of threatening events that from an evolutionary point of view should be rehearsed most frequently. Consequently, the threat-simulation theory provides us with the most parsimonious explanation of dreaming, because different kinds of dreams can be explained by referring to a single mechanism, the operation of the threat-simulation system. Different dream events can be ordered on a single continuum according to the different degrees of threat they contain, and their appearance in dreams can be explained by pointing to the relative salience of the memory traces and threat scripts that the dreams are composed of.

Furthermore, several sleep disorders, such as night terrors, sleepwalking, nocturnal wandering, and REM sleep behavior disorder (RBD), can be seen as inappropriate over-activation of the threat-simulation mechanisms. If they are activated during NREM sleep, then night terrors, sleepwalking, or nocturnal wandering may result, where the subject tries to escape a simulated threat in an altered state of consciousness, a mixture of wakefulness and NREM sleep. If they are overly activated during REM sleep without atonia, then RBD results, where the dreamer acts out his threat-avoidance behaviors (for vivid examples of such cases, see chapter 23).

The Mechanisms behind Posttraumatic Nightmares

Persistent posttraumatic nightmares are produced by the threat-simulation mechanisms when a set of memory traces is associated with an overwhelming charge of threatening emotional content. This set of memory traces thus becomes overly salient for the dream production mechanisms and, in the absence of serious competitors, tends to be selected over and over again. The salience of the memory trace should normally slowly wear off, but in some cases the threat simulations themselves (as well as waking flashbacks) may reactivate the memory traces so often that they remain highly salient for extended periods of time.

Any procedure that decreases the emotional charge associated with the memory traces should render them less salient for dream production. There is evidence that recording one's nightmares and rehearsing them with a changed ending, or thinking about them in a relaxed state (desensitization), leads to significant decreases in nightmare frequency among chronic nightmare sufferers (Krakow, Kellner, Pathak, & Lambert, 1995, 1996; Neidhardt, Krakow, Kellner, & Pathak, 1992; Kellner, Neidhardt, Krakow, & Pathak, 1992). These techniques probably decrease the negative emotional charge associated with the memory traces involved in nightmare generation, thus directly decreasing their salience for dream production. Efficient methods for manipulating the salience of the traces will obviously be clinically useful in the treatment of disturbing threat simulations (i.e., recurrent nightmares).

Threat Simulation as a Biological Defense System

It is illuminating to compare the threat-simulation mechanism with other biological defense mechanisms. The immune system has evolved to protect us from microscopic pathogens, whereas the dream production system (along with a number of other systems) has evolved to protect us from dangerous macroscopic enemies and events in the environment. When a pathogen has invaded the host, an appropriate immune response is elicited, and when the antigen has been removed from the system, the immune response switches off because it is no longer required, and the immune system is restored to a resting state. Certain parts of the immune system, however, "remember" the infectious agent, and are now better prepared to fight it next time. Analogously, when a threatening event is encountered in the real world, a threat-simulation response is elicited by the dream-production system, and when the response in completed after repeated threat simulations, the individual will be better prepared to cope with similar threats in the future. If real threats are completely removed from the individual's environment, the threat-simulation system gradually returns to a "resting state" where the content of dreams becomes more heterogeneous and less troubled.

Even when the immune system is in the resting state, large numbers of leukocytes continue to be produced. For example, millions of granulocytes are released from the bone marrow every minute, even in the absence of acute inflammation (Roitt, Brostoff, & Male, 1998). These cells only live for 2 to 3 days; thus, if the individual is saved from infection for some time, astronomical numbers of granulocytes live and die without ever realizing their biological function at all. One may ask, But what is the biological function of all *those* granulocytes that never took part in any immune response? They must have some hidden function since they are so numerous and are produced so regularly. This question implies a misunderstanding of the biological functionality of the immune system. Similarly, to insist that all those dreams that do *not* simulate threats must have some hidden function of their own is to misunderstand the biological function of dreaming. Exactly as the evolved biological function of the immune system is to elicit appropriate immune responses when triggered by antigens, the evolved biological function of the dream-production system is to construct appropriate threat simulations when triggered by real threats. If no antigens are encountered and recognized within the organism, the immune system remains in a resting state, but it nevertheless continues to produce leukocytes; if no traces of threat-related experiences are encountered during regular dream production, the system nevertheless always ends up producing some kinds of dreams.

Furthermore, biological adaptations often have features that appear nonfunctional or even dysfunctional. Immune responses frequently occur in an exaggerated or inappropriate form (Roitt et al., 1998). Type I hypersensitivity—a typical allergic reaction—is an immune response caused by harmless antigens (e.g., pollen). In the worst cases it can lead to a generalized anaphylaxis and even death. Another example of an extremely harmful immune response is autoimmunity, where the immune system attacks the individual's own tissue. A highly efficient immune system may thus be prone to false alarms, but probably is also more efficient when it is really needed. As long as the net result is that those of our ancestors equipped with an operational immune system were more likely to reproduce successfully than those without, the system is biologically functional, even if negative side effects sometimes occur.

Therefore, we should not be surprised to learn that efficient threat simulation sometimes may have harmful side effects. A highly sensitive threat-simulation system may erroneously treat horror films or TV news as cues about threats in the environment, and consequently construct threat simulations—terrible nightmares—around themes that are completely fictional or about events taking place on the other side of the globe. Furthermore, subjects suffering from acute or chronic nightmares typically complain of sleep disturbances: for example, fear of going to sleep, awakening from sleep, restless sleep, insomnia, and daytime fatigue (Inman, Silver, & Doghramji, 1990; Krakow, Tandberg, Scriggins, & Barey, 1995) It is unclear to what extent ancestral humans might have suffered from sleep disturbances due to intensive threat simulations. If some of them sometimes did, that would have constituted a negative side effect of threat simulation, but—like an allergic reaction—one whose costs would not typically have been too high compared with the benefits. However, ancestral humans were psychologically adapted to the types of threats that were ever-present in their environment. Their life was in this respect rather predictable and stable. The typical ancestral threats and dangers were a normal part of their lives, whereas the events that in the modern population cause post-traumatic symptoms are usually extraordinary, unpredictabble events that happen to people who normally live in a relatively safe environment.

My conclusion is that the dream-production system can be seen as an ancestral defense mechanism comparable to other biological defense mechanisms whose function is to automatically elicit efficient protective responses when the appropriate cues are encountered. The concept of "inducible defense mechanism" in biology refers to defense mechanisms whose efficiency gradually increases when the mechanisms are activated by appropriate threats to the organism. Hence, threat simulation during dreaming constitutes an inducible defense mechanism.

The Threat-Simulation Theory Tested

To test the predictions of the theory systematically and quantitatively, we have developed a method for quantifying threatening content in dream reports. In the first of a series of studies, we identified all threatening events in almost 600 home-based dream reports from fifty-two subjects and then analyzed their content by using the Dream-Threat Rating Scale (Revonsuo & Valli, 2000).

We predicted that if the threat-simulation hypothesis has any truth to it, then we should find a relatively high frequency of threatening events in the dreams of normal subjects, and the content of threatening events in dreams should reflect the original function of this system as a threat simulator. Therefore, we hypothesized that normal subjects should encounter severe, life-threatening dangers with a higher frequency in dreams than in real life; that the dreamed threats should predominantly threaten the dream self and the people closest to and most significant for the dreamer in real life; that dream threats should be relatively realistic; and that the dream self should be likely to take at least some defensive action against the impending threats.

The main results were fully consistent with the predictions of the threat-simulation theory. Threatening events in dreams were found to be surprisingly frequent: on average there was about one threatening event per dream report, although some dreams contained multiple threats and others none at all. However, nearly 70% of the reports contained at least one threatening event.

Aggression was the most common type of threatening event in dreams. If escapes and pursuits are also regarded as a form of aggression, then aggression accounted for 42% of threatening events in the data. Failures, accidents, and misfortunes were also quite frequent, whereas disease and disasters are relatively rare types of threatening event in dreams.

We found that threatening events in dreams include a substantial proportion of severe and even fatally dangerous situations. Over 20% of the dream threats consisted of life-threatening situations or situations which, should they happen in real life, could cause serious damage to the physical well-being of the self. Since there was on average about one threat per dream report, then about every fifth dream includes a mortal threat. An average normal subject would thus experience several life-threatening situations in their dreams within a few days or weeks, whereas comparable situations are, fortunately, much less frequent in waking life. Events such as being assaulted, stabbed, shot at, pursued by strangers or animals, or participating in combat must be extremely rare or nonexistent in the waking lives of average Finnish university students, but are not very uncommon in their dream lives. Therefore, severe threats are grossly overrepresented in dream life.

Threatening events were found to be quite heavily self-centered, which makes sense in the light of the threat-simulation function. If the point of the system is to simulate real-life threats critical to the survival and reproductive success of the individual, then it is expected to simulate threats in which the self is often directly jeopardized, and people important to the reproductive success of the self are also often involved. In earlier studies it has been found that, first, the dreamer is more often the victim than the aggressor in aggressive interactions; second, that in 70% of cases the misfortunes in dreams happen to the dreamer (Domhoff, 1996); and third, that the dream self is also nearly always the victim in nightmares (Hartmann, 1993). Indeed, threatening events in dreams are predominantly directed at the dream self. Obviously, the simulation of threatening events only targeted at strangers or insignificant physical resources would not be relevant to the future survival of the self and thus could not serve as a rehearsal of the dreamer's threat-perception and threat-avoidance skills.

Threatening events in dreams were found to be based on relatively realistic rather than fantastic information. A threatening event in a dream is not a simple replay of the fictional threats that we regularly encounter in movies and television. In those imaginary cases, the threat is very often remote from everyday life (a comet hitting the Earth; a remote war; a space battle; fighting off vampires, aliens, or other supernatural intruders; witnessing rare natural disasters; fictitious crimes, etc.) and certainly not self-centered: our own personal well-being is not threatened by what goes on in a movie. In TV and movies we often see strangers threatened by exotic threats, whereas in dreams it is typical that we ourselves and our closest ones are most often threatened by familiar and realistic dangers.

In most cases the self is an active participant in the threatening event, and when the self in some way reacts to the situation, it is likely to react in a relevant way. Remarkably, if the threatening event is lethal, then the self is significantly more likely to show appropriate defensive responses than if the situation is less dangerous. These observations are consistent with the predictions of the threat-simulation hypothesis: if threat-avoidance behavior is being rehearsed during dreaming, then the dream self needs to be active, especially when its own life is directly in danger.

Taken together, the findings of the first empirical study directly testing the threat-simulation theory (Revonsuo & Valli, 2000) turned out to be in harmony with the theory's predictions. In our ongoing studies (Valli, Revonsuo, Pälkäs, Ismail, Ali, & Punamäki, 2005) we have analyzed dream reports from Kurdish and Palestinian children who have lived in traumatizing, warlike conditions, and personally witnessed or experienced violence and death. The results show that, exactly as the theory predicts, these children have a significantly higher frequency of threats in dreams, and their dream threats are more dangerous and severe than those of children living in more peaceful conditions.

For example, traumatized Kurdish children had threats in 80% of their dream reports, whereas Finnish children living in safe conditions experienced threatening events in only 30% of dreams. Furthermore, the Kurdish children's dream threats were much more severe and life-threatening than those of the Finnish group. Interestingly, exposure to real-life threats not only increases the proportion of threatening dreams, it also increases *dreaming per se* (or at least dream memory and reporting): traumatized children report significantly more dreams than nontraumatized ones.

The threat-simulation theory is empirically testable. Its predictions are currently being tested in a number of studies that look at threat simulation in recurrent dreams, nightmares, in traumatized children and adults, and in relation to real-life threats (e.g., see Desjardins & Zadra, 2004; A. Zadra, Desjardins, & Marcotte, in press). Although the threat-simulation theory's predictions are in harmony with most of the empirical findings so far, further exploration and testing are required to establish the scope and the limits of the dreaming brain as a threat-simulation mechanism.

Summary

Converging evidence from a wide variety of sources supports the view that the nocturnal world simulation we know as "dreaming" is functionally specialized in the simulation of dangers and threatening events. This view explains several prominent features of our ordinary dreams, children's dreams, typical and universal dream themes, recurrent dreams, bad dreams and nightmares, night terrors, posttraumatic dreams, and the deep impact of real-life threats to dream content. In the biological research program on consciousness, dreaming thus turns out to be an evolved, automatically programmed world simulation during sleep. During threat-simulation dreams the brain prepares itself to rapidly recognize and evaluate approaching dangers, and to swiftly compute safe trajectories in risky situations where navigation in the world is particularly unsafe and one's future reproductive success is at stake.

The phenomenal world simulation in the brain thus plays an indispensable functional role for the organism. During wakefulness, the brain sets and monitors current behavioral trajectories by largely relying on the internal world simulation. Consciousness provides a unified phenomenal model of the spatial distribution of the goal objects that surround the organism, and simultaneously presents the adaptive value of each object by connecting the simulated objects to semantic-conceptual knowledge and affective or emotional valence. During dreaming, the brain constructs emergency rehearsals within the world-simulation mechanism to practice rapid and efficient escapes from potential threats in the real world. Thus, the phenomenal *world-for-me* turns out to be, in terms of its role in organism-environment interaction, a navigational mechanism in the brain (or a crucial component of such mechanisms).

Biological realism has thereby good grounds for rejecting epiphenomenalism. Phenomenal consciousness, the world simulation in the brain, constitutes an inner beacon, guiding the physical body of flesh and bones to trajectories across the physical world that tend to lead to survival and future reproductive success. The function of the inner phenomenal beacon is to contribute in that way to the continued existence of the world-for-me—until the inevitable day when the phenomenal lights go out for good and *nothing-for-me* shall reign once more.

Notes

Chapter 1

1. Here I follow Niiniluoto (2002, p. 26) who formulates ontological dependence thus: A is ontologically dependent on B if A could not exist without B existing. To test A's independence of B, ask whether A could still exist in a world where B has disappeared.

2. What is the relationship between multilevel explanation and traditional metaphysical functionalism and computationalism, the leading explanatory strategies in classical cognitive science and perhaps also in modern philosophy of mind? Functionalism and computationalism seem to focus on only specific parts of the full multilevel explanation. Traditional metaphysical functionalism concentrates on the *contextual* explanation of a phenomenon. A functionalistic explanation of mind defines the relation of a mental phenomenon to its typical causes (e.g., sensory input, other mental phenomena) and its typical causal effects (e.g., further mental phenomena, motor output). Functionalists in philosophy of mind believe that when these input-output relations are fully specified, then the mental phenomenon has been fully explained. Computationalism in cognitive science concentrates on specifying the input-output transformations in terms of computations (algorithms) and implies that when these have been fully specified, then the phenomenon has been fully explained: they are the *ultimate* explanations of mental phenomena. By contrast, multilevel explanation in biology sees functional and computational explanations as only *parts* of the whole story. (For a discussion of the differences in explanatory strategies in cognitive science and neuroscience, see Revonsuo 2001a.)

Chapter 2

1. There is a modern approach to consciousness called "neurophenomenology" (Lutz & Thompson, 2003) that may be more promising for the empirical scientist than old continental philosophy. But there are some problems with this approach, too (see chapter 8). Daniel Dennett (1991) has proposed that phenomenology should be construed as "heterophenomenology," but what he means by that is the study of the verbal (and other) reports or "texts" produced by any intentional systems, without assuming that there is any real inner subjective experience that originally caused the subject to produce the report. So, at bottom, a heterophenomenologist studies verbal reports and the behaviors that produce such reports, not inner subjective experience.

2. Lewis's account of qualia further included the ideas that qualia are ineffable (not linguistically describable), atomic, unanalyzable, and reidentifiable properties of experience. Many philosophers have attacked these ideas. In the light of empirical evidence, it is now clear that the qualities of experience are not reidentifiable, because our discriminative sensory abilities are far greater than our recognition capacity that relies on memories of past experiences. When I use the notion of "qualities of experience," I do not mean to subscribe to every aspect of the classic notion of qualia formulated by Lewis.

3. To say that phenomenal consciousness involves the *having* of patterns of subjective experience however, seems to imply that there is some entity *external* to the patterns of experience who *has* them (say, the "self" or the "subject"). Still, it is entirely possible to formulate the idea of primary or phenomenal consciousness

without such an implication. Phenomenal consciousness just means there being at least some patterns of subjective experience present in the organism's mind-brain. It is an open theoretical question whether there is an "I," who literally *has* the experiences but is separate from them, or whether we should construe the situation the other way round: the experiences have (or rather constitute) an "I" or a "self" (more on this in chapter 7).

4. The relationship between attention and consciousness remains controversial. Many cognitive scientists hold that attention is *necessary* for consciousness; that is, that there is no form of consciousness before or outside attentional selection. But it is at least equally plausible to hold that phenomenal consciousness is independent of attentional selection (see Lamme 2003). More on this in chapter 15.

5. On other higher-order forms of consciousness: There are other concepts that also refer to special forms of higher-order consciousness. In psychology such terms as "phonological awareness" and "linguistic awareness" are not uncommon. The basic idea behind such terms is reflective consciousness as applied to a specific content of primary consciousness. The emergence of phonological awareness, for example, requires that the child becomes aware of phonemes as components of language. Becoming aware of them requires that one learns to selectively attend to single phonemes in words, and thus take phonemes as objects in reflective consciousness. One may then manipulate phonemes in working memory or report the first or the last phoneme in a word, and so on. Attentional selection of an entity, reflective operations or cognitive manipulation in working memory over it, and ability to give descriptive reports about it are usually required to show awareness of the entity. "X-awareness" in general is thus the ability to apply reflective consciousness to entities of type X.

6. The representational criterion can be used to determine whether a given state is an "altered" state of consciousness or not. In hypnosis research there is a persistent controversy over whether or not hypnosis produces an ASC. This controversy could be solved by using the multilevel approach and the representational criterion of ASC. In Kallio and Revonsuo (2003) we outline this type of new framework for hypnosis research. We suggest that hypnosis may involve an ASC in only a small subgroup of people, called "hypnotic virtuosos," who experience dramatic changes in consciousness (e.g., vivid hallucinations) during hypnosis. Therefore, they should be the principal model system for any empirical tests concerning the existence of an ASC in hypnosis. In other people, the effects of hypnotic induction and suggestion can probably be explained without reference to an ASC.

Chapter 4

1. Also Bertrand Russell (1927b) made a clear distinction between the phenomenal body known through direct experience and its external physical counterpart. The phenomenal body is known to us only through sensations: it is nothing but a complex, unified bundle of sensations, and therefore quite different from what physics calls a body.

Chapter 6

1. Contemporary theorists who have developed ideas similar to the world-simulation metaphor include Max Velmans (1996, 2000), Thomas Metzinger (2003), and Steve Lehar (2003a).

2. Incidentally, the window-on-world organization seems to be assumed when consciousness is described as a "mental screen" that some internal mental eye or homunculus is watching. Antonio Damasio (1999) talks about the movie-in-the-brain and the self as an observer of that movie (but he does say that the appearance of an observer is generated within the movie, which would capture the "self-in-world" structure of consciousness). It is indeed incorrect to talk about a mental screen in the brain because it makes a misleading metaphor of consciousness. There is no such thing as an internal mental screen, because the phenomenal level is not organized in that way.

3. For more information on the Cybersphere, see http://www.vr-systems.ndtilda.co.uk/sphere1.htm#Information

4. What does this grainlessness reveal about the phenomenal level of organization? It reveals that phenomenal features exist in a fieldlike format at the phenomenal level, so that the property of color, for example, fills in the shape of an object entirely, smoothly, and continuously rather than discontinuously pixel by pixel (or voxel by voxel). Pixels or voxels do not exist at the phenomenal level (but note that this does not exclude pixel-

like organization from the underlying nonphenomenal levels of organization). This observation supports the Gestalt psychology view of consciousness as a field and undermines the structuralist view of consciousness as composed of "elements" or "atoms" of simple sensations.

Chapter 7

1. Representative realism is a thesis which (unlike representationalism) does not confuse the phenomenal content of consciousness with its representational content. Phenomenal content of consciousness is constituted by the surrogates at the phenomenal level; representational content is constituted by the *relationship* between the surrogate and its external causes or correlates.

2. J. R. Smythies has defended representative realism against such accusations in numerous writings since the 1950s (see, e.g., J. R. Smythies 1965, 1994a; for related arguments, see Fox 1994), and I am following his line of argumentation here.

3. The *representational* contents, of course, can be "right" or "wrong" in the sense that they may represent the physical environment either correctly or incorrectly. To say that patterns of phenomenal features are "right" or "wrong" is to *relate* those patterns to something outside of themselves, for example, to the external stimulus environment. Thus, the *representational* content of primary consciousness can be evaluated as "correctly representing" or "misrepresenting," but the phenomenal content by itself, primary consciousness per se, is neither "right" nor "wrong."

4. John Foster (2000) advocates a variety of sense-datum theory which illustrates some of the additional difficulties of that approach. He takes the (visual) sense-data themselves to be purely two-dimensional: spatial arrangements of color in a flat, 2D field. Somehow this flat field is "interpreted" or "attributed" the third dimension of depth: "In short, the only way in which we can think of a visual sense-datum as genuinely structured in depth is by supposing that it exists in an external space, and that its various parts stand, within that space, in certain distance relations to the subject" (p. 159). Thus, according to this story, somehow the sense-data are externalized into the external physical space surrounding the organism in order to account for its 3D structure. Foster (2000) denies the possibility that the sense-data themselves could be three-dimensional, because he believes that a sense-datum internal to awareness cannot stand in a relation to the subject or stand at a certain distance from him. It seems to me that Foster here confuses the *biological organism* (the body of flesh and bones) in the external physical space and the spatial relations it bears to external physical objects, with the *phenomenal body image* and the phenomenal spatial relations it bears to other phenomenal entities surrounding it in virtual space. He does not seem to realize that the so-called subject in front of whom the "sense-data" appear in 3D space is *not* the physical organism but the phenomenal body image, and that the space in which they appear is *not* the external physical space surrounding the organism. Thus, he resorts to the solution that 2D sense-data have to be projected out of the mind and superimposed somehow on the external 3D space surrounding the organism. This confusion is precisely the mistake that the great Gestalt psychologist Wolfgang Köhler warned us against back in the 1920s. According to the world-simulation metaphor, three-dimensionality of phenomenal depth is an intrinsic feature of the phenomenal level of organization.

5. Philosophers traditionally distinguish between primary and secondary qualities. Do the internal phenomenal features include both types of qualities? In other words, is it only the secondary qualities (such as colors) of objects that are located in the world-for-me in the brain, or are the primary qualities (such as shape, spatiality) supposed to be there as well? In this issue I agree with the Gestalt psychologist Wolfgang Köhler: ". . . it was a great step when man began to ask questions about the nature of seeing, feeling and hearing. And it was a revolution when he found that colors, noises, smells, etc., were merely products of influences excerted on him by the surroundings. Still, these surroundings seemed to subsist in their *primary* characteristics and to remain "the real world." When those *secondary* qualities were subtracted as purely subjective ingredients, the *primary* qualities seemed to remain directly given as characteristics of reality. But eventually the *primary* qualities of naive realism turned out to be just as subjective as their *secondary* comparisons: the form, the weight, and the movement of things had to be given the same interpretation as colors and sounds; they, too, depended on the experiencing organism and were merely end results of complicated processes in its interior. What was left? The answer was that, henceforth, *no* phase of immediate experience could be regarded as part of the real world. . . . As a result, science had to construct an objective and independent world of physical things, physical space, physical time and physical movement, and had to maintain that this world appears at no point in direct experience." (Köhler 1947, pp. 6–7)

Chapter 8

1. A Dennettian heterophenomenologist would see dream content analysis not as the study of the virtual world at the phenomenal level of organization in the brain, but as the study of words in dream reports (and perhaps of the entirely fictional, unreal world that can be read into those words). Note that in such a case there is a crucial failure to distinguish *data* from *phenomena.* For a biological realist, dream reports are the data, but the phenomenal level of organization is the phenomenon that is being studied. If dream research is construed as the study of words in dream reports, then EEG research should not be seen as the study of electrophysiological events inside the brain but as the study of ink curves printed on paper or of patterns of luminous phosphor displayed on computer screens, for those are the only things the EEG researchers are directly in touch with. For biological realism, the natural phenomena being studied are not to be identified with the data, whether words or curves or colorful topographical maps. The phenomena of interest to biological realism are hidden *behind* the data; the data *inform* us about the phenomena.

2. Noë and Thompson (2004) respond in the following way to the accusation that their doctrine locates consciousness outside the head: "It is *not* our view that consciousness is outside the head, but rather that some of the causal substrates of consciousness *might* be. Whether or not the vehicles of consciousness cross the skull boundary is an empirical question whose answer has not yet been decided. . . . Neural states may not be sufficient for human and animal experience, but they surely are necessary (i.e. they surely make a contribution to the determination of consciousness)." (p. 93) If I understand them correctly, their view is that we do not yet *know* where the "causal substrates" (or "vehicles") of consciousness are located in the physical world, and that it is a viable empirical possibility that some of them at least are outside the skull. By contrast, I do not think that the location of consciousness or its constitutive basis is an open empirical question anymore: the evidence from dreaming, reviewed at length in this book, establishes that the internal mechanisms of the brain are sufficient for consciousness and that consciousness is thus located within the confines of the brain.

3. In philosophy, the terms *intentional* and *intentionality* do not mean the same as in everyday language (i.e., "deliberately" or "purposely"). Instead, they refer to a *relation* between two entities (e.g., a "mental act" and its "object," or a "vehicle of representation" and its "content") such that the first entity is *directed at,* or *about,* or *referring to,* the second one. "Intentionality" is thus also called "aboutness" or "directedness." Thought is regarded as intentional in exactly this sense: when we think about the sun, for example, we perform a *mental act* that is directed at the giant physical body at the center of our solar system, which is the *object* or *content* of our thought.

4. As this discussion suggests, I accept John Searle's (1992) idea of intrinsic intentionality as the basic, genuine form of intentionality.

5. A particularly clear formulation of externalist representationalism can be found in Skokowski (2002): "As a materialist, I want to say that my experiential states are in my brain. But as an externalist, I want to point out that the *contents* of these states . . . are generally to be found *outside* the brain. My mental states are, in short, intentional. . . . The contents of my experiences are properties in the world. Thus my experiences are about external properties. These properties are the contents of my experiences. These properties are qualia" (pp. 3–4).

6. To what extent does the world simulation metaphor of consciousness, the "world-for-me," involve a kind of "self-representational" approach to consciousness? First, the "world-for-me" does not necessarily involve any explicit representation of the self or any reflective awareness of the self. The "me" in the "world-for-me" is the "subject," and the "subject" is nothing over and above (or outside) the global bundle of co-conscious experiences. So, the "world-for-me" is really a "world-for-itself," a world of simple phenomenal presence. However, as phenomenal presence is taken to be "self-presenting," does this notion of "self-presentation" invoke a kind of primitive self-awareness, comparable to the "pre-reflective self-consciousness" of neurophenomenology? It seems not, as the latter is understood to involve a tacit reference to *bodily* self-awareness, a pre-reflective experience of bodily subjectivity (Lutz & Thompson, 2003), whereas the self-presentation of simple phenomenality in the philosophy of presence involves no necessary reference, either implicitly or explicitly, to a body or embodiment.

7. There are many different versions of higher-order theories of consciousness. According to some, the higher-order mental state directed at the first-order state is a perceptual state (higher-order perception or HOP theory). This version is defended, for example, by William G. Lycan. According to others, the higher-order state is a thought (HOT theory). The best known supporter of HOT theory is David Rosenthal. Space

does not permit me to go into the details of the many versions of HOT and HOP theories currently found in the literature, or to distinguish between the subtle differences that different theorists hold.

8. The HOT-theorist Rocco Gennaro (1996), for example, believes that there are "nonconscious phenomenal states" which can be defined as "phenomenal states without their qualitative properties." He argues that what justifies us in treating a state as a nonconscious *phenomenal* state (e.g., a nonconscious pain) is that the state shows a similar functional-behavioral role as a conscious state and that the system is capable of conscious phenomenal states of the same type. According to this conception, phenomenality is constituted by something else than qualitative experiences, because a state can lose all its qualities but remain a phenomenal state. By contrast, according to my view phenomenality is constituted by the existence of qualitative experiences, it is nothing over and above them; therefore, if the qualities of experience are subtracted from a mental state, nothing worthy of the label "phenomenal" remains.

9. If HOT theorists believe that the nonconscious mental states are at bottom neurophysiological states, then does the difference between biological realism and HOT theory disappear? I fear not, because their ontological commitments are so different. According to biological realism, the mental realm is constituted by phenomenality, and phenomenality in turn must be explained by a microlevel of nonphenomenal and nonmental neurophysiology. The microlevel mechanism of phenomenal consciousness cannot (and should not) be described in mental terms; the downward-looking explanation is a neural level of description. By contrast, according to HOT theorists, the mental realm is NOT constituted by phenomenality, but by what they take to be more fundamental forms of mentality, namely nonconscious intentional mental states. The lower-level mechanism that explains phenomenal consciousness is a mental level and thus described in psychological terms (nonconscious sensations, thoughts, perceptions). Only if these psychological terms were taken by HOT theorists as mere observer-relative labels of what in reality are purely neurophysiological mechanisms might biological realism and HOT theory approach each other to some extent.

10. The discussion of direct realism is partly derived from Revonsuo, A. (2001). Putting color back where it belongs. *Consciousness and Cognition, 10*(1), 78–84, with the permission of Academic Press, Elsevier Inc.

11. The discussion of panpsychism is drawn from Revonsuo, A. (2003). Consciousness as phenomenal ether? *Behavioral and Brain Sciences, 26*(4), 422–423, with the permission of Cambridge University Press.

12. For those who are unfamiliar with the philosophy of science, *instrumentalism* and *realism* are two opposing metaphysical views. The former says that scientific theories are mere instruments for predicting future observations, but we should not believe that the theoretical entities postulated by the theories (electrons, black holes, atoms, the big bang, and so on) *really* exist. Perhaps they do, perhaps they don't: for science, all that matters is that the theories yield accurate predictions. The theoretical entities are just human concepts rather than realities somewhere out there. Scientific realism, by contrast, is committed to the view that the theoretical entities postulated by the best available theories in science really do exist out there. There is such a reality as described by science, even if we can never directly observe it, but only infer the theoretical entities indirectly from our experiences and observations.

Chapter 9

1. A more specific hypothesis concerning the way in which neural activity might use the unity of physical space-time to realize globally unified phenomenality is the *electromagnetic field theory* of consciousness. This theory comes in a variety of forms and has historical (Köhler [1929] 1930) as well as modern proponents (Pockett, 2000, 2002; McFadden, 2002; John, 2002; Searle, 2000). Wolfgang Köhler ([1930] 1971) wrote: ". . . all these sensory processes, wherever they start on the periphery of our organism, are finally conducted to one common final field inside the brain, the distribution in which determines the spatial properties of all sensory experience" (p. 246). Susan Pockett (2000, 2002) formulates the central idea of electromagnetic field theory in this way: consciousness (qualia) is identical with certain yet-undefined spatiotemporal patterns in the electromagnetic field. I am sympathetic toward these field theories and I hope they will develop to a stage where their statements can be put to direct empirical tests. In any case, if we use the classification of theories introduced by Searle (2000), biological realism coupled with the world-simulation metaphor of consciousness surely counts as a "unified field theory" rather than a "building block theory" of consciousness. What sets my theory apart from the other field theories is that in my view the physical field involved is not identical with consciousness. The field is a subphenomenal physical entity that supports (rather than is) the spatial features of the phenomenal consciousness we directly experience.

2. Dainton (2003) agrees that this solution narrows the explanatory gap: "For Revonsuo, the fact that experiences occur in a phenomenal void is a positive boon. It means that it makes sense to suppose that our experiences inherit their spatial characteristics (their extensions, their spatial relations) from a physical field of a kind which is not, in general, phenomenal in nature. This at least narrows the explanatory gap, and does so while minimizing the risk of panpsychism. It may well be that our brains generate coherent spatially extended fields. If these fields are (in some manner) imbued with localized patterns of phenomenal properties by neural activity, we have a direct link between phenomenal and physical space. In fact, we have an identity: phenomenal space *is* physical space, albeit field-filled physical space. Of course, there is still a good deal to be explained: how, exactly, does a physical field come to carry or be imbued with phenomenal properties as a consequence of neural activity? Even so, progress has been made, the gap between the phenomenal and the physical is less wide than it was" (p. 17).

Chapter 10

1. Semir Zeki (2003) has recently expressed a similar idea of different hierarchical levels of consciousness. He distinguishes three levels of consciousness: (1) microconsciousnesses (simple qualitative features), (2) macroconsciousness (perceptual objects constituted by microconsciousnesses coherently bound together), and (3) unified consciousness (including the self as the perceiving person).

2. Damasio is here talking about *neural* patterns that represent self, object, and their relationship as necessary for consciousness. If I understand him correctly, those neural representations must bring about *phenomenal* images where the self is related to the object. Thus, for Damasio, the bridge across the gap from the neural level to the phenomenal level rests on the simultaneous representation of self-object relations at both levels (neural and phenomenal). If my interpretation is correct, then Damasio's theory predicts that selfless experiences are impossible. In a selfless experience the representation of the organism itself, as well as the self-object relationship, is absent from both neural and phenomenal levels. And when those things are absent, no consciousness should be possible at all. The evidence from dreaming shows otherwise, however.

3. This particular dream report went on like this: "The sleep technician, who was skilled in interviewing subjects on their awakening from REM sleep, tried to get him to volunteer more information, but in vain. All that Mr. R. was able to report was the one word, carbide. He added that it was "some kind of smelly gas." Carbide does have a particularly pungent smell which can usually be detected after the oxy-acelytene welding of metal. Mr. R. rejected the possibility that he had ever worked in this particular field at any time during his life. He knew what carbide was but could think of no reason why that particular word had appeared in his REM sleep. Three days after Mr. R.'s sleep test, on December 3, the worst industrial accident in history took place in Bhopal, India. In an explosion at a chemical plant, more than four thousand people lost their lives and a further twenty thousand were injured. The plant was owned by an American company called Union Carbide. I can still remember my shock when I heard the news over the radio" (Lavie, 1996, p. 96)

4. This explains why the visual world is not just a grand illusion as has been claimed, based on the phenomenon of change blindness (see chapter 15 on the relationship between attention and consciousness). This also explains Dennett's (1991) puzzle about the wallpaper covered with hundreds of identical photographs of Marilyn. After examining a few of them, the brain uses its built-in Ockham's razor and simply gives the same semantic interpretation to all of the potential Marilyns that were not actually looked at, but if they were, would likely turn out to be exactly like the ones that were. The very same semantic window is open to all those similar-looking patches unless contrary evidence arises. And usually in such situations contrary evidence does not turn up (unless the wallpaper is a practical joke or a clever experiment), so Ockham's razor is a practical and usually correct way of handling the situation.

Chapter 11

1. This chapter is drawn partly from Revonsuo, A. (1999). Binding and the phenomenal unity of consciousness. *Consciousness and Cognition, 8*(2), 173–185, with the permission of Academic Press, Elsevier Inc.

2. Several theorists have argued recently that there is no (phenomenal) binding problem (e.g., Garson, 2001; O'Regan & Noe, 2001). Their arguments usually try to show that our idea of the phenomenal unity of consciousness rests on a confusion or is an illusion or intellectual error. Thus, for them the problem of the unity

of consciousness is just a "pseudoproblem" that need not be solved; it only needs to be "dissolved." The underlying motivation for denying the unity of phenomenal consciousness is in many cases the denial of the whole notion (and reality) of phenomenal consciousness itself.

Chapter 12

1. Color opponency may not be a law applying to the phenomenal level, after all. In some exceptional circumstances, subjects report seeing reddish greens or bluish yellows. Billock and Tsou (2004) report that in their experiments, when they presented a retinally stabilized bipartite field of opponent colors, subjects reported "forbidden" colors: "The border collapsed completely and the two colored sides appeared to run together, like diffusing inks or melting waxes, creating new color combinations undreamt of in Hering's philosophy. In some cases these manifest as a gradient which ran from red on one side to green on the other, with every possible shade of reddish green in between. In other cases, subjects report seeing a spatially homogeneous reddish green, the red and green components of which were as compelling as the red and blue components of purple" (pp. 87–88). If reddish greens and bluish yellows are possible at the phenomenal level, then the microlevel constitutive mechanisms of *phenomenal* red and green or *phenomenal* blue and yellow are not absolutely mutually exclusive but can coexist and blend into each other, thus creating the "forbidden" colors. If that is the case, then the true source of color opponency must reside *outside* the phenomenal level (somewhere along the etiological pathway). That arrangement would make reddish greens and bluish yellows only extremely unlikely to arise at the phenomenal level, but not impossible.

2. Dennett (1991) argued that apparent motion phenomena show that there is no Cartesian theater in the brain. If two lights of different color are used, the moving light changes color midway on its trajectory between the lights. Dennett thought it would be impossible to explain how one can see a red light moving and turning green *before* the actual green flash occurs. But the notion "the actual green flash" is ambiguous, for there are two separate events it could refer to: the onset of the second (the physically green) light in the external stimulus field, or the perceptual experience of the phenomenally green spot in its final position in the phenomenal visual field. Of course, the experience of the motion and the change of the seen color (which are events at the phenomenal level in the brain) cannot take place before the physical onset of the second light in the external stimulus field has occurred. It takes time for the brain to construct the coherence and dynamics of the phenomenal world simulation in the brain and, necessarily, the simulated events lag behind in time from their physical causes in the external world. (For a more detailed analysis of why Dennett is wrong in his interpretation of the color-phi experiment, see Revonsuo 1993).

Chapter 13

1. Russell (1948) argued that spatial relations given in sensation are always between data of the same sense, and the conception of one unitary space must be abandoned. To say that a visual and a tactile experience are in the same place is not strictly accurate; we should say instead that they are in correlated places in two different spaces, visual and tactile. The various spaces created by relations of unimodal sensory fields can be bound into one space by correlations; experience of correlations is necessary to create this single unified space. Russell's idea seems to be that consciousness is first disunified or comes in several separate spaces and only after we have repeatedly experienced the correlations between a visual and a tactile experience (e.g., pinpricks on the body surface) do those separate spaces blend together. The inability of the simultanagnosic patient to locate visual objects with respect to his own body may be explained also by saying that it is not possible anymore to correlate the contents of visual awareness and the contents of bodily awareness; they remain as if in separate spaces. However, it seems there has to be some *deeper* unity of experience that has *not* been lost. Otherwise it would be difficult to explain how a correlation between the two sensations in different modalities could be experienced by *the same subject.* How could they be phenomenal events in a single subject's experience in the first place, unless at some deeper level they occurred in the same sphere of experience to begin with? Learning through experienced correlation may be the key to creating spatial *coherence* and organization between different experiences, but in order for a single subject to experience any correlations at all, the distinct experiences must already belong to a single sphere of experience or be coconscious. The phenomenal coordinate system, shared by the unimodal spatial maps in a single subject's brain, enables the experience of correlation between sensations in different modalities, and therefore contributes to the

development of coherent spatial organization at the phenomenal level. If coconsciousness is totally missing (as seems to be the case for lateralized stimuli in split-brain patients) no correlations will be experienced and the two experiences remain in distinct phenomenal coordinate systems. If the location map that is damaged in simultanagnosia concerns visual modality only, then the simultanagnosic patient should still be able to spatially localize *auditory* phenomena, such as the chirping of a bird. Auditory phenomenology should still create a phenomenal background space, where different sounds come from different directions and locations. If this is accurate, then it would be interesting to know whether multisensory stimuli (say the singing bird) could still be spatially integrated and localized across the modalities. The preserved auditory space might help to place the visual percept in the context of the auditorily experienced location and thus relate it to the auditory phenomenal background.

Chapter 14

1. But there is a neurological disorder of vision called *palinopsia,* where a single visual object multiplies in the phenomenal visual field and gets copied and inserted into several locations in the phenomenal visual field, usually after the original stimulus is long gone. The previous dream with the multiplying pills or watercolors is to some extent reminiscent of palinopsia.

2. Dream characters have also been studied in detail by David Kahn who found that 62% of characters known to the dreamer were inaccurately portrayed in the dream, the most typical source for this being the character's behavior (Kahn, Pace-Schott, & Hobson, 2002). Kahn and Hobson (2003) reported that 47% of dream characters were found to have at least one implausible feature, whereas 53% were judged to be normal by the dreamers themselves. However, during dreaming only 15% of the characters were noticed to have an implausible feature. This shows that reflective consciousness is suppressed during dreaming. In general, Kahn's findings are in harmony with ours, although the studies have some methodological differences.

Chapter 15

1. If attention biases competition between representations, how could the difference between simultanagnosia and neglect be explained? In neglect, the phenomenal sphere for one half of space exists; therefore the objects (or half-objects) in that space can be accessed by attentional biasing, whereas nothing in the neglected side of space can reach that level due to lack of activation of the entire background space. In simultanagnosia, there is *no competition between the two sides* of background space, because *neither side exists* at the phenomenal level anymore. Thus, now a single but *whole* object representation alone may be selected to win the competition for highest level of activity. Neither half of the object is any longer masked by the unevenly distributed activation of the hemifields of background space.

2. The world-simulation metaphor is also consistent with the view that there is a phenomenal background field present for the subject but that the field is not properly updated without attention, and therefore the critical stimuli in CB and IB are not experienced by the subjects. In this case, attention is necessary for the *representational contents* of consciousness. Outside the location of attention in the subjective visual field, visual phenomenology is not updated and does not covary with the stimulus field—new stimulus information cannot reach the phenomenal level there. But still, attention is not necessary for the *phenomenal contents* of consciousness to *exist*—a background field of phenomenal consciousness surely still *exists* even if not being properly updated by concurrent stimuli. By contrast, the radical version states that attention is necessary both for the representational and the phenomenal contents of consciousness, a view in direct conflict with the world-simulation metaphor.

Chapter 18

1. This chapter is drawn partly from Revonsuo, A. (2001). Can functional brain imaging discover consciousness in the brain? *Journal of Consciousness Studies, 8*(3), 3–23; and Revonsuo, A. (2001). Discovering the mechanisms of consciousness. *Journal of Consciousness Studies, 8*(3), 44–50: with the permission of Imprint Academic.

Chapter 19

1. This chapter is drawn partly from Revonsuo, A. (2001). Can functional brain imaging discover consciousness in the brain? *Journal of Consciousness Studies, 8*(3), 3–23; and Revonsuo, A. (2001). Discovering the mechanisms of consciousness. *Journal of Consciousness Studies, 8*(3), 44–50: with the permission of Imprint Academic.

2. The ability of conscious information to spread widely in the cognitive system has been called "global broadcasting" by Baars (1988) and "access consciousness" by Block (1995).

3. The rate of phenomenal reorganization should not be confused with the *delay* between stimulus onset and onset of the experience at the phenomenal level. We do not know exactly how long it takes before a proximal visual stimulus in the retina causes the corresponding experience at the phenomenal level; estimates vary from 150 to 500 ms. Since the speed of neural activations is limited, the phenomenal level should be always a little late in modeling external physical events (see Bachmann 2000). In our own studies, we have observed the first EEG responses specifically correlating with phenomenal awareness of visual stimuli arising around 150 ms and peaking around 200 to 300 ms from stimulus onset (Vanni, Revonsuo, Saarinen, & Hari, 1996; Koivisto & Revonsuo, 2003; Wilenius-Emet, Revonsuo, & Ojanen, 2004). The slowness of the phenomenal level is compensated by the much faster reactions of nonconscious visuomotor action guiding systems, which keep track of changes faster than those that the phenomenal level can handle. If you have ever played badminton or tennis, you must have noticed how you sometimes can hit the ball instinctively even if it's moving too fast to be seen. How is this possible? At least two explanations can be offered. First, there is evidence that fast visuomotor zombie systems can direct eye movements and pointing or reaching arm movements independently of visual awareness and even without the subject knowing anything about the involvement of such nonconscious guiding. It has been found that pointing movements to targets remain accurate even if the target suddenly jumps during a saccade without the subject noticing it. This happens even in the dark where only the target is lit. The subjects cannot see their own hands moving and are never aware of the target jump; still, their pointing hand correctly changes its trajectory in response to a target jump. Furthermore, the visuomotor delay is only about 110 milliseconds, which is considerably faster than response times to consciously perceived stimuli (Rossetti, 1998). Second, there may be mechanisms that compensate for the slowness of conscious visual perception and correct for the expected lag of the perceived position of rapidly moving visual objects (Nijhawan & Khurana, 2000). Thus, although many philosophers have argued that consciousness is too slow to be of any use for the organism, it is obvious that the phenomenal level, in interaction with fast visuomotor zombie systems and corrective movement perception mechanisms, can keep the organism out of harm's way even in an environment involving rapidly moving objects.

4. This critique of Zeki and Bartels may be somewhat outdated. Semir Zeki (2003) has recently developed his view and now he postulates not only the multiple microconsciousnesses but also macroconsciousness and the global unity of consciousness as higher levels of consciousness. His latest model thus takes the constraint of unity into account.

Chapter 20

1. This chapter is drawn partly from Revonsuo, A. (2001). Can functional brain imaging discover consciousness in the brain? *Journal of Consciousness Studies, 8*(3), 3–23; and Revonsuo, A. (2001). Discovering the mechanisms of consciousness. *Journal of Consciousness Studies, 8*(3), 44–50: with the permission of Imprint Academic.

2. I have chosen to evaluate the above methods (single-cell recordings, EEG, MEG, PET, fMRI) because they are the ones most often used in studies of the neural correlates of consciousness. Several other methods exist that should be briefly mentioned. For example, it is possible to measure not only single-cell activity but also *multiple unit activity* (MUA) and *local field potentials* (LFPs) with invasive microelectrodes. LFPs indicate the *average activity of postsynaptic signals* on dendrites and somata near the electrode tip (within 1 mm of it), and contain the synchronized components at the *inputs* of the local neural population. MUA contains the synchronized components at the *outputs* of a local population and gives an *estimate of average spike activity* near the electrode tip (Eckhorn, 1994). These averaged measures can detect oscillatory synchrony in local cortical cell populations, which is a highly interesting spatial scale, but the signals depicted in the

recordings do not reveal the organized patterns of synchronicity within the cell population; they only depict the changes in the averaged amplitude at a chosen frequency band. Also, a variety of optical imaging methods exist (for a review, see Bonhoeffer & Grinvald 1996). Visible or infrared light reflection from the exposed surface of the cortex can be photographed. The sources of the optical signals originate in changes in blood volume and changes in the oxygen saturation level of hemoglobin. Thus, optical imaging captures basically the same type of phenomena as PET and fMRI, but with better spatial resolution. Therefore, the same limitations also apply: Optical images are not images of electrophysiological phenomena but of levels of blood flow and oxygen consumption in neural tissue. The images reflect the spatial distribution of neural activity (or the average rate of firing within neural populations) with high spatial resolution, but cannot reveal the patterns of neural synchronicity. Furthermore, the technique has the practical limitation that the skull must be opened to expose the surface of the cortex. Recently, however, noninvasive optical imaging through the human skull has become possible (Villringer & Chance, 1997).

Chapter 21

1. As Woody (2000) observes, the extra information contained in a lower-level description can be a double-edged sword. The failure of lower-level descriptions to truly account for or describe higher-level phenomena becomes apparent already at the chemical levels of organization. Quantum mechanics is incapable of providing descriptions of chemical reality that would be even remotely practical or useful: "While in principle a wavefunction is a precise and definite description, it cannot be recognized as such by humans; the information it contains stays coyly out of sight, and sadly out of mind. . . . [T]here is no obvious way to capture traditional categories of chemical practice from the set of wavefunctions specified by these calculations. . . . These are practical difficulties, but underneath is a more fundamental one, namely, whether types, and their tokens, can be explicitly represented in the scheme or whether we are limited to particulars. . . . There is no underlying *aufbau,* no line of reasoning to aid further theory development. While chemists can think of CO_2 and SO_2 as having significantly related reactive properties, wavefunction representations do not explicitly acknowledge such facts nor is it clear how they could capture this information." (Woody, 2000, p. S618)

2. Harnad (2000) complains that there is a long litany of "self-x" terms (self-awareness, self-representation, self-reference) that are meant to illuminate consciousness, but in reality merely rename it. Could the same complaint be raised against "self-presentation"? Only in case "self-presentation" or "inner presence" cannot be translated into a lower-level mechanism that specifies how a bioelectrical phenomenon could become present for itself in a qualitatively unique manner. At some level, there must be a set of micromechanisms that accounts for the direct inner presence (or self-presence) of phenomenal consciousness in the brain, just like there is at some subcellular microlevel a set of mechanisms that accounts for the ability of whole biological organisms to reproduce or self-replicate.

Chapter 22

1. This chapter is drawn partly from Revonsuo, A., Johanson, M., Wedlund, J. E., & Chaplin, J. (2000). The zombies among us: Consciousness and automatic behavior. In Y. Rossetti & A. Revonsuo (Eds.), *Beyond dissociations: Interaction between dissociated implicit and explicit processing.* (pp. 331–351). Amsterdam: John Benjamins, with permission of the publisher.

Chapter 23

1. This chapter is drawn in part from Revonsuo, A., & Rossetti, Y. (2000). Dissociation and interaction: Windows to the hidden mechanisms of consciousness. In Y. Rossetti & A. Revonsuo (Eds.), *Beyond dissociations: Interaction between dissociated implicit and explicit processing* (pp. 353–367). Amsterdam: John Benjamins, with permission of the publisher.

Chapter 24

1. Parts of this chapter are reprinted in modified form from Revonsuo, A. (2000). The reinterpretation of dreams: An evolutionary hypothesis of the function of dreaming. *Behavioral and Brain Sciences, 23*(6), 877–901, with the permission of Cambridge University Press.

2. For the full original formulation of the theory presented in this chapter, see Revonsuo (2000b), and for my reply to a wide variety of peer commentaries and criticisms, see Revonsuo (2000a). These original papers are also reprinted in E. Pace-Schott, M. Solms, M. Blagrove, & S. Harnad (Eds.). *Sleep and dreaming, scientific advances and reconsiderations,* New York: Cambridge University Press 2003. In this chapter, only the main points of the theory are summarized.

3. Schredl and Doll (1998), however, found a balanced ratio of positive and negative emotions in diary dreams, but only when the dream emotions were self-rated by the dreamers rather than by external raters. Still, emotions explicitly mentioned in dream reports (i.e., the ones available for external raters) are predominantly negative.

References

Aldrich, M. (1993). Sleep paralysis. In M. A. Carskadon (Ed.), *Encyclopedia of sleep and dreaming* (pp. 569–570). New York: Macmillan.

Alkire, M. T., Haier, R. J., & Fallon, J. H. (2000). Toward a unified theory of narcosis: Brain imaging evidence for a thalamocortical switch as the neurophysiologic basis of anesthetic-induced unconsciousness. *Consciousness and Cognition, 9*(3), 370–386.

Amzica, F., & Steriade, M. (1996). Progressive cortical synchronization of ponto-geniculo-occipital potentials during rapid eye movement sleep. *Neuroscience, 72*(2), 309–314.

Armstrong, D. M. (1961). *Perception and the physical world.* London: Routledge & Kegan Paul.

Baars, B. J. (1988). *A cognitive theory of consciousness.* New York: Cambridge University Press.

Baars, B. J. (1997). *In the theater of consciousness: The workspace of the mind.* New York: Oxford University Press.

Baars, B. J. (1998). Metaphors of consciousness and attention in the brain. *Trends in Neurosciences, 21,* 58–62.

Baars, B. J. (2003). The double life of B.F. Skinner: Inner conflict, dissociation and the taboo against consciousness. *Journal of Consciousness Studies, 10*(1), 5–25.

Bachmann, T. (2000). *Microgenetic approach to the conscious mind.* Amsterdam: John Benjamins.

Backhaus, W. (1998). Conscious and unconscious color vision in man and animals. In C. Taddei-Ferretti & C. Musio (Eds.), *Downward processes in the perception representation mechanisms* (pp. 373–389). Singapore: World Scientific.

Barbur, J. L., Watson, J. D. G., Frackowiak, R. S. J., & Zeki, S. (1993). Conscious visual perception without V1. *Brain, 116,* 1293–1302.

Baron-Cohen, S., Burt, L., Smith-Laittan, F., Harrison, J., Bolton, P. (1996). Synaesthesia: Prevalence and familiality. *Perception, 25*(9), 1073–1079.

Barrett, D. (Ed.). (1996). *Trauma and dreams.* Cambridge, MA: Harvard University Press.

Bauer, R. M. (1984). Autonomic recognition of names and faces in prosopagnosia: A neuropsychological application of the guilty knowledge test. *Neuropsychologia, 22,* 457–469.

Bechtel, W. (1994). Levels of description and explanation in cognitive science. *Minds and Machines, 4,* 1–25.

Bechtel, W., & Abrahamsen, A. (1991). *Connectionism and the mind.* Cambridge, MA: Blackwell.

Bechtel, W., & Richardson, R. C. (1992). Emergent phenomena and complex systems. In A. Beckermann, H. Flohr, & J. Kim (Eds.), *Emergence or reduction? Essays on the prospects of nonreductive physicalism* (pp. 257–288). Berlin: de Gruyter.

Bechtel, W., & Richardson, R. C. (1993). *Discovering complexity. Decomposition and localization as strategies in scientific research.* Princeton, NJ: Princeton University Press.

Beckers, G., & Zeki, S. (1995). The consequences of inactivating areas V1 and V5 on visual motion perception. *Brain, 118,* 49–60.

Beran, R. G. (1992). Automatisms—the current legal position related to clinical practice and medicolegal interpretation. *Clinical and Experimental Neurology, 29,* 81–91.

Berti, A., & Rizzolatti, G. (1992). Visual processing without awareness: Evidence from unilateral neglect. *Journal of Cognitive Neuroscience, 4,* 345–351.

Biederman, I. (1990). Higher-level vision. In D. N. Osherson, S. M. Kosslyn, & J. M. Hollerbach (Eds.), *Visual cognition and action* (pp. 41–72). Cambridge, MA: MIT Press.

Billock, V. A., & Tsou, B. H. (2004). What do catastrophic visual binding failures look like? *Trends in Neurosciences, 27*(2), 84–89.

Bilu, Y. (1989). The other as a nightmare: The Israeli-Arab encounter as reflected in children's dreams in Israel and the West Bank. *Political Psychology, 10*(3), 365–389.

Blackmore, S. J. (1992). *Beyond the body. An investigation of out-of-the-body experiences.* Chicago: Academy Chicago Publishers.

Blagrove, M. (1996). Problems with the cognitive psychological modeling of dreaming. *Journal of Mind and Behavior, 17,* 99–134.

Block, N. (1995). On a confusion about a function of consciousness. *Behavioral and Brain Sciences, 18,* 227–247.

Block, N. (2001). Paradox and cross purposes in recent work on consciousness. *Cognition, 79,* 197–219.

Boeve, B. F., Silber, M. H., Ferman, T. J., et al. (1998). REM sleep behavior disorder and degenerative dementia: An association likely reflecting Lewy body disease. *Neurology, 51,* 363–370.

Bonhoeffer, T., & Grinvald, A. (1996). Optical imaging based on intrinsic signals. The methodology. In A. W. Toga & J. C. Mazziotta (Eds.), *Brain mapping, The methods* (pp. 55–97). San Diego: Academic Press.

Borbély, A. (1984). Schlafgewohnheiten, Schlafqualität und Schlafmittelkonsum der Schweizer Bevölkerung. Ergebnisse einer Repräsentativumfrage. *Schweizerische Aerztezeitung, 65*(34), 1606–1613.

Braun, A. R., Balkin, T. J., Wesensten, N. J., et al. (1998). Dissociated pattern of activity in visual cortices and their projections during human rapid eye movement sleep. *Science, 279,* 91–95.

Breger, L. (1967). Function of dreams. *Journal of Abnormal Psychology, 72*(5), 1–28.

Bridgeman, B. (2000). Interactions between vision for perception and vision for behavior. In Y. Rossetti & A. Revonsuo (Eds.), *Beyond dissociation: Interaction between dissociated implicit and explicit processing* (pp. 17–40). Amsterdam: John Benjamins.

Broad, C. D. (1925). *The mind and its place in nature.* London: Routledge & Kegan Paul.

Bruyer, R. (1991). Covert face recognition in prosopagnosia: A review. *Brain and Cognition, 15,* 223–235.

Busch, N. A., Debener, S., Kranczioch, C., Engel, A. K., & Herrmann, C. S. (2004). Size matters: Effects of stimulus size, duration and eccentricity on the visual gamma-band response. *Clinical Neurophysiology, 115*(8), 1810–1820.

Bulkeley, K. (2003). *Dreams of healing. Transforming nightmares into visions of hope.* New York: Paulist Press.

Campbell, A. (1999). Staying alive: Evolution, culture, and women's intrasexual aggression. *Behavioral and Brain Sciences, 22,* 203–252.

Chalmers, D. J. (1996). *The conscious mind.* Oxford: Oxford University Press.

Chalmers, D. J. (2000). What is a neural correlate of consciousness? In T. Metzinger (Ed.), *Neural correlates of consciousness* (pp. 17–39). Cambridge, MA: MIT Press.

Cherry, S. R., & Phelps, M. E. (1996). Imaging brain function with positron emission tomography. In A. W. Toga & J. C. Mazziotta (Eds.), *Brain mapping: The methods* (pp. 191–221). San Diego: Academic Press.

Clark, A. (1993). *Sensory qualities.* Oxford: Oxford University Press.

Clark, A. (1996). True theories, false colors. *Philosophy of Science, 63* (Suppl.), S143–150.

Clark, A. (2000). *A theory of sentience.* Oxford: Oxford University Press.

Cole, J., & Paillard, J. (1995). Living without touch and peripheral information about body position and movement: Studies with deafferented subjects. In J. L. Bermudez, A. Marcel, & N. Eilan (Eds.), *The body and the self* (pp. 245–266). Cambridge, MA: MIT Press.

Comella, C. L., Nardine, T. M., Diederich, N. J., & Stebbins, G. T. (1998). Sleep-related violence, injury, and REM sleep behavior disorder in Parkinson's disease. *Neurology, 51,* 526–529.

Cosmides, L., & Tooby, J. (1995). From function to structure: The role of evolutionary biology and computational theories in cognitive neuroscience. In M. S. Gazzaniga (Ed.), *The cognitive neurosciences* (pp. 1199–1210). Cambridge, MA: MIT Press.

Cowey, A., & Stoerig, P. (1992). Reflections on blindsight. In A. D. Milner & M. D. Rugg (Eds.), *The neuropsychology of consciousness* (pp. 11–37). London: Academic Press.

Craver, C. F. (2001). Role functions, mechanisms, and hierarchy. *Philosophy of Science, 68,* 53–74.

Craver, C. F., & Darden, L. (2001). Discovering mechanisms in neurobiology: The case of spatial memory. In P. Machamer, R. Grush, & P. McLaughlin (Eds.), *Theory and method in the neurosciences* (pp. 112–137). Pittsburgh: University of Pittsburgh Press.

Crick, F. (1994). *The astonishing hypothesis.* London: Simon & Schuster.

Crick, F., & Koch, C. (1990). Towards a neurobiological theory of consciousness, *Seminars in the Neurosciences, 2,* 273–304.

Crick, F., & Koch, C. (1995). Are we aware of neural activity in primary visual cortex? *Nature, 375,* 121–123.

Crick, F., & Koch, C. (1998). Consciousness and neuroscience. *Cerebral Cortex, 8,* 97–107.

Crick, F., & Koch, C. (2003). A framework for consciousness. *Nature Neuroscience, 6*(2), 119–126.

Cytowic, R. E. (1993). *The man who tasted shapes.* London: Abacus.

Dainton, B. (2000). *Stream of consciousness.* London: Routledge.

Dainton, B. (2003). Unity in the void: Reply to Revonsuo. *Psyche, 9*(08). Retrieved 15 September 2004, from http://psyche.csse.monash.edu.au/symposia/dainton/rev-r.pdf

Damasio, A. R. (1989). Time-locked multiregional retroactivation: A systems-level proposal for the neural substrates of recall and recognition. *Cognition, 33,* 25–62.

Damasio, A. R. (1999). *The feeling of what happens.* New York: Harcourt Brace.

DeDuve, C. (1991). *Blueprint for a cell: The nature and origin of life.* Burlington, NC: Neil Patterson.

Dehaene, S., & Naccache, L. (2001). Towards a cognitive neuroscience of consciousness: Basic evidence and a workspace framework. *Cognition, 79,* 1–37.

Del Re, G. (1998). Ontological status of molecular structure. *HYLE—An International Journal for the Philosophy of Chemistry, 4*(2), 81–103.

Dement, W. C. (1972). *Some must watch while some must sleep.* New York: Norton.

Dennett, D. C. (1976). Are dreams experiences? *Philosophical Review, 73,* 151–171.

Dennett, D. C. (1987). *The intentional stance.* Cambridge, MA: MIT Press.

Dennett, D. C. (1991). *Consciousness explained.* Boston: Little, Brown.

Deouell, L. Y. (2002). Pre-requisities for conscious awareness: Clues from electrophysiological and behavioral studies of unilateral neglect patients. *Consciousness and Cognition, 11,* 546–567.

Desjardins, S., & Zadra, A. (2004). Threat simulation in nightmares (abstract). *Sleep, 27,* A61.

Domhoff, G. W. (1996). *Finding meaning in dreams. A quantitative approach.* New York: Plenum.

Dretske, F. (1995). *Naturalizing the mind.* Cambridge, MA: MIT Press.

Driver, J., & Vuilleumier, P. (2001). Perceptual awareness and its loss in unilateral neglect and extinction. *Cognition, 79,* 39–88.

Duong, T. Q., Kim, D. S., Ugurbil, K., & Kim, S. G. (2000). Spatiotemporal dynamics of the BOLD fMRI signals: Toward mapping submillimeter cortical columns using the early negative response. *Magnetic Resonance in Medicine, 44,* 231–242.

Dyken, M. E., Lin-Dyken, D. C., Seaba, P., & Yamada, T. (1995). Violent sleep-related behavior leading to subdural hemorrhage. *Archives of Neurology, 52,* 318–321.

Eckhorn, R. (1994). Oscillatory and non-oscillatory synchronizations in the visual cortex and their possible roles in associations of visual features. In J. van Pelt, M. A. Corner, H. B. M. Uylings, & F. H. Lopes da Silva (Eds.), *Progress in brain research* (Vol. 102, pp. 405–426). Amsterdam: Elsevier.

Edelman, D. B., Baars, B. J., & Seth, A. K. (2005). Identifying hallmarks of consciousness in nonmammalian species. *Consciousness and Cognition, 14,* 169–187.

Edelman, G. M. (1989). *The remembered present.* New York: Basic Books.

Edelman, G. M., & Tononi, G., (2000). *A universe of consciousness.* New York: Basic Books.

Eilan, N., Marcel, A., & Bermudez, J. L. (1995). Self-consciousness and the body: An interdisciplinary introduction. In J. L. Bermudez, A. Marcel, & N. Eilan (Eds.), *The body and the self* (pp. 1–28). Cambridge, MA: MIT Press.

Ellis, A. W., & Young, A. W. (1988). *Human cognitive neuropsychology.* Hove, UK: Lawrence Erlbaum.

Engel, A. K., Fries, P., König, P., Brecht, M., & Singer, W. (1999). Temporal binding, binocular rivalry, and consciousness. *Consciousness and Cognition, 8*(2), 128–151.

Engel, A. K., & Singer, W. (2001). Temporal binding and the neural correlates of sensory awareness. *Trends in Cognitive Sciences, 5,* 16–25.

Ernst, T., & Henning, J. (1994). Observation of a fast response in functional MR. *Magnetic Resonance in Medicine, 32,* 146–149.

Farah, M. J. (1990). *Visual agnosia.* Cambridge, MA: MIT Press.

Farah, M. J. (1994). Visual perception and visual awareness after brain damage: A tutorial overview. In C. Umiltá & M. Moscovitch (Eds.), *Attention and performance XV, Conscious and nonconscious information processing* (pp. 37–76). Cambridge, MA: MIT Press.

Farah, M. J. (2000). *The cognitive neuroscience of vision.* Oxford: Blackwell.

Farthing, W. G. (1992). *The psychology of consciousness.* New York: Prentice Hall.

Feyerabend, P. (1995). *Killing time, The autobiography of Paul Feyerabend.* Chicago: University of Chicago Press.

ffytche, D. H., Howard, R. J., Brammer, M. J., David, A., Woodruff, P., & Williams, S. (1998). The anatomy of conscious vision: An fMRI study of visual hallucinations. *Nature Neuroscience, 1,* 738–742.

Flanagan, O. (1995). Deconstructing dreams: The spandrels of sleep. *Journal of Philosophy, 92,* 5–27.

Flohr, H. (2000). NMDA receptor–mediated computational processes and phenomenal consciousness. In T. Metzinger (Ed.), *Neural correlates of consciousness* (pp. 245–258). Cambridge, MA: MIT Press.

Fodor, J. A. (1983). *The modularity of mind.* Cambridge, MA: MIT Press.

Fookson, J., & Antrobus, J. (1992). A connectionist model of bizarre thought and imagery. In J. Antrobus & M. Bertini (Eds.), *Neuropsychology of sleep and dreaming* (pp. 197–214). Hillsdale, NJ: Lawrence Erlbaum.

Foster, J. (2000). *The nature of perception.* Oxford: Oxford University Press.

Fotheringhame, D. K., & Young, M. P. (1997). Neural coding schemes for sensory representation: Theoretical proposals and empirical evidence. In M. D. Rugg (Ed.), *Cognitive neuroscience* (pp. 47–76). Cambridge, MA: MIT Press.

Foulkes, D. (1982). *Children's dreams: Longitudinal studies.* New York: Wiley.

Foulkes, D. (1985). *Dreaming: A cognitive-psychological analysis.* Hillsdale, NJ: Lawrence Erlbaum.

Foulkes, D. (1994). Point of view in spontaneous waking thought. *Perceptual and Motor Skills, 78,* 681–682.

Foulkes, D. (1999). *Children's dreaming and the development of consciousness.* Cambridge, MA: Harvard University Press.

Foulkes, D., & Kerr, N. H. (1994). Point of view in nocturnal dreaming. *Perceptual and Motor Skills, 78,* 690.

Foulkes, D., Sullivan, B., Kerr, N. H., & Brown, L. (1988). Appropriateness of dream feelings to dreamed situations. *Cognition and Emotion, 2*(1), 29–39.

Fox, I. (1994). Our knowledge of the internal world. *Philosophical Topics, 22,* 59–106.

Fries, P., Roelfsema, P. R., Engel, A. K., König, P., & Singer, W. (1997). Synchronization of oscillatory responses in visual cortex correlates with perception in interocular rivalry. *Proceedings of the National Academy of Sciences, USA, 94,* 12699–12704.

Friston, K. J., & Frackowiak, R. S. J. (1997). Images of the future: A philosophical coda. In R. S. J. Frackowiak, K. J. Friston, C. D. Frith, R. J. Dolan, & J. C. Mazziotta (Eds.), *Human brain function* (pp. 487–517). San Diego: Academic Press.

Frith, C. D., Blakemore, S. J., & Wolpert, D. M. (2000). Abnormalities in the awareness and control of action. *Philosophical Transactions of the Royal Society of London. Series B: Biological Sciences, 355,* 1771–1788.

Garfield, P. (2001). *The universal dream key. The 12 most common dream themes around the world.* New York: Harper Collins.

Garson, J. W. (2001). Dissolving the binding problem. *Philosophical Psychology, 14*(4), 515–533.

Gazzaniga, M. S. (1995a). Consciousness and the cerebral hemispheres. In M. S. Gazzaniga (Ed.), *The cognitive neurosciences* (1391–1400), Cambridge, MA: MIT Press.

Gazzaniga, M. S. (1995b). Preface to the cognitive neurosciences. In M. S. Gazzaniga (Ed.), *The cognitive neurosciences.* Cambridge, MA: MIT Press.

Gazzaniga, M. S., Ivry, R. B., & Mangun, G. R. (2002). *Cognitive neuroscience. The biology of the mind* (2nd ed.). New York: Norton.

Gennaro, R. J. (1996). *Consciousness and self-consciousness.* Amsterdam: John Benjamins.

Germain, A., Nielsen, T. A., Zadra, A., & Montplaisir, J. (2000). The prevalence of typical dream themes challenges the specificity of the threat simulation theory. *Behavioral and Brain Sciences, 23*(6), 940–941.

Gibson, J. J. (1979). *The ecological approach to visual perception.* Boston: Houghton Mifflin.

Giere, R. N. (1988). *Explaining science.* Chicago: University of Chicago Press.

Gillet, G. R., & McMillan, J. (2001). *Consciousness and intentionality.* Amsterdam: John Benjamins.

Goodale, M. A., & Milner, A. D. (1992). Separate visual pathways for perception and action. *Trends in Neurosciences, 15,* 20–25.

Gray, C. M. (1999). The temporal correlation hypothesis of visual feature integration: Still alive and well. *Neuron, 24,* 31–47.

Gregor, T. (1981). A content analysis of Mehinaku dreams. *Ethos, 9,* 353–390.

Grossenbacher, P. G., & Lovelace, C. T. (2001). Mechanisms of synesthesia: Cognitive and physiological constraints. *Trends in Cognitive Sciences, 5*(1), 36–41.

Guilleminault, C., Moscovitch, A., & Leger, D. (1995). Forensic sleep medicine: Nocturnal wandering and violence. *Sleep, 18,* 740–748.

Hall, C. S. (1955). The significance of the dream of being attacked. *Journal of Personality, 24,* 164–180.

Hall, C. S., & Domhoff, G. W. (1963). Aggression in dreams. *International Journal of Social Psychiatry, 9,* 259–267.

Hall, C. S., & Domhoff, G. W. (1964). Friendliness in dreams. *Journal of Social Psychology, 62,* 309–314.

Hall, C. S., & Van de Castle, R. L. (1966). *The content analysis of dreams.* New York: Appleton-Century-Crofts.

Hall, R. J. (1996). The evolution of color vision without colors. *Philosophy of Science, 63* (Suppl.), S125–133.

Halligan, P. W., & Marshall, J. C. (Eds.). (1996). *Method in madness.* Hove, UK: Psychology Press.

Hameroff, S. R., & Scott, A. C. (1998). A Sonoran afternoon: A discussion of the relevance of quantum theory to consciousness. In S. R. Hameroff, A. W. Kaszniak, & A. C. Scott (Eds.), *Toward a science of consciousness II* (pp. 635–644). Cambridge, MA: MIT Press.

Hamad, S. (2000). Correlation vs. causality. How/why the mind-body problem is hard. *Journal of Consciousness Studies, 7,* 54–61.

Hartmann, E. (1984). *The nightmare: The psychology and biology of terrifying dreams.* New York: Basic Books.

Hartmann, E. (1993). Nightmares. In M. Carskadon (Ed.), *Encyclopedia of sleep and dreaming* (pp. 406–408). New York: Macmillan.

Hartmann, E. (1996). Outline for a theory on the nature and functions of dreaming. *Dreaming, 6,* 147–170.

Hartmann, E. (1998). *Dreams and nightmares.* New York: Plenum.

Heilman, K. M., Watson, R. T., & Valenstein, E. (2000). Neglect I: Clinical and anatomical issues. In M. J. Farah & T. E. Feinberg (Eds.), *Patient-based approaches to cognitive neuroscience* (pp. 115–123). Cambridge, MA: MIT Press.

Heim, M. (1998). *Virtual realism.* New York: Oxford University Press.

Heiss, W. D., Pawlik, G., Herholz, K., Wagner, R., & Wienhard, K. (1985). Regional cerebral glucose metabolism in man during wakefulness, sleep, and dreaming. *Brain Research,* 327(1–2), 362–366.

Heywood, C. A., & Cowey, A. (1999). Cerebral achromatopsia. In G. W. Humphreys (Ed.), *Case studies in the neuropsychology of vision* (pp. 17–39). Hove, UK: Psychology Press.

Heywood, C. A., & Zihl, J. (1999). Motion blindness. In G. W. Humphreys (Ed.), *Case studies in the neuropsychology of vision* (pp. 1–16). Hove, UK: Psychology Press.

Hobson, J. A. (1988). *The dreaming brain.* New York: Basic Books.

Hobson, J. A. (1992). A new model of brain-mind state: Activation level, input source, and mode of processing (AIM). In J. S. Antrobus & M. Bertini (Eds.), *The neuropsychology of sleep and dreaming* (pp. 227–246). Hillsdale, NJ: Lawrence Erlbaum.

Hobson, J. A. (1997). Dreaming as delirium: A mental status exam of our nightly madness. *Seminars in Neurology, 17,* 121–128.

Hobson, J. A. (1999). *Consciousness.* New York: Scientific American Library.

Hobson, J. A. (2001). *The dream drugstore. Chemically altered states of consciousness.* Cambridge, MA: MIT Press.

Hobson, J. A., Pace-Schott, E. F., & Stickgold, R. (2000). Dream science 2000: A response to commentaries on dreaming and the brain. *Behavioral and Brain Sciences, 23*(6), 1019–1035.

Hut, P., & Shepard, R. N. (1996). Turning "the hard problem" upside down & sideways. *Journal of Consciousness Studies, 3*(4), 313–329.

Inman, D. J., Silver, S. M., & Doghramji, K. (1990). Sleep disturbance in post traumatic stress disorder: A comparison with non-PTSD insomnia. *Journal of Traumatic Stress,* 3, 429–437.

Intraub, H. (1999). Understanding and remembering briefly glimpsed pictures: Implications for visual scanning and memory. In V. Coltheart (Ed.), *Fleeting memories: Cognition of brief visual stimuli* (pp. 47–70). Cambridge, MA: MIT Press.

Jackson, F. (1986). What Mary didn't know. *Journal of Philosophy, 83,* 291–295.

James, W. [1890] (1950). *The principles of psychology* (Vols. 1–2). Reprint, New York: Dover.

John, E. R. (2002). The neurophysics of consciousness. *Brain Research Reviews, 39,* 1–28.

Johanson, M., Revonsuo, A., Chaplin, J., & Wedlund, J. E. (2003). Level and content of consciousness in connection with partial epileptic seizures. *Epilepsy and Behavior, 4*(3), 283–288.

Jones, E. G. (2001). The thalamic matrix and thalamocortical synchrony. *Trends in Neurosciences, 24*(10), 595–601.

Jouvet, M. (1993). Metabolic control of REM sleep. In M. A. Carskadon (Ed.), *Encyclopedia of sleep and dreaming* (pp. 369–370). New York: Macmillan.

Kahn, D., & Hobson, J. A. (2003). State dependence of character perception. *Journal of Consciousness Studies, 10*(3), 57–68.

Kahn, D., Pace-Schott, E. F., & Hobson, J. A. (1997). Consciousness in waking and dreaming: The roles of neuronal oscillation and neuromodulation in determining similarities and differences. *Neuroscience, 78*(1), 13–38.

Kahn, D., Pace-Schott, E. & Hobson, J. A. (2002). Emotion and cognition: Feeling and character identification in dreaming. *Consciousness and Cognition, 11,* 34–50.

Kallio, S., & Revonsuo, A. (2003). Hypnotic phenomena and altered states of consciousness: A multilevel framework of description and explanation. *Contemporary Hypnosis, 20*(3), 111–164.

Kallio, S., & Revonsuo, A. (2005). Altering the state of the altered state debate: Reply to commentaries. *Contemporary Hypnosis, 22,* 44–55.

Kanwisher, N. (2001). Neural events and perceptual awareness. *Cognition, 79,* 89–113.

Kapur, N. (1997). *Injured brains of medical minds, views from within.* Oxford: Oxford University Press.

Karlsson, L. (2001). *Dream experience: Phenomenology meets cognitive neuroscience.* Lund, Sweden: Lund University.

Karnath, H. O., Ferber, S., & Himmelbach, M. (2001). Spatial awareness is a function of the temporal not the posterior parietal lobe. *Nature, 411(6840),* 950–953.

Karnath, H. O., & Hartje, W. (1987). Residual information processing in the neglected visual half-field. *Journal of Neurology, 234,* 180–184.

Karnath, H. O., Himmelbach, M., & Rorden, C. (2002). The subcortical anatomy of human spatial neglect: Putamen, caudate nucleus and pulvinar. *Brain, 125*(Pt. 2), 350–360.

Kellner, R., Neidhardt, J., Krakow, B., & Pathak, D. (1992). Changes in chronic nightmares after one session of desensitization or rehearsal instructions. *American Journal of Psychiatry, 149,* 659–663.

Kerr, N. H. (1993). Dreams of the blind. In M. A. Carskadon (Ed.), *Encyclopedia of sleep and dreaming* (pp. 79–80). New York: Macmillan.

Kim, J. (1992). "Downward causation" in emergentism and nonreductive physicalism. In A. Beckermann, H. Flohr, & J. Kim (Eds.), *Emergence or reduction? Essays on the prospects of nonreductive physicalism* (pp. 119–138). Berlin: de Gruyter.

Kim, J. (1998). *Mind in a physical world.* Cambridge, MA: MIT Press.

Köhler, S., & Moscovitch, M. (1997). Unconscious visual processing in neuropsychological syndromes: A survey of the literature and evaluation of models of consciousness. In M. D. Rugg (Ed.), *Cognitive neuroscience* (pp. 305–373). Cambridge, MA: MIT Press.

Köhler, W. [1929] (1971). An old pseudoproblem. (E. Goldmeier, Trans.). In M. Henle (Ed.), *The selected papers of Wolfgang Köhler* (pp. 125–141). Reprinted, New York: Liveright.

Köhler, W. [1930] (1971). The new psychology and physics. In M. Henle (Ed.), *The selected papers of Wolfgang Köhler* (pp. 237–251). Reprint, New York: Liveright.

Köhler, W. (1947). *Gestalt psychology.* New York: Liveright.

Koivisto, M., & Revonsuo, A. (2003). An ERP study of change detection, change blindness and visual awareness. *Psychophysiology, 40,* 423–429.

Koivisto, M., & Revonsuo, A. (2004). Preconscious analysis of global structure: Evidence from masked priming. *Visual Cognition, 11*(1), 105–127.

Koivisto, M., Revonsuo, A., Hyönä, J., Bergman, M., & Kallio, S. (submitted). Cueing helps to recover from inattentional blindness.

Koivisto, M., Revonsuo, A., & Lehtonen, M. (in press). Independence of visual awareness from the scope of attention: An electrophysiological study. *Cerebral Cortex.*

Koivisto, M., Revonsuo, A., & Salminen, N. (2005). Electrophysiological brain responses reveal the independence of visual awareness from attention at early processing stages. *Neuroreport, 16,* 817–821.

Kostopoulos, G. K. (2001). Involvement of the thalamocortical system in epileptic loss of consciousness. *Epilepsia, 42*(Suppl. 3), 13–19.

Krakow, B., Kellner, R., Pathak, D., & Lambert, L. (1995). Imagery rehearsal treatment for chronic nightmares. *Behaviour Research and Therapy, 33,* 837–843.

Krakow, B., Kellner, R., Pathak, D., & Lambert, L. (1996). Long term reduction of nightmares with imagery rehearsal treatment. *Behavioural and Cognitive Psychotherapy, 24,* 135–148.

Krakow, B., Tandberg, D., Scriggins, L., & Barey, M. (1995). A controlled comparison of self-rated sleep complaints in acute and chronic nightmare sufferers. *Journal of Nervous and Mental Disease, 183,* 623–627.

Kushida, C. A., Clerk, A. A., Kirsch, C. M., Hotson, J. R., & Guilleminault, C. (1995). Prolonged confusion with nocturnal wandering arising from NREM and REM sleep: A case report. *Sleep, 18,* 757–764.

LaBerge, S. (1990). Psychophysiological studies of consciousness during sleep. In R. R. Bootzin, J. F. Kihlstrom, & D. L. Schacter (Eds.), *Sleep and cognition* (pp. 109–126). Washington, DC: American Psychological Association.

LaBerge, S., Nagel, L. E., Dement, W. C., & Zarcone, V. P. (1981). Lucid dreaming verified by volitional communication during REM sleep. *Perceptual and Motor Skills, 52,* 727–732.

Ladavas, E., Berti, A., & Farne, A. (2000). Dissociation between conscious and non-conscious processing in neglect. In Y. Rossetti & A. Revonsuo (Eds.), *Beyond dissociations* (pp. 175–193). Amsterdam: John Benjamins.

Lahav, R. (1993). What neuropsychology tells us about consciousness. *Philosophy of Science, 60,* 67–85.

Lamme, V. A. (2000). Neural mechanisms of visual awareness: A linking proposition. *Brain and Mind, 1,* 385–406.

Lamme, V. A. (2003). Why visual awareness and attention are different. *Trends in Cognitive Sciences, 7,* 12–18.

Lamme, V. A., & Roelfsema, P. R. (2000). The distinct modes of vision offered by feedforward and recurrent processing. *Trends in Neurosciences, 23*(11), 71–579.

Landers, J. (1992). Reconstructing ancient populations. In S. Jones, R. Martin, & D. Pilbeam (Eds.), *The Cambridge encyclopedia of human evolution* (pp. 402–405). New York: Cambridge University Press.

Lavie, P. (1996). *The enchanted world of sleep.* New Haven, CT: Yale University Press.

Lehar, S. (2003a). Gestalt isomorphism and the primacy of subjective conscious experience: A Gestalt bubble model. *Behavioral and Brain Sciences, 26,* 375–444.

Lehar, S. (2003b). *The world in your head.* Mahwah, NJ: Lawrence Erlbaum.

Levine, J. (1983). Materialism and qualia: The explanatory gap. *Pacific Philosophical Quarterly, 64,* 354–361.

Levine, J. (1993). On leaving out what it's like. In M. Davies & G. W. Humphreys (Eds.), *Consciousness* (pp. 121–136). Oxford: Blackwell.

Levine, J. (2001). *Purple haze. The puzzle of consciousness.* New York: Oxford University Press.

Levine, J. B. (1991). The role of culture in the representation of conflict in dreams. A comparison of Bedouin, Irish, and Israeli children. *Journal of Cross-Cultural Psychology, 22*(4), 472–490.

Lewis, C. I. [1929] (1956). *Mind and the world order.* Reprint, New York: Dover.

Lhermitte, F. (1986). Human autonomy and the frontal lobes. Part II: Patient behavior in complex and social situations: The "environmental dependency syndrome." *Annals of Neurology, 19,* 335–343.

Lhermitte, F., Pillon, B., & Serdaru, M. (1986). Human autonomy and the frontal lobes. Part I: Imitation and utilization behavior: A neuropsychological study of 75 patients. *Annals of Neurology, 19,* 326–334.

Lippman, C. W. (1953). Hallucinations of physical duality in migraine. *Journal of Nervous and Mental Disease, 117,* 345–350.

Llinás, R. R. (2001). *I of the vortex: From neurons to self.* Cambridge, MA: MIT Press.

Llinás, R. R., & Paré, D. (1991). Of dreaming and wakefulness. *Neuroscience, 44,* 521–535.

Llinás, R. R., & Paré, D. (1996). The brain as a closed system modulated by the senses. In R. Llinas & P. S. Churchland (Eds.), *The mind-brain continuum* (pp. 1–18). Cambridge, MA: MIT Press.

Llinás, R. R., & Ribary, U. (1993). Coherent 40-Hz oscillation characterizes dream state in humans. *Proceedings of the National Academy of Sciences, USA, 90*(5), 2078–81.

Llinás, R., & Ribary, U. (1994). Perception as an oneiric-like state modulated by the senses. In C. Koch & J. L. Davis (Eds.), *Large-scale neuronal theories of the brain* (pp. 111–124). Cambridge, MA: MIT Press.

Llinás, R., Ribary, U., Contreras, D., & Pedroarena, C. (1998). The neuronal basis for consciousness. *Philosophical Transactions of the Royal Society of London. Series B: Biological Sciences, 353,* 1841–1849.

Lloyd, D. (1997). Consciousness and its discontents. *Communication & Cognition, 30*(3-4), 273–284.

Logothetis, N. K., & Wandell, B. A. (2004). Interpreting the BOLD signal. *Annual Review of Physiology, 66,* 735–769.

Louie, K., & Wilson, M. A. (2001). Temporally structured replay of awake hippocampal ensemble activity during rapid eye movement sleep. *Neuron, 29,* 145–156.

Lutz, A., & Thompson, E. (2003). Neurophenomenology: Integrating subjective experience and brain dynamics in the neuroscience of consciousness. *Journal of Consciousness Studies, 10* (9-10), 31–52.

Lutzenberger, W., Pulvermueller, F., Elbert, T., & Birbaumer, N. (1995). Local 40 Hz-activity in human cortex induced by visual stimulation. *Neuroscience Letters, 183,* 1–4.

Machamer, P., Darden, L., & Craver, C. F. (2000). Thinking about mechanisms. *Philosophy of Science, 67,* 1–25.

Mack, A., & Rock, I. (1998). *Inattentional blindness.* Cambridge, MA: MIT Press.

Mahowald, M. W. (1993). Sleepwalking. In M. Carskadon (Ed.), *Encyclopedia of sleep and dreaming* (pp. 578–579). New York: Macmillan.

Mahowald, M. W., Bundlie, S. R., Hurwitz, T. D., & Schenck, C. H. (1990). Sleep violence—Forensic science implications: Polygraphic and video documentation. *Journal of Forensic Sciences, 35,* 413–432.

Mahowald, M. W., & Schenck, C. H. (1992). Dissociated states of wakefulness and sleep. *Neurology, 42*(Suppl. 6), 44–52.

Mahowald, M. W., Woods, S. R., & Schenck, C. H. (1998). Sleeping dreams, waking hallucinations, and the central nervous system. *Dreaming, 8,* 89–102.

Maienschein, J. (1991). From presentation to representation in E.B. Wilson's *The Cell. Biology and Philosophy, 6,* 227–254.

Malcolm, N. (1959). *Dreaming.* London: Routledge & Kegan Paul.

Mallon, B. (2002). *Dream time with children.* London: Jessica Kingsley.

Maloney, K. J., Cape, E. G., Gotman, J., & Jones, B. E. (1997). High-frequency gamma electroencephalogram activity in association with sleep-wake states and spontaneous behaviors in the rat. *Neuroscience, 76*(2), 541–555.

Mangan, B. (1993). Taking phenomenology seriously: The "fringe" and its implications for cognitive research. *Consciousness and Cognition, 2,* 89–108.

Maquet, P., Peters, J. M., Aerts, J., et al. (1996). Functional neuroanatomy of human rapid-eye-movement sleep and dreaming. *Nature, 383,* 163–166.

Marcel, A. J. (1983). Conscious and unconscious perception: An approach to the relations between phenomenal experience and perceptual processes. *Cognitive Psychology, 15,* 238–300.

Marks, G. A. (1993). PGO waves. In M. A. Carskadon (Ed.), *Encyclopedia of sleep and dreaming* (pp. 447–448). New York: Macmillan.

Marks, I. M., & Nesse, R. M. (1994). Fear and fitness: An evolutionary analysis of anxiety disorders. *Ethology and Sociobiology, 15,* 247–261.

Marshall, J. C., & Halligan, P. W. (1988). Blindsight and insight in visuo-spatial neglect. *Nature, 336,* 766–767.

Maselli, R. A., Rosenberg, R. S., & Spire, J. P. (1988). Episodic nocturnal wanderings in non-epileptic young patients. *Sleep, 11,* 156–161.

Mayr, E. (1982). *The growth of biological thought.* Cambridge, MA: Belknap / Harvard University Press.

Mayr, E. (1996). *This is biology.* Cambridge, MA: Belknap / Harvard University Press.

Mazziotta, J. C. (1996). Time and space. In A. W. Toga & J. C. Mazziotta (Eds.), *Brain mapping, the methods* (pp. 389–406). San Diego: Academic Press.

McFadden, J. (2002). Synchronous firing and its influence on the brain's electromagnetic field. *Journal of Consciousness Studies, 9*(4), 23–50.

McFarlane, A. C. (1987). Posttraumatic phenomena in a longitudinal study of children following a natural disaster. *Journal of the American Academy of Child and Adolescent Psychiatry, 26*(5), 764–769.

McGinn, C. (1991). *The problem of consciousness.* Oxford: Blackwell.

McGinn, C. (1999). *The mysterious flame.* New York: Basic Books.

McGlinchey-Berroth, R., Milberg, W. P., Verfaellie, M., Alexander, M., & Kilduff, P. T. (1993). Semantic processing in the neglected visual field: Evidence from a lexical decision task. *Cognitive Neuropsychology, 10,* 79–108.

McLaughlin, B. P. (1992). The rise and fall of British emergentism. In A. Beckermann, H. Flohr, & J. Kim (Eds.), *Emergence or reduction? Essays on the prospects of nonreductive physicalism* (pp. 49–93). Berlin: de Gruyter

Meindl, R. S. (1992). Human populations before agriculture. In S. Jones, R. Martin, & D. Pilbeam (Eds.), *The Cambridge encyclopedia of human evolution* (pp. 406–410). New York: Cambridge University Press.

Menon, R. S., & Kim, S-G. (1999). Spatial and temporal limits in cognitive neuroimaging with fMRI. *Trends in Cognitive Sciences, 3,* 207–216.

Metzinger, T. (1995a). Faster than thought. In T. Metzinger (Ed.), *Conscious experience* (pp. 425–461). Thorverton, UK: Imprint Academic.

Metzinger, T. (1995b). The problem of consciousness. In T. Metzinger (Ed.), *Conscious experience* (pp. 3–37). Thorverton, UK: Imprint Academic.

Metzinger, T. (1998). Präsentationaler Gehalt. In F. Esken & D. Heckmann (Eds.), *Bewusstsein und Repräsentation* (pp. 377–405). Paderborn, Germany: Ferdinand Schöningh.

Metzinger, T. (2000). The subjectivity of subjective experience: A representationalist analysis of the first-person perspective. In T. Metzinger (Ed.), *Neural correlates of consciousness* (pp. 285–306). Cambridge, MA: MIT Press.

Metzinger, T. (2003). *Being no one. The self-model theory of subjectivity.* Cambridge, MA: MIT Press.

Milner, A. D., & Goodale, M. A. (1995). *The visual brain in action.* Oxford: Oxford University Press.

Money, J. (1960). Phantom orgasm in the dreams of paraplegic men and women. *Archives of General Psychiatry, 3,* 373–382.

Morrison, A. R. (1983). A window on the sleeping brain. *Scientific American, 248,* 86–94.

Näätänen, R., Ilmoniemi, R. J., & Alho, K. (1994). Magnetoencephalography in studies of human cognitive brain function. *Trends in Neurosciences, 17,* 389–395.

Nader, K. (1996). Children's traumatic dreams. In D. Barrett (Ed.), *Trauma and dreams* (pp. 9–24). Cambridge, MA: Harvard University Press.

Nader, K., Pynoos, R., Fairbanks, L., & Frederick, C. (1990). Children's PTSD reactions one year after a sniper attack at their school. *American Journal of Psychiatry, 147,* 1526–1530.

Nagel, T. (1974). What is it like to be a bat? *Philosophical Review, 83,* 435– 450.

Neidhardt, E. J., Krakow, B., Kellner, R., & Pathak, D. (1992). The beneficial effects of one treatment session and recording of nightmares on chronic nightmare sufferers. *Sleep, 15,* 470–473.

Newcombe, F., Young, A. W., & de Haan, E. H. F. (1989). Prosopagnosia and object agnosia without covert recognition. *Neuropsychologia, 27,* 179–191.

Newman, J. (1995). Thalamic contributions to attention and consciousness. *Consciousness and Cognition, 4*(2),172–93.

Newman, J., & Grace, A. A. (1999). Binding across time: The selective gating of frontal and hippocampal systems modulating working memory and attentional states. *Consciousness and Cognition, 8,* 196–212.

Nielsen, T. A. (2000). Covert REM sleep effects on REM mentation: Further methodological considerations and supporting evidence. *Behavioral and Brain Sciences, 23*(6), 1040–1057.

Niiniluoto, I. (2002). *Critical scientific realism.* Oxford: Oxford University Press.

Nijhawan, R., & Khurana, B. (2000). Conscious registration of continuous and discrete visual events. In T. Metzinger (Ed.), *Neural correlates of consciousness* (pp. 203–219). Cambridge, MA: MIT Press.

Noë, A., & Thompson, E. (2004a). Are there neural correlates of consciousness? *Journal of Consciousness Studies, 11* (1), 3–28.

Noë, A., & Thompson, E. (2004b). Sorting out the neural basis of consciousness. *Journal of Consciousness Studies, 11*(1), 87–98.

Nunez, P. L. (1990). Physical principles and neurophysical mechanisms underlying event related potentials. In J. Rohrbaugh, R. Johnson, & R. Parasuraman (Eds.), *Event-related potentials of the brain* (pp. 19–36). New York: Oxford University Press.

Nunez, P. L. (1995). *Neocortical dynamics and human EEG rhythms.* New York: Oxford University Press.

Ojanen, V., Revonsuo, A., & Sams, M. (2003). Visual awareness of low-contrast stimuli is reflected in event-related brain potentials. *Psychophysiology, 40,* 192–197.

O'Regan, J. K., & Noë, A. (2001). A sensorimotor account of vision and visual consciousness. *Behavioral and Brain Sciences, 24*(5), 939–1031.

Oswald, I., & Evans, J. (1985). On serious violence during sleep-walking. *British Journal of Psychiatry, 147,* 688–691.

Paillard, J., Michel, F., & Stelmach, G. (1983). Localization without content: A tactile analogue of blind sight. *Archives of Neurology, 40,* 548–551.

Pallis, C. A. (1955). Impaired identification of faces and places with agnosia for colours. *Journal of Neurology, Neurosurgery and Psychiatry, 18,* 218–224.

Palmer, S. E. (1999). *Vision science.* Cambridge, MA: MIT Press.

Palmini, A. L., Gloor, P., & Jones-Gotman, M. (1992). Pure amnestic seizures in temporal lobe epilepsy. Definition, clinical symptomatology and functional anatomical considerations. *Brain, 115,* 749–769.

Panksepp, J. (1998). *Affective neuroscience.* New York: Oxford University Press.

Parker, S., Mitchell, R. W., & Boccia, M. L. (Eds.). (1994). *Self-awareness in animals and humans.* Cambridge: Cambridge University Press.

Penfield, W. (1975). *The mystery of the mind.* Princeton, NJ: Princeton University Press.

Penrose, R. (1989). *The emperor's new mind.* New York: Oxford University Press.

Pisella, L., & Rossetti, Y. (2000). Interaction between conscious identification and non-conscious sensorimotor processing. In Y. Rossetti & A. Revonsuo (Eds.), *Beyond dissociation* (pp. 129–152). Amsterdam: John Benjamins.

Pivik, R. T. (1991). Tonic states and phasic events in relation to sleep mentation. In S. J. Ellman & J. S. Antrobus (Eds.), *The mind in sleep. Psychology and psychophysiology* (pp. 214–247). New York: Wiley.

Place, U. T. (2000). Consciousness and the zombie within. In Y. Rossetti & A. Revonsuo (Eds.), *Beyond dissociation* (pp. 295–329). Amsterdam: John Benjamins.

Plazzi, G., Tinuper, P., Montagna, P., Provini, F., & Lugaresi, E. (1995). Epileptic nocturnal wanderings. *Sleep, 18,* 749–756.

Pockett, S. (2000). *The nature of consciousness: A hypothesis.* New York: Writers Club Press.

Pockett, S. (2002). Difficulties with the electromagnetic field theory of consciousness. *Journal of Consciousness Studies, 9*(4), 51–56.

Pollen, D. (1999). On the neural correlates of visual perception. *Cerebral Cortex, 9,* 4–19.

Pöppel, E., Held, R., & Frost, D. (1973). Residual visual function after brain wounds involving the central visual pathways in man. *Nature, 243,* 295–296.

Posner, M. I., & Raichle, M. E. (1994). *Images of mind.* New York: Scientific American Library.

Punamäki, R-L. (1997). Determinants and mental health effects of dream recall among children living in traumatic conditions. *Dreaming,* 7, 235–263.

Raffman, D. (1995). On the persistence of phenomenology. In T. Metzinger (Ed.), *Conscious experience* (pp. 293–308). Paderborn, Germany: Ferdinand Schöning.

Rainville, R. E. (1994). The role of dreams in the rehabilitation of the adventitiously blind. *Dreaming, 4*(3), 155–164.

Rechtschaffen, A. (1978). The single-mindedness and isolation of dreams. *Sleep, 1,* 97–109.

Rechtschaffen, A., & Buchignani, C. (1992). The visual appearance of dreams. In J. S. Antrobus & M. Bertini (Eds.), *The neuropsychology of sleep and dreaming* (pp. 143–155). Hillsdale, NJ: Lawrence Erlbaum.

Rechtschaffen, A., & Foulkes, D. (1965). Effect of visual stimuli on dream content. *Perceptual and Motor Skills, 20,* 1149–1160.

Reinsel, R., Antrobus, J., & Wollman, M. (1992). Bizarreness in dreams and waking fantasy. In J. S. Antrobus & M. Bertini (Eds.), *The neuropsychology of sleep and dreaming* (pp. 157–184). Hillsdale, NJ: Lawrence Erlbaum.

Reitmaa, I., Vanhala, J., Kauttu, A., & Antila, M. (1995). *Virtuaaliympäristöt* [Virtual Environments]. Reports from the Finnish Technology Development Center No. 45. Helsinki: TEKES.

Renault, B., Signoret, J. L., Debruille, B., Breton, F., & Bolger, F. (1989). Brain potentials reveal covert facial recognition in prosopagnosia. *Neuropsychologia, 27,* 905–912.

Revonsuo, A. (1993). Is there a ghost in the cognitive machinery? *Philosophical Psychology, 6,* 387–405.

Revonsuo, A. (1994a). The fragile smell of rose, the peculiar aboutness of thought, and the elusive subject of conscious experience. In A. Revonsuo & M. Kamppinen (Eds.), *Consciousness in philosophy and cognitive neuroscience* (pp, 105–114). Hillsdale, NJ: Lawrence Erlbaum.

Revonsuo, A. (1994b). In search of the science of consciousness. In A. Revonsuo & M. Kamppinen (Eds.), *Consciousness in philosophy and cognitive neuroscience* (pp. 249–285). Hillsdale, NJ: Lawrence Erlbaum.

Revonsuo, A. (1995a). Conscious and nonconscious control of action. *Behavioral and Brain Sciences, 18,* 265–266.

Revonsuo, A. (1995b). Consciousness, dreams, and virtual realities. *Philosophical Psychology, 8,* 35–58.

Revonsuo, A. (1995c). Words interact with colors in a globally aphasic patient: Evidence from a Stroop-like task. *Cortex, 31,* 377–386.

Revonsuo, A. (1999). Binding and the phenomenal unity of consciousness. *Consciousness and Cognition, 8*(2), 173–185.

Revonsuo, A. (2000a). Did ancestral humans dream for their lives? *Behavioral and Brain Sciences, 23*(6), 1063–1082.

Revonsuo, A. (2000b). The reinterpretation of dreams: An evolutionary hypothesis of the function of dreaming. *Behavioral and Brain Sciences, 23*(6), 877–901.

Revonsuo, A. (2001a). On the nature of explanation in neurosciences. In P. Machamer, R. Grush, & P. McLaughlin (Eds.), *Theory and method in the neurosciences* (pp. 45–69). Pittsburgh: University of Pittsburgh Press.

Revonsuo, A. (2001b). Putting color back where it belongs. *Consciousness and Cognition, 10,* 78–84.

Revonsuo, A. (2003a). Consciousness as phenomenal ether? *Behavioral and Brain Sciences 26*(4), 422–423.

Revonsuo, A. (2003b). The contents of phenomenal consciousness: One relation to rule them all and in the unity bind them. *Psyche, 9*(8). Retrieved 14 September 2004, from http://psyche.csse.monash.edu.au/v9/psyche-9-08-revonsuo.html

Revonsuo, A., & Laine, M. (1996). Semantic processing without conscious understanding in a case of global aphasia: Evidence from auditory event-related brain potentials. *Cortex, 32,* 29–48.

Revonsuo, A., & Salmivalli, C. (1995). A content analysis of bizarre elements in dreams. *Dreaming, 5*(3), 169–187.

Revonsuo, A., & Tarkko, K. (2002). Binding in dreams. *Journal of Consciousness Studies, 9*(7), 3–24.

Revonsuo, A., & Valli, K. (2000). Dreaming and consciousness: Testing the threat simulation theory of the function of dreaming. *Psyche,* 6. Retrieved 14 September 2004, from http://psyche.cs.monash.edu.au/v6/psyche-6-08-revonsuo.html

Revonsuo, A., Wilenius-Emet, M., Kuusela, J., & Lehto, M. (1997). The neural generation of a unified illusion in human vision. *NeuroReport, 8*(18), 3867–3870.

Rheingold, H. (1991). *Virtual reality.* New York: Simon & Schuster.

Riddoch, G. (1917). Dissociation of visual perception due to occipital injuries, with especial reference to appreciation of movement. *Brain, 40,* 15–57.

Rittenhouse, C. D., Stickgold, R., & Hobson, A. (1994). Constraint on the transformation of characters, objects, and settings in dream reports. *Consciousness and Cognition, 3,* 100–113.

Rizzo, M., Hurtig, R., & Damasio, A. R. (1987). The role of scanpaths in facial recognition and learning. *Annals of Neurology, 22,* 41–45.

Rizzolatti, G., Riggio, L., & Sheliga, B. M. (1994). Space and selective attention. In C. Umiltá & M. Moscovitch (Eds.), *Attention and performance XV, Conscious and nonconscious information processing* (pp. 231–265). Cambridge, MA: MIT Press.

Robbins, P., & Houshi, F. (1983). Some observations on recurrent dreams. *Bulletin of the Menninger Clinic, 47,* 262–265.

Robertson, L., Treisman, A., Friedman-Hill, S., & Grabowecky, M. (1997). The interaction of spatial and object pathways: Evidence from Balint's syndrome. *Journal of Cognitive Neuroscience, 9*(3), 295–317.

Robertson, L. C. (1999). What can spatial deficits teach us about feature binding and spatial maps? *Visual Cognition, 6*(3–4), 409–430.

Robertson, L. C. (2003). Binding, spatial attention and perceptual awareness. *Nature Reviews Neuroscience, 4,* 93–102.

Rodriguez, E., George, N., Lachaux, J. P., Martinerie, J., Renault, B., & Varela, F. J. (1999). Perception's shadow: Long-distance synchronization of human brain activity. *Nature, 397*(6718), 430–433.

Roelfsema, P. R., Engel, A. K., König, P., & Singer, W. (1996). The role of neuronal synchronization in response selection: A biologically plausible theory of structured representations in the visual cortex. *Journal of Cognitive Neuroscience, 8*(6), 603–625.

Roelfsema, P. R., & Singer, W. (1998). Detecting connectedness. *Cerebral Cortex, 8,* 385–396.

Roitt, I., Brostoff, J., & Male, D. (1998). *Immunology* (5th ed.). London: Mosby.

Ross, P. W. (2001). The location problem for color subjectivism. *Consciousness and Cognition, 10,* 42–58.

Rossetti, Y. (1998). Implicit short-lived representations of space in brain damaged and healthy subjects. *Consciousness and Cognition, 7,* 520–558.

Rossetti, Y., & Revonsuo, A. (Eds.). (2000). *Beyond dissociation: Interaction between dissociated implicit and explicit processing.* Amsterdam: John Benjamins.

Rossetti, Y., Rode, G., & Boisson, D. (1995). Implicit processing of somaesthetic information: A dissociation between where and how? *NeuroReport, 6,* 506–510.

Russell, B. (1927a). *The analysis of matter.* London: Routledge.

Russell, B. (1927b). *Philosophy.* New York: Norton

Russell, B. (1948). *Human knowledge: Its scope and limits.* New York: Simon and Schuster.

Sacks, O. (1985). *The man who mistook his wife for a hat.* London: Picador.

Sacks, O. (1995). *An anthropologist on Mars.* London: Picador.

Saffran, E. M., & Schwartz, M. F. (1994). Of cabbages and things: Semantic memory from a neuropsychological perspective—A tutorial review. In C. Umiltá, & M. Moscovitch (Eds.), *Attention and performance XV: Conscious and nonconscious information processing* (pp. 507–536). Cambridge, MA: MIT Press.

Saint-Denys, H. de [1867] (1982). *Dreams and how to guide them* (M. Schatzman, Ed. & Trans.). Reprint, London: Duckworth.

Sajama, S., & Vihjanen, S. (1993). Representation and reality. In M. Kamppinen (Ed.), *Consciousness, cognitive schemata, and relativism* (pp. 171–228). Dordrecht, Netherlands: Kluwer.

Salmon, W. C. (1989). Four decades of scientific explanation. In P. Kitcher & W. C. Salmon (Eds.), *Scientific explanation. Minnesota studies in the philosophy of science* 13 (pp. 3–195). Minneapolis: University of Minnesota Press.

Sauve, K. (1999). Gamma-band synchronous oscillations: Recent evidence regarding their functional significance. *Consciousness and Cognition, 8*(2), 213–224.

Schacter, D. L. (1996). *Searching for memory.* New York: Basic Books.

Schacter, D. L., McAndrews, M. P., & Moscovitch, M. (1988). Access to consciousness: Dissociations between implicit and explicit knowledge in neuropsychological syndromes. In L. Weiskrantz (Ed.), *Thought without language* (pp. 242–278). Oxford: Oxford University Press.

Schenck, C. H. (1993). REM sleep behavior disorder. In M. A. Carskadon (Ed.), *Encyclopedia of sleep and dreaming* (pp. 499–505). New York: Macmillan.

Schenck, C. H., Bundlie, S. R., Ettiger, M. G., & Mahowald, M. W. (1986). Chronic behavioral disorders of human REM sleep: A new category of parasomnia. *Sleep, 9,* 293–308.

Schenck, C. H., & Mahowald, M. W. (1995). A polysomnographically documented case of adult somnambulism with long-distance automobile driving and frequent nocturnal violence: Parasomnia with continuing danger as a noninsane automatism? *Sleep, 18,* 765–772.

Schredl, M., & Doll, E. (1998). Emotions in diary dreams. *Consciousness and Cognition, 7,* 634–646.

Schwartz, S., & Maquet, P. (2002). Sleep imaging and the neuropsychological assessment of dreams. *Trends in Cognitive Sciences, 6*(1), 23–30.

Searle, J. R. (1992). *The rediscovery of the mind.* Cambridge, MA: MIT Press.

Searle, J. R. (2000). Consciousness. *Annual Review of Neuroscience, 23,* 557–578.

Seth, A. K., Baars, B. J., & Edelman, D. B. (2005). Criteria for consciousness in humans and other mammals. *Consciousness and Cognition, 14,* 119–139.

Sheinberg, D. L., & Logothetis, N. K. (1997). The role of temporal cortical areas in perceptual organization. *Proceedings of the National Academy of Sciences, USA, 94,* 3408–3413.

Sherrington, C. S. (1935). Santiago Ramón y Cajal 1852–1934. *Obituary Notes of the Royal Society, 4,* 425–441.

Shuren, J. E., Brott, T. G., Scheft, B. K., & Houston, W. (1996). Preserved color imagery in an achromatopsic. *Neuropsychologia, 34,* 485–489.

Siewert, C. P. (1998). *The significance of consciousness.* Princeton, NJ: Princeton University Press.

Simons, J. (2000). Attentional capture and inattentional blindness. *Trends in Cognitive Sciences, 4*(4), 147–155.

Singer, W. (1994). The organization of sensory motor representations in the neocortex: A hypothesis based on temporal coding. In C. Umilta & M. Moscovitch (Eds.), *Attention and performance XV, Conscious and nonconscious information processing* (pp. 77–107). Cambridge, MA: MIT Press.

Singer, W. (1999). Neuronal synchrony: A versatile code for the definition of relations? *Neuron, 24,* 49–65.

Singer, W. (2000). Phenomenal awareness and consciousness from a neurobiological perspective. In T. Metzinger (Ed.), *Neural correlates of consciousness* (pp. 121–137). Cambridge, MA: MIT Press.

Singer, W., & Gray, C. M. (1995). Visual feature integration and the temporal correlation hypothesis. *Annual Review of Neuroscience, 18,* 555–586.

Skokowski, P. (2002). I, zombie. *Consciousness and Cognition, 11,* 1–9.

Smythies, J. (1994a). Requiem for the identity theory. *Inquiry, 37,* 311329.

Smythies, J. (1994b). *The walls of Plato's cave.* Aldershot, UK: Avebury.

Smythies, J. (1996). A note on the concept of the visual field in neurology, psychology, and visual neuroscience. *Perception, 25,* 369–371.

Smythies, J. (2003). Space, time and consciousness. *Journal of Consciousness Studies, 10*(3), 47–56.

Smythies, J. R. (1965). The representative theory of perception. In J. R. Smythies (Ed.), *Brain and mind* (pp. 241–264). London: Routledge & Kegan Paul.

Snyder, F. (1970). The phenomenology of dreaming. In L. Madow & L. H. Snow (Eds.), *The psychodynamic implications of the physiological studies on dreams* (pp. 124–151). Springfield, IL: Charles S Thomas.

Snyder, T. J., & Gackenbach, J. (1988). Individual differences associated with lucid dreaming. In: J. Gackenbach & S. LaBerge (Eds.), *Conscious mind, sleeping brain.* (pp. 221–259). New York: Plenum.

Solms, M. (1997). *The neuropsychology of dreams.* Mahwah, NJ: Lawrence Erlbaum.

Sperling, G. (1960). The information available in brief visual presentations. *Psychological Monographs, 74,* 1–29.

Squires, E. J. (1998). Why are quantum theorists interested in consciousness? In S. R. Hameroff, A. W. Kaszniak, & A. C. Scott (Eds.), *Toward a science of consciousness II* (pp. 609–618). Cambridge, MA: MIT Press.

Steriade, M. (2001). *The intact and sliced brain.* Cambridge, MA: MIT Press.

Stoddard, F. J., Chedekel, D. S., & Shakun, L. (1996). Dreams and nightmares of burned children. In D. Barrett (Ed.), *Trauma and dreams* (pp. 25–45). Cambridge, MA: Harvard University Press.

Strauch, I. (1996). Animal characters in dreams and fantasies of children. *ASD Newsletter, 13*(1), 11–13.

Strauch, I., & Meier, B. (1996). *In search of dreams. Results of experimental dream research.* New York: SUNY Press.

Strawson, G. (1994). *Mental reality.* Cambridge, MA: MIT Press.

Stubenberg, L. (1998). *Consciousness and qualia.* Amsterdam: John Benjamins.

Stufflebeam, R. S., & Bechtel, W. (1997). PET: Exploring the myth and the method. *Philosophy of Science, Proceedings, 64,* 95–106.

Stuss, D. T., Shallice, T., Alexander, M. P., & Picton, T. W. (1995) A multidisciplinary approach to anterior attentional functions. *Annals of the New York Academy of Sciences,* 769. 191–211.

Tallon, C., Bertrand, O., Bouchet, P., & Pernier, J. (1995). Gamma-range activity evoked by coherent visual stimuli in humans. *European Journal of Neuroscience, 7,* 1285–1291.

Tallon-Baudry, C. (2003). Oscillatory synchrony and human visual cognition. *Journal of Physiology, Paris, 97*, 355–363.

Tallon-Baudry, C., & Bertrand, O. (1999). Oscillatory gamma activity in humans and its role in object representation. *Trends in Cognitive Sciences, 3,* 151–162.

Tallon-Baudry, C., Bertrand, O., Delpuech, C., & Pernier, J. (1996). Stimulus specificity of phase-locked and non-phase locked 40 Hz visual responses in human. *Journal of Neuroscience, 16,* 4240–4249.

Tallon-Baudry, C., Bertrand, O., Delpuech, C., & Pernier, J. (1997). Oscillatory gamma-band (30–70 Hz) activity induced by a visual search task in humans. *Journal of Neuroscience, 17,* 722–734.

Taylor, J. G. (2001). The central role of the parietal lobes in consciousness. *Consciousness and Cognition, 10,* 379–417.

Terr, L. (1990). *Too scared to cry.* New York: Basic Books.

Thompson, E. (2001). Empathy and consciousness. *Journal of Consciousness Studies, 8*(5–7), 1–32.

Thompson, E., & Varela, F. J. (2001). Radical embodiment: neural dynamics and consciousness. *Trends in Cognitive Sciences, 5*(10), 418–425.

Titchener, E. B. (1896). *An outline of psychology.* New York: Macmillan.

Toga, A. W., & Mazziotta, J. C. (1996). *Brain mapping.* San Diego: Academic Press.

Tong, F. (2003). Primary visual cortex and visual awareness. *Nature Reviews Neuroscience, 4,* 219–229.

Tong, F., Nakayama, K., Vaughan, J. T., & Kanwisher, N. (1998). Binocular rivalry and visual awareness in human extrastriate cortex. *Neuron, 21,* 753–759.

Tononi, G., Srinivasan, R., Russell, D. P., & Edelman, G. M. (1998). Investigating neural correlates of conscious perception by frequency-tagged neuromagnetic responses. *Proceedings of the National Academy of Sciences, USA, 95*(6), 3198–203.

Tooby, J., & Cosmides, L. (1992). The psychological foundations of culture. In J. Barkow, L. Cosmides, & J. Tooby (Eds.), *The adapted mind: Evolutionary psychology and the generation of culture* (pp. 19–136). New York: Oxford University Press.

Tooby, J., & Cosmides, L. (1995). Mapping the evolved functional organization of mind and brain. In M. S. Gazzaniga (Ed.), *The cognitive neurosciences* (pp. 1185–1197). Cambridge, MA: MIT Press.

Tranel, D., & Damasio, A. R. (1985). Knowledge without awareness: An autonomic index of facial recognition by prosopagnosics. *Science, 228,* 1453–1454.

Tranel, D., & Damasio, A. R. (1988). Non-conscious face recognition in patients with face agnosia. *Behavioural Brain Research, 30,* 235–249.

Treisman, A. (1988). Features and objects: The Fourteenth Bartlett Memorial Lecture. *Quarterly Journal of Experimental Psychology, 40A,* 201–237.

Treisman, A. (1994). Modularity and attention: Is the binding problem real? *Visual Cognition, 2,* 303–311.

Treisman, A. (1996). The binding problem. *Current Opinion in Neurobiology, 6,* 171–178.

Treisman, A. (1999). Solutions to the binding problem: Progress through controversy and convergence. *Neuron, 24,* 105–110.

Treisman, A. (2003). Consciousness and perceptual binding. In A. Cleeremans (Ed.), *The unity of consciousness* (pp. 95–113). Oxford: Oxford University Press.

Treisman, A. M., & Schmidt, H. (1982). Illusory conjunctions in the perception of objects. *Cognitive Psychology, 14,* 107–141.

Tulving, E. (1985). Memory and consciousness. *Canadian Psychology— Psychologie Canadienne 26*(1), 1–12.

Turner, R., Howseman, A., Rees, G., & Josephs, O. (1997). Functional imaging with magnetic resonance. In R. S. Fracowiak, K. J. Friston, C. D. Frith, R. J. Dolan, & J. C. Mazziotta (Eds.), *Human brain function* (pp. 467–486). San Diego: Academic Press.

Tye, M. (1995). *Ten problems of consciousness. A representational theory of the phenomenal mind.* Cambridge, MA: MIT Press.

Ullman, S. (1996). *High-level vision.* Cambridge, MA: MIT Press.

Umiltá, C. (2001). Mechanisms of attention. In: B. Rapp (Ed.), *The handbook of cognitive neuropsychology* (pp. 135–158). Hove, UK: Psychology Press.

Uslar, D. von (1990). *Der Traum als Welt.* Stuttgart: Hirzel.

Valberg, A. (2001). Unique hues: An old problem for a new generation. *Vision Research, 41,* 1645–1657.

Vallar, G. (1997). Spatial frames of reference and somatosensory processing: a neuropsychological perspective. *Philosophical Transactions of the Royal Society of London. Series B: Biological Sciences, 352,* 1401–1409.

Vallar, G. (1998). Spatial hemineglect in humans. *Trends in Cognitive Sciences, 2,* 87–97.

Valli, K., Revonsuo, A., Pälkäs, O., Ismail, K. H., Ali, K. J., & Punamäki, R. L. (2005). The threat simulation theory of the evolutionary function of dreaming: Evidence from dreams of traumatized children. *Consciousness and Cognition, 14,* 188–218.

Van de Castle, R. L. (1970). *The psychology of dreaming.* New York: General Learning Press.

Van de Castle, R.L. (1983). Animal figures in fantasy and dreams. In A. H. Katcher & A. M. Beck (Eds.), *New perspectives on our lives with companion animals* (pp. 148–173). Philadelphia: University of Pennsylvania Press.

Van Eeden, F. [1913] (1990). A study of dreams. In C. T. Tart (Ed.), *Altered states of consciousness* (pp. 175–190). Reprint, New York: Harper Collins.

Van Orden, G. C., & Paap, K. R. (1997). Functional neuroimages fail to discover pieces of mind in the parts of the brain. *Philosophy of Science, Proceedings, 64,* 85–94.

Vanni, S., Revonsuo, A., Saarinen, J., & Hari, R. (1996). Visual awareness of objects correlates with activity of right occipital cortex, *NeuroReport, 8,* 183–186.

Velmans, M. (1996). What and where are conscious experiences? In M. Velmans (Ed.), *The science of consciousness* (pp. 181–196). London: Routledge.

Velmans, M. (2000). *Understanding consciousness.* London: Routledge.

Velmans, M. (2003). Is the world in the brain, or the brain in the world? *Behavioral and Brain Sciences, 26*(4), 427–429.

Villringer, A., & Chance, B. (1997). Non-invasive optical spectroscopy and imaging of human brain function. *Trends in Neurosciences, 20*(10), 435–442.

Vogel, G. W. (1993). Incorporation into dreams. In M. A. Carskadon (Ed.), *Encyclopedia of sleep and dreaming* (pp. 297–298). New York: Macmillan.

Volpe, B. T., Ledoux, J. E., & Gazzaniga, M. S. (1979). Information processing of visual stimuli in an extinguished field. *Nature, 282,* 722–724.

Weiskrantz, L. (1992). Introduction: Dissociated issues. In A. D. Milner & M. D. Rugg (Eds.), *The neuropsychology of consciousness* (pp. 1–10). New York: Academic Press.

Weiskrantz, L. (1997). *Consciousness lost and found.* Oxford: Oxford University Press.

Weiskrantz, L., Warrington, E. K., Sanders, M. D., & Marshall, J. (1974). Visual capacity in the hemianopic field following a restricted occipital ablation. *Brain, 97,* 709–728.

Whitehead, A. N. [1925] (1997). *Science and the modern world.* Reprint, New York: Free Press.

Wilenius-Emet, M., Revonsuo, A., & Ojanen, V. (2004). An electrophysiological correlate of human visual awareness. *Neuroscience Letters, 354,* 38–41.

Wilmer, H. A. (1996). The healing nightmare: War dreams of Vietnam veterans. In D. Barrett (Ed.), *Trauma and dreams* (pp. 85–99). Cambridge, MA: Harvard University Press.

Wolfe, J. M. (1999). Visual search: Preattentive processing and the guidance of visual attention. In C. Taddei-Ferretti & C. Musio (Eds.), *Neuronal bases and psychological aspects of consciousness* (pp. 144–164). Singapore: World Scientific.

Wolfe, J. M., & Cave, K. R. (1999). The psychophysical evidence for a binding problem in human vision. *Neuron, 24,* 11–17.

Wolpert, D. M., Goodbody, S. J., & Husain, M. (1998). Maintaining internal representations: The role of the human superior parietal lobe. *Nature Neuroscience, 1,* 529–533.

Woody, A. I. (2000). Putting quantum mechanics to work in chemistry: The power of diagrammatic representation. *Philosophy of Science, Proceedings, 67,* 612–627.

Wrangham, R., & Peterson, D. (1996). *Demonic males. Apes and the origins of human violence.* New York: Houghton Mifflin.

Wright, E. (1993). More qualia trouble for functionalism: The Smythies TV-hood analogy. *Synthese, 97,* 365–382.

Wu, M. F. (1993). Sensory processing and sensation during sleep. In M. A. Carskadon (Ed.), *Encyclopedia of sleep and dreaming* (pp. 533–535). New York: Macmillan.

Young, A. W. (1994a). Conscious and nonconscious recognition of familiar faces. In C. Umiltá, & M. Moscovitch (Eds.), *Attention and performance XV, Conscious and nonconscious information processing* (pp. 153–178). Cambridge, MA: MIT Press.

Young, A. W. (1994b). Neuropsychology of awareness. In A. Revonsuo, & M. Kamppinen (Eds.), *Consciousness in philosophy and cognitive neuroscience* (pp. 173–203). Hillsdale, NJ: Lawrence Erlbaum.

Young, A. W., & de Haan, E. H. F. (1990). Impairments of visual awareness. *Mind & Language, 5,* 29–48.

Young, A. W., & Ellis, H. D. (2000). Overt and covert face recognition. In Y. Rossett & A. Revonsuo (Eds.), *Beyond dissociation* (pp. 195–219). Amsterdam: John Benjamins.

Zadra, A., Desjardins, S., & Marcotte, E. (in press). Evolutionary function of dreams: A test of the threat simulation theory in recurrent dreams. *Consciousness and Cognition.*

Zadra, A., & Donderi, D. C. (2000). Threat perceptions and avoidance in recurrent dreams. *Behavioral and Brain Sciences, 23*(6), 1017–1018.

Zadra, A. L. (1996). Recurrent dreams: Their relation to life events. In D. Barrett (Ed.), *Trauma and dreams* (pp. 231–247). Cambridge, MA: Harvard University Press.

Zadra, A. L., Nielsen, T. A., & Donderi, D. C. (1998a). Prevalence of auditory, olfactory, and gustatory experiences in home dreams. *Perceptual and Motor Skills, 87*(3, Pt. 1), 819–826.

Zadra, A. L., Nielsen, T. A., Germain, A., Lavigne, G., & Donderi, D. C. (1998b). Pain in dreams. *Pain Research and Management, 3*(3), 155–161.

Zeki, S. (1992). *A vision of the brain.* Oxford: Blackwell.

Zeki, S. (2003). The disunity of consciousness. *Trends in Cognitive Sciences, 7*(5), 214–218.

Zeki, S., & Bartels, A. (1999). Towards a theory of visual consciousness. *Consciousness and Cognition, 8*(2), 225–259.

Zihl, J., von Cramon, D., & Mai, N. (1983). Selective disturbance of movement vision after bilateral brain damage. *Brain, 106,* 313–340.

The zombie within (1998). *New Scientist,* 5 September, 31.

Author Index

Subject Index